Diagnosis and Management of Head and Face Pain

James Y. Suen • Erika Petersen
Editors

Diagnosis and Management of Head and Face Pain

A Practical Approach

Springer

Editors
James Y. Suen
Department of Otolaryngology-HNS
University of Arkansas for
Medical Sciences
Little Rock, AR
USA

Erika Petersen
Department of Neurosurgery
University of Arkansas for
Medical Sciences
Little Rock, AR
USA

ISBN 978-3-030-08153-9 ISBN 978-3-319-90999-8 (eBook)
https://doi.org/10.1007/978-3-319-90999-8

Printed on acid-free paper

This Springer imprint is published by the registered company Springer International Publishing AG, part of Springer Nature
The registered company address is: Gewerbestrasse 11, 6330 Cham, Switzerland

To our residents, nurses, and assistants who work with me—without their help, I could not do what I do to help patients.
And to my family: Karen, Brent and Constance, Tiffany, Bradley and Jessica, Brennan, and to my wonderful grandchildren, Sophia, Vivian, and Ethan James. They are my joy outside of work!

James Y. Suen

To my husband, Shane Estep, my partner and love.
To my son Ethan, who teaches me to look at the puzzles of life with fresh curiosity.
To my sister, Aili, and my father, Karl, and all my family for all their support and love.
In loving memory of Elisabeth Saranec Petersen, who launched me on the way.

Erika Petersen

Preface

Millions of people throughout the world suffer with pain of the face and head. The costs of these problems are tremendous and include medical treatment, lost wages, and lost productivity. Problems with opioid addiction and the emotional distress existing in patients and their families are often under-recognized in these patients.

Many physicians do not like dealing with patients who have facial and head pain, because they feel they have little to offer them except medications. With the opioid crisis in the United States, physicians are becoming reluctant to prescribe narcotics, even when many times these may be the only drugs that help patients tolerate their pain. Patients with uncontrolled facial and head pain are desperate and feel helpless, and often the clinicians treating them are limited in the possible treatment options to consider.

We accepted the task of editing this textbook on the treatment of facial and head pain because we know there are many options for treating these patients besides medications, such as narcotics. As a head and neck surgeon, I have seen many patients with severe pain from cancer or trauma. Rather than sending these patients to other physicians, I would think of ways to try to stop pain in these patients. Dr. Petersen, in her neurosurgical practice, has also seen patients whose options required exploring less familiar alternatives to address refractory symptoms. With this experience, we have seen and operated on most nerves innervating the head and neck. This has proven to be an advantage in knowing where the cranial and cervical nerves are located and what areas they innervate. We have found that doing nerve blocks and/or removing the peripheral nerves has helped many patients with face and head pain. In some instances, the appropriate neurosurgical, neuromodulation, or dental procedure has been the key.

Because of this success in helping patients with face and head pain, we have had many referrals from neurologists, neurosurgeons, pain specialists, and dentists. This has given us a major learning experience over the past 10 years, and sharing this experience can give guidance to other clinicians on how to manage patients with face and head pain.

The treatment of head and face pain benefits from a multidisciplinary approach. Similarly, we have gathered a group of experts from multiple specialties—neurology, neurosurgery, anesthesiology, interventional pain, psychiatry, psychology, dentistry, otolaryngology, plastic surgery, neuroradiology, radiation oncology—to contribute to this textbook. We have tried to make this as comprehensive as possible and as practical as possible.

From our experience, we feel that the majority of face and head pain is the result of problems with the peripheral nerves of the trigeminal nerve and the cervical nerves. Most of these nerves are accessible for nerve blocks, or for decompression or resection, when indicated. Diagnosis depends on a good knowledge of anatomy of the nerves innervating the head and face, and on the understanding of the differential diagnosis based on obtaining a good history. The key to treatment is arriving at the correct diagnosis.

This textbook is divided into four parts. The first part covers the clinical fundamentals: etiology, pathophysiology, anatomy, and nomenclature. The second part covers evaluation and diagnosis, where diagnostic nerve blocks are discussed in detail. These blocks should be considered a crucial part of the evaluation. The third part discusses management and treatment options, and the fourth part presents representative clinical cases and the management. Overall there are 42 chapters which give a comprehensive overview of face and head pain.

We hope this textbook gives clinicians a systematic approach to treating face and head pain. It reviews the more standard methods of treatment and introduces some newer methods.

Little Rock, AR, USA James Y. Suen
Little Rock, AR, USA Erika Petersen

Acknowledgments

We wish to thank all the contributors who took time from their busy practices to write chapters. This group of contributors, who are each considered experts in their field, helped to make this a comprehensive textbook on facial and head pain. This was a team effort that we hope will provide the reader with new insights to the diagnosis and treatment of face and head pain.

Also we want to thank Leslie Norris who did the medical illustrations for our chapters. Our special thanks goes to Joni Fraser, Development Editor at Springer Publishers, who provided wonderful assistance throughout this effort.

We would like to thank all those clinicians who have influenced our practice and specifically our approach to head and facial pain.

Finally, we offer our gratitude to patients that we have treated over the years who suffer with head and face pain. Thank you for trusting us to find treatments for you. We hope this textbook will offer hope and treatment to all patients who suffer from similar conditions.

Contents

Part III Management and Treatment

Part IV Representative Clinical Cases

Contributors

Vikas Agarwal, MD Department of Radiology, University of Pittsburgh Medical Center, Pittsburgh, PA, USA

Ruben G. Alexander, MD Department of Anesthesiology, Emory University School of Medicine, Atlanta, GA, USA

William G. Austen Jr., MD Division of Plastic and Reconstructive Surgery, Harvard Medical School, Massachusetts General Hospital, Boston, MA, USA

Sharona Ben-Haim, MD Department of Neurosurgery, University of California San Diego, La Jolla, CA, USA

William J. Binder, MD Department of Head and Neck Surgery, University of California-Los Angeles, Los Angeles, CA, USA

David Geffen School of Medicine, Los Angeles, CA, USA

Andrew Blitzer, MD, DDS Department of Otolaryngology-Head and Neck Surgery, Columbia University College of Physicians and Surgeons, New York, NY, USA

Department of Otolaryngology, Icahn School of Medicine at Mt. Sinai, New York, NY, USA

New York Center for Voice and Swallowing Disorders, New York, NY, USA

Rutgers New Jersey Medical School, Newark, NJ, USA

Head and Neck Surgical Group, New York, NY, USA

Tyler Burns, MD Department of Anesthesiology, University of Arkansas for Medical Sciences, Little Rock, AR, USA

Tsinsue Chen, MD Victor Horsley Department of Neurosurgery, National Hospital of Neurology and Neurosurgery, London, UK

Division of Neurosurgery, Barrow Neurological Institute, St. Joseph's Hospital and Medical Center, Phoenix, AR, USA

Leanne R. Cianfrini, PhD The Doleys Clinic, Birmingham, AL, USA

Shannon W. Clark, MD Department of Neurological Surgery, Thomas Jefferson University, Philadelphia, PA, USA

Matthew D. Cox, MD Division of Otology/Neurotology, Department of Otolaryngology/Head and Neck Surgery, University of Arkansas for Medical Sciences, Little Rock, AR, USA

John Diaz Day, MD Department of Neurosurgery, University of Arkansas for Medical Sciences, Little Rock, AR, USA

Daniel M. Doleys, PhD The Doleys Clinic, Birmingham, AL, USA

Yuanxu Dong, MD Department of Pediatric Anesthesiology, Arkansas Children's Hospital, Little Rock, AR, USA

John L. Dornhoffer, MD Division of Otology/Neurotology, Department of Otolaryngology/Head and Neck Surgery, University of Arkansas for Medical Sciences, Little Rock, AR, USA

Christopher S. Fiedorek, Md, MTh Department of Anesthesiology, University of Arkansas for Medical Sciences, Little Rock, AR, USA

Ryan T. Fitzgerald, MD Department of Radiology, University of Arkansas for Medical Sciences, Little Rock, AR, USA

Harold W. Goforth, MD Lerner College of Medicine, Cleveland Clinic Foundation, Center for Neurological Restoration, Section of Headache Medicine, Cleveland, OH, USA

Center for Neurological Restoration, Neurological Institute, Cleveland Clinic, Cleveland, OH, USA

Johnathan H. Goree, MD Department of Anesthesiology, University of Arkansas for Medical Sciences, Little Rock, AR, USA

Matthew Helton, MD Department of Neurosurgery, University of Arkansas Medical Sciences, Little Rock, AR, USA

Byron Hills, MD Department of Neurosurgery, University Hospitals Cleveland Medical Center, University Heights, OH, USA

Anthony F. Jahn, MD Professor of Clinical Otolaryngology, Icahn School of Medicine at Mount Sinai, New York, NY, USA

John K. Jones, MD, DMD Department of Otolaryngology/Head and Neck Surgery/Oral and Maxillofacial Surgery, University of Arkansas for Medical Sciences, Little Rock, AR, USA

Rachel Kaye, MD New York Center for Voice and Swallowing Disorders, New York, NY, USA

Rutgers New Jersey Medical School, Newark, NJ, USA

Andre Machado, MD, PhD The Cleveland Clinic, Center for Neurological Restoration, Cleveland, OH, USA

Jordan Taylor MacNeil, Bachelor of Science (Hon), MD Department of Anesthesiology, University of Arkansas for Medical Sciences, Little Rock, AR, USA

Manjit Matharu, BSc, MBChB, PhD Department of Neurology, National Hospital of Neurology and Neurosurgery, London, UK

UCL Institute of Neurology and The National Hospital for Neurology and Neurosurgery, Headache Group, London, UK

Jonathan P. Miller, MD Department of Neurological Surgery, University Hospitals Cleveland Medical Center, Case Western Reserve University, Cleveland, OH, USA

Julien Arden Norton, MD Department of Otolaryngology/Head and Neck Surgery, University of Arkansas for Medical Sciences, Little Rock, AR, USA

Trusharth Patel, MD Division of Pain Medicine, Department of Anesthesiology, Emory University School of Medicine, Atlanta, GA, USA

José A. Peñagarícano, MD Department of Radiation Oncology, University of Arkansas for Medical Sciences, Little Rock, AR, USA

Erika A. Petersen, MD Department of Neurosurgery, University of Arkansas for Medical Sciences, Little Rock, AR, USA

Ahmed M. Raslan, MD, FAANS Department of Neurological Surgery, OHSU, Portland, OR, USA

Maricruz Rivera, PhD Case Western Reserve University, School of Medicine, Cleveland, OH, USA

Joshua M. Rosenow, MD Department of Neurosurgery, Northwestern Memorial Hospital, Chicago, IL, USA

Taylor E. Rush, PhD Center for Neurological Restoration, Neurological Institute, Cleveland Clinic, Cleveland, OH, USA

Nathaniel M. Schuster, MD Center for Pain Medicine, Department of Anesthesiology, University of California, San Diego, La Jolla, CA, USA

Ashwini Sharan, MD, FACS Department of Neurological Surgery, Thomas Jefferson University, Philadelphia, PA, USA

Vinita Singh, MD Department of Anesthesiology, Emory University School of Medicine, Atlanta, GA, USA

Konstantin V. Slavin, MD Department of Neurosurgery, University of Illinois at Chicago, Chicago, IL, USA

Chelsey Smith, MD ENTcare, Dothan, AL, USA

Boris Spektor, MD Department of Anesthesiology, Emory University School of Medicine, Atlanta, GA, USA

Michael D. Staudt, MD, MSc Department of Neurological Surgery, Case Western Reserve University, University Hospitals Cleveland Medical Center, Cleveland, OH, USA

Natalie Strickland, MD Department of Anesthesiology, University of Arkansas Medical Sciences, Little Rock, AR, USA

James Y. Suen, MD Department of Otolaryngology—Head and Neck Surgery, University of Arkansas for Medical Sciences, Little Rock, AR, USA

Jennifer A. Sweet, MD Department of Neurosurgery, Case Western Reserve University, University Hospitals Cleveland Medical Center, Cleveland, OH, USA

Rabia Tari, MD Department of Neurosurgery, University of Illinois at Chicago, Chicago, IL, USA

Taylor Anne Wilson, MD, MS Department of Neurosurgery, University of Arkansas for Medical Sciences, Little Rock, AR, USA

Eric J. Wright, MD Division of Plastic and Reconstructive Surgery, Department of Surgery, University of Arkansas for Medical Sciences, Little Rock, AR, USA

Chengyuan Wu, MD, MSBmE Department of Neurological Surgery, Thomas Jefferson University, Philadelphia, PA, USA

Ludvic Zrinzo, MD, PhD, FRCS Victor Horsley Department of Neurosurgery, National Hospital of Neurology and Neurosurgery, London, UK

Unit of Functional Neurosurgery, Department of Movement Disorders, UCL Institute of Neurology, University College London, London, UK

Part I
Clinical Fundamentals

Chapter 1
Applied Neuroanatomy of the Face and Head

Chelsey Smith and James Y. Suen

Introduction

Comprehensive knowledge of the neuroanatomy of the head, neck, and face is paramount to the treatment of pain located in these areas. In the arenas of both otolaryngology and neurosurgery, we encounter these nerves and their landmarks daily just by the nature of our surgical expertise, and this becomes a valuable tool when evaluating and treating the facial and head pain patient. When facial and head pain is seen through the lens of anatomy rather than the serpentine tunnel of conditions of chronicity, the assessments and plans become more efficient and concise. It can even eliminate the use of imaging modalities, including ultrasound (often used to aid in finding peripheral nerves for nerve injections). Knowing the nerve anatomy can help the physician determine the nerves which may be triggering the patient's pain or headache on the initial visit.

Overview of the Head, Face, and Neck Dermatomes

Three specific nerve groups are the treatment focus for facial and head pain: the trigeminal nerve, the upper cervical plexus, and the greater occipital nerve. Comprehension of these three neuroanatomical structures allows for diagnostic and

C. Smith
ENTcare, Dothan, AL, USA

J. Y. Suen (✉)
Department of Otolaryngology—Head and Neck Surgery,
University of Arkansas for Medical Sciences, Little Rock, AR, USA
e-mail: suenjamesy@uams.edu

J. Y. Suen, E. Petersen (eds.), *Diagnosis and Management of Head and Face Pain*, https://doi.org/10.1007/978-3-319-90999-8_1

potentially therapeutic pain relief in all head and face dermatome distributions. Knowing the dermatomes will aid in determining a patient's "trigger" point(s) and localizes pain distribution so that a specific nerve(s) can be targeted for therapy. It is simple mapping that both the patient and the physician can refer.

Figure 1.1 depicts the dermatomes of the head and neck. The three anterior zones correlate with the distal sensory nerve innervations of the three trigeminal nerve divisions. The upper cervical plexus dermatome is depicted by the region from the upper anterior neck around the lower earlobe and over the parotid and angle of jaw areas. Lastly, the greater occipital nerve supplies the posterior scalp from the vertex of the skull down to the upper posterior neck.

Each of these three anatomical positions will be described in the following text.

It is important to understand that pain in one nerve dermatome distribution can cause pain in the other branches of that division and even into the other divisions. Also pain in the trigeminal nerve branches can trigger pain in the lesser or greater occipital nerves through a connection in the brain stem called the trigeminocervical complex, and vice versa, the occipital nerve pain can trigger trigeminal nerve pain.

Trigeminal Nerve

The trigeminal nerve arises from the Pons and goes into Meckel's cave in the cavernous sinus where the trigeminal ganglion is located. This ganglion contains the cell bodies for the afferent sensory nerve fibers of the trigeminal nerve's three divisions, the ophthalmic, the maxillary, and the mandibular divisions, commonly referred to as V1, V2, and V3 [1].

It is important to know the branches of each of these three divisions and where they innervate the face and head (Fig. 1.2).

The first division, V1, is the ophthalmic branch. It enters the orbit through the superior orbital fissure and has several nerves to eye structures, to the internal upper nose, and then further divides into the supraorbital, supratrochlear, and infratrochlear nerve branches as it exits the orbit. *The supraorbital nerve* exits the orbit through the supraorbital notch or foramen, and it supplies the upper eyelid and the ipsilateral forehead to the vertex of the scalp. The notch or foramen can be a place where the supraorbital nerve can be compressed. A notch occurs about 83% of the time and is usually encircled by a ligamentous fascial band which encircles the nerve [2]. The *supratrochlear nerve* exits at the superior-medial part of the orbit near the bridge of the nose and supplies the skin of the forehead near the midline (Fig. 1.3). Pain in V1 can be in the eyelid, the forehead, or the top of the head and can trigger headaches, commonly diagnosed as migraine headaches.

The *infratrochlear nerve* supplies the skin over the bridge of the nose and the medial part of the lower eyelid.

The second division, V2, is the maxillary branch, and it is primarily sensory in function. It is more complex and takes more study to understand the innervation and where pain from V2 can elicit. The main nerve of V2 is the *infraorbital nerve* which

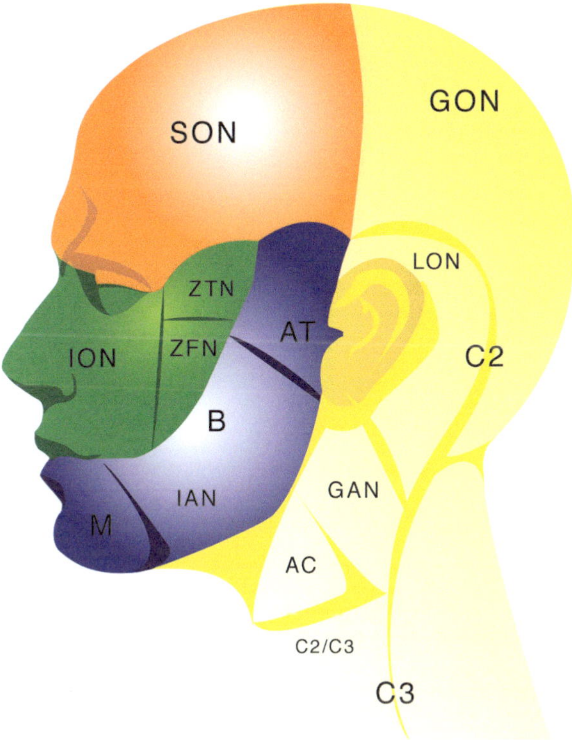

Fig. 1.1 Dermatomes of the trigeminal nerves to the face and of the upper cervical plexus and greater occipital nerves to the back of the head and upper neck. Orange ophthalmic division of trigeminal; green maxillary division of trigeminal; purple mandibular division; yellow upper cervical plexus and greater occipital nerves

goes in a groove in the floor of the orbit and exits through the infraorbital foramen and supplies the midface. There are two other branches of this nerve which are important to know. One is the *posterior superior alveolar nerve* (Fig. 1.2) which comes off the V2 after it exits the foramen rotundum and wraps around the posterior-lateral wall of the maxilla where it enters the underlying bone and innervates the posterior upper teeth. It is common for pain in this nerve to be diagnosed as dental pain and result in dental extractions with no pain relief.

The second important branch is the *zygomaticotemporal nerve* (ZTN) which leaves the infraorbital nerve in the floor of the orbit and goes into the zygoma bone and exits just lateral to or through the bone of the lateral orbital rim and goes to the anterior temporalis muscle area (Fig. 1.3). The foramen where the ZTN exits the zygoma is about 7 mm lateral to the lateral orbital rim and about 8 mm cranial to the lateral canthus. It goes into the temporalis muscle or just superficial to it. Sometimes the ZTN comes out just lateral to the lateral orbital rim. Pain in this nerve is quite common and can cause temporal headaches which are commonly called migraine headaches.

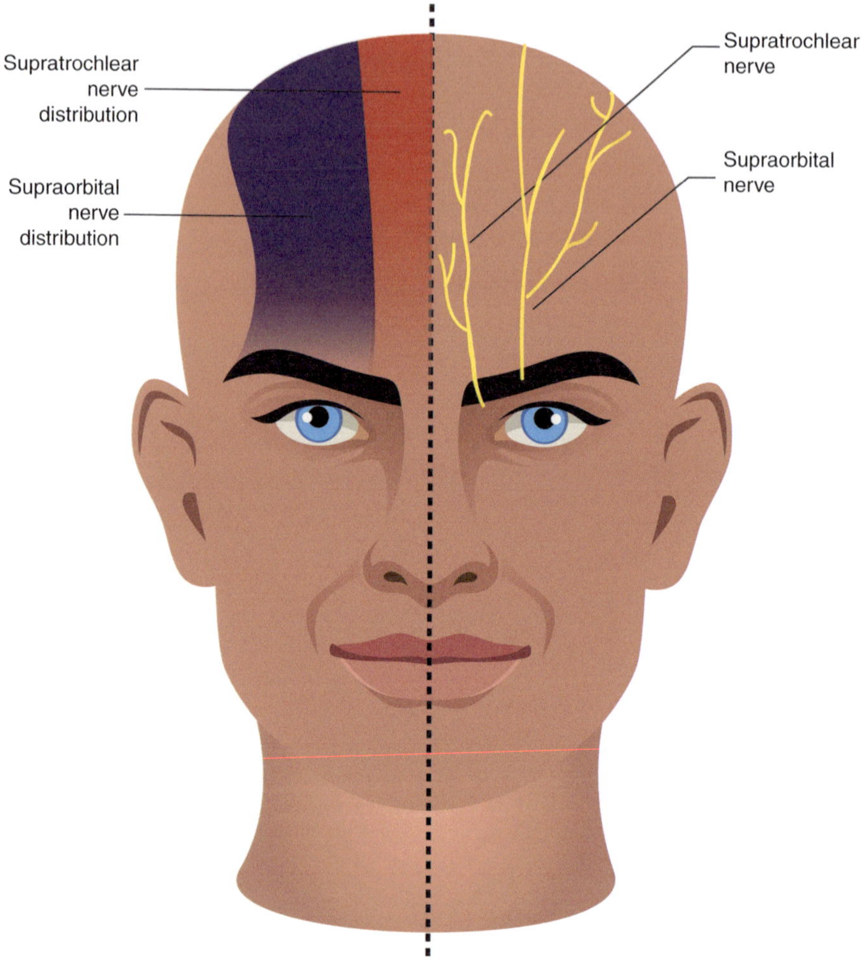

Fig. 1.2 The trigeminal nerve ganglion with the three major divisions: ophthalmic, maxillary, and mandibular

The third division, V3, is called the mandibular branch (Fig. 1.2), and it has both sensory and motor function. The motor part supplies the muscles of mastication. The sensory branches go to three main areas: *the lingual nerve* to the tongue, the *inferior alveolar nerve* into the mandible in the ascending ramus and supplying the lower jaw teeth and exiting the mental foramen to supply the chin and lower lip, and the third branch, the *auriculotemporal nerve* (*ATN*), which exits just posterior to the mandibular condyle and goes superiorly to the area of the temple and above the ear (Fig. 1.1). Pain can occur in one or all of these branches. We feel the auriculotemporal nerve can also trigger migraine headaches.

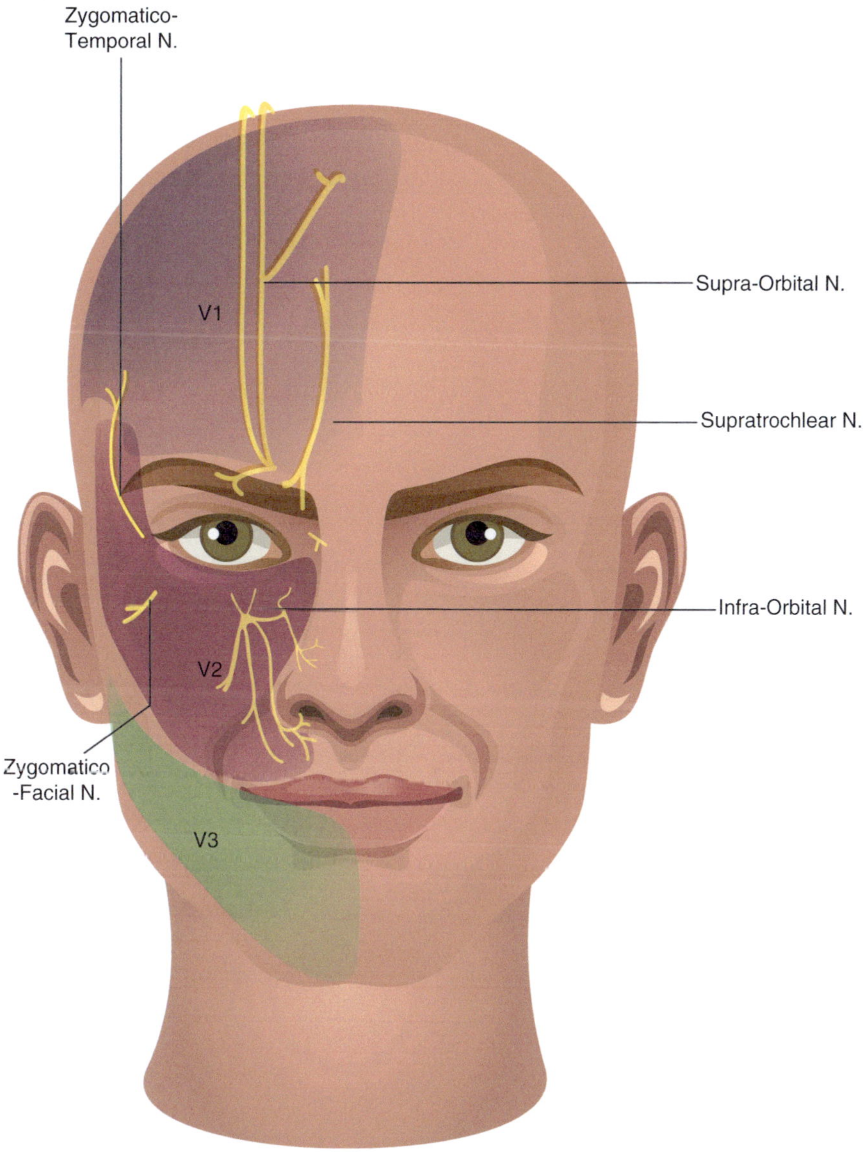

Fig. 1.3 The supraorbital and supratrochlear nerves innervate the forehead to the vertex of the scalp. This also illustrates the location of the zygomaticotemporal nerve branch of the maxillary division of the trigeminal nerve

Upper Cervical Plexus

Neuritis originating from the upper cervical plexus is commonly encountered during the work-up of the head and neck pain patient. Consisting of both motor (ansa cervicalis) and sensory components, its distal reaches are wide and disperse. For the purposes of this chapter, the focus will be on the sensory portions only [2]. Origins for the cervical plexus begin deep to the sternocleidomastoid muscle (SCM) formed by the ventral rami of C2, C3, and C4. After emanating from deep to the SCM, the sensory branches route just above the midpoint of the posterior border of the SCM and then scatter to their distal destinations. *Branches of the upper cervical plexus nerves include the lesser occipital, greater auricular, and the transverse cervical nerves* (Fig. 1.4).

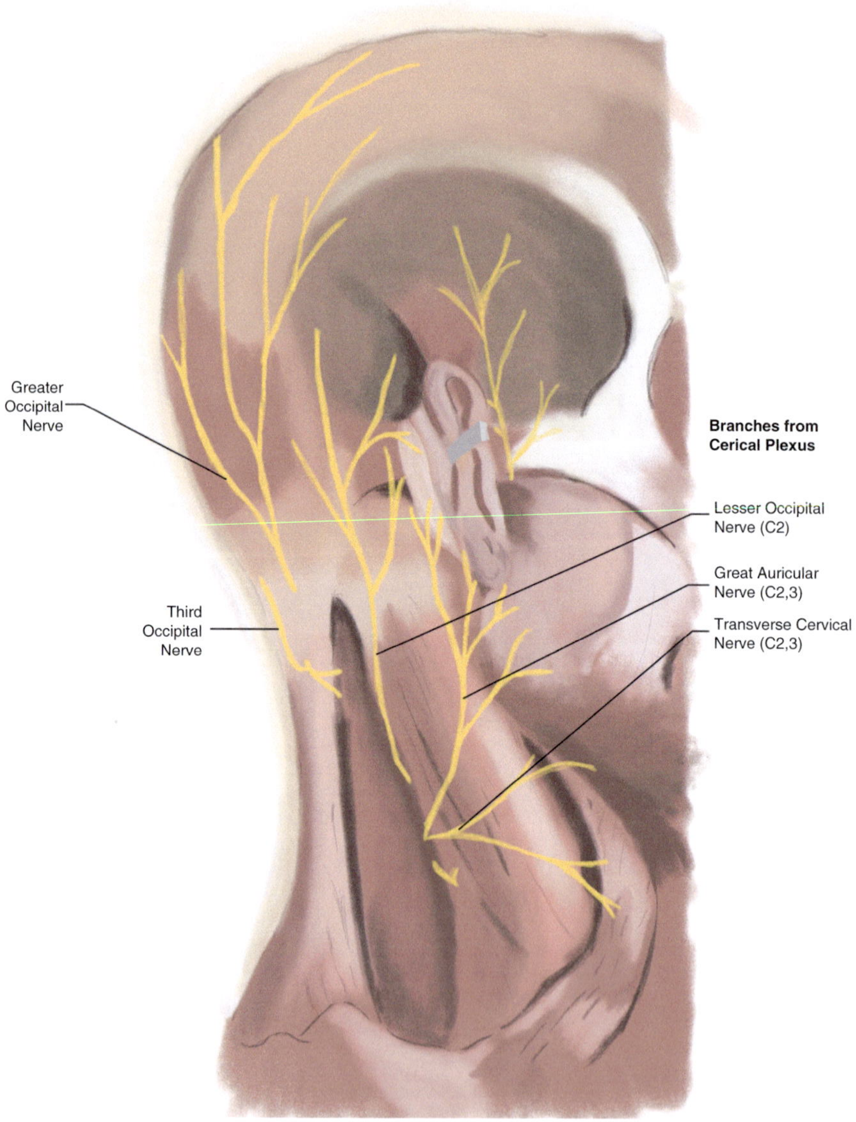

Fig. 1.4 Upper cervical plexus nerves include the lesser occipital, greater auricular, and transverse cervical nerves from C2 to C3

It is important to understand the anatomical location at which the nerves emerge from the posterior border of the SCM as this is the location for insertion of the needle for clinical nerve blocks. We use the definition of "Erb's point" to aid in localizing the site of emergence as being approximately halfway between the mastoid process and the clavicle along the posterior edge of the SCM. From this point, 1–2 cm superior to this location along the posterior border of the SCM is considered Erb's point. This is considered the "sweet spot" for cervical plexus nerve blocks and is where the main branches of the upper cervical plexus are in close proximity before they separate and go to different areas (Fig. 1.4).

Lesser Occipital Nerve: the lesser occipital nerve is a sensory nerve that is derived from the ventral rami of C2 and C3. After passing over the posterior border of the SCM muscle, it usually ascends along the posterior border of the SCM but may go deep to the muscle and surface over the mastoid process and supplies sensory innervation posterior to the ear, and up to the temple area above the ear. This is important to know because pain above the ear can be related to the lesser occipital nerve.

Greater Auricular Nerve: ventral rami C2 and C3 also give rise to the greater auricular nerve fibers. Exiting the posterior border of the SCM, this nerve proceeds toward the lower earlobe as it crosses the SCM. It innervates the lower part of the ear, the skin overlying the tail of the parotid gland and over the angle of the mandible (Fig.1.4).

Transverse Cervical Nerve: similar to the lesser occipital and greater auricular nerves, the transverse cervical nerve also arises from the C2 and C3 ventral rami. After passing over the posterior border of the SCM, it continues anteriorly in a horizontal fashion and innervates the skin along the jaw line.

Greater Occipital Nerve

The greater occipital nerve can be a common source for severe head and neck pain, frequently described as "tension headaches" [3]. Fortunately, it is easily accessible for clinical treatment. The dorsal ramus of C2 is the source of this nerve. It pierces the suboccipital triangle between the obliquus capitis inferior muscle and the semispinalis capitis muscle. As it ascends superficial to the semispinalis and deep to the trapezius, it eventually pierces through the superior portion of the trapezius at the level of the nuchal line [4] (Fig. 1.4). The nuchal line is an excellent landmark for finding the appropriate latitude of the greater occipital nerve and where it begins its course into the subcutaneous scalp. Other helpful landmarks include the posterior midline sulcus of the neck and the occipital protuberance (Fig. 1.5). From this midline site, the occipital nerves can be found approximately 1.5–2.5 cm laterally. Once the greater occipital nerve commences its subcutaneous course, it ascends and innervates the skin of the posterior scalp to the level of the vertex.

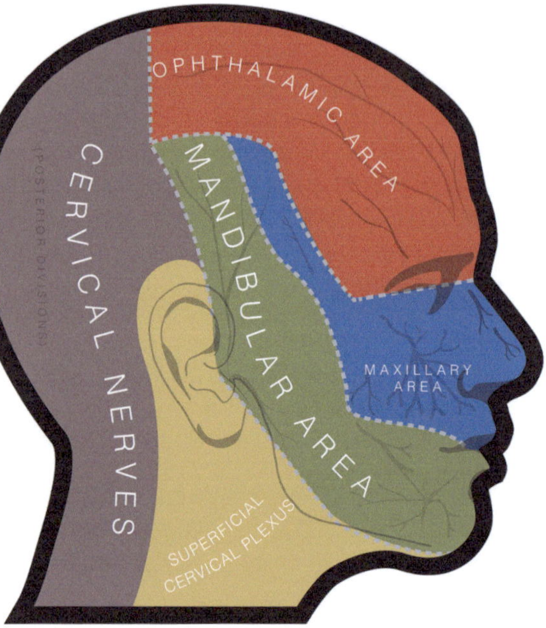

Fig. 1.5 The terminal branches of the greater occipital nerves and the lesser occipital nerves in relationship to the occipital protuberance and mastoid landmarks

Conclusion

The trigeminal nerve, the upper cervical plexus nerves, and the greater occipital nerves are the primary nerves which causes head and face pain. It is important to learn the dermatomes that these nerves innervate. All these nerves are accessible in multiple ways for pain treatment modalities. This will be the focus of the remaining portions of this text.

The sensory neuroanatomy of the head and neck is unparalleled in its detail and elegance, but when dissected down to its fundamentals, it can be a straightforward way to think about the diagnosis and treatment of facial pain. Concise medical comprehension of these nerves and dermatomes can be the intersection between physician assessment and patient understanding, leading to satisfying clinical encounters concerning head and face pain. Anatomic knowledge is a pillar of punctual and accurate diagnosis in this arena.

References

1. Norton NS. Netter's head and neck anatomy for dentistry. 2nd ed. Amsterdam: Elsevier. p. 176–8.
2. Fallucco M, Janis JE, Hagan RR. The anatomical morphology of the supraorbital notch: clinical relevance to the surgical treatment of migraine headaches. Plast Reconstr Surg. 2012;130:1227–33.

3. Norton NS. Netter's head and neck anatomy for dentistry. 2nd ed. Amsterdam: Elsevier. 2012: p. 131, 144, 159.
4. Ducic I, Moriarty M, Al-Attar A. Anatomical variations of the greater occipital nerve: implications for the etiology of chronic headaches. Plast Reconst Surg. 2009;123:859–63, discussion 864.

Chapter 2
Etiology of Head Pain

Trusharth Patel and Tyler Burns

Introduction

Cranial neuralgias represent a group of more common forms of head and facial pain. The etiology can usually be narrowed down to one specific cranial nerve or a branch of a cranial nerve. Imaging, at times, can help with making the diagnosis, but many times astute history taking and examination will confirm a correct diagnosis. Important information to extract from the patient regarding pain includes onset, location, radiation pattern, aggravating factors such as chewing, mouth opening, associated symptoms such as history of multiple sclerosis or previous herpes zoster flare, risk factors for neoplasm, and alleviating factors [1]. This chapter attempts to describe the etiology of the more common types of head and facial pain to help the clinician understand the complexity of these problems and recognize presenting symptoms.

Trigeminal Neuralgia

Trigeminal neuralgia represents one of the most common cranial neuralgia conditions seen for head and face pain. The incidence is 4.7 per 100,000 per year in men and 7.2 per 100,000 per year in women [1]. There is increased incidence beyond the

T. Patel (✉)
Division of Pain Medicine, Department of Anesthesiology,
Emory University School of Medicine, Atlanta, GA, USA
e-mail: trusharth.patel@emory.edu

T. Burns
Department of Anesthesiology, University of Arkansas for Medical Sciences,
Little Rock, AR, USA
e-mail: ltburns@uams.edu

J. Y. Suen, E. Petersen (eds.), *Diagnosis and Management of Head and Face Pain*, https://doi.org/10.1007/978-3-319-90999-8_2

age of 50 [2]. The distinction between typical and atypical forms of trigeminal neuralgia is based on the constellation of symptoms rather than etiology [2]. It is typically precipitated by light touch or temperature changes of sensitive areas of the face. The most common etiology is compression of the trigeminal nerve root at the entry point into the pons. Most cases, 80–90%, result from compression by vasculature and characterize classic or idiopathic trigeminal neuralgia. Benign neoplasms of the posterior fossa, such as acoustic neuroma, meningioma, and epidermoid cysts, account for 10–20% of compressive cases [3]. The pathophysiology in compressive lesions is thought to be from indentation of the nerve tract at the site of compression resulting in demyelination of sensory fibers in the root entry zone as seen on pathological specimens [4]. The demyelination results in dysregulation of incoming signal transduction as well as spontaneously evoked aberrant discharge in response to an innocuous stimulus [2]. In the absence of vascular loops causing neurovascular compression, trigeminal neuralgia is characterized as secondary or symptomatic. In addition to benign tumors, multiple sclerosis and brainstem infarction fall into this latter category [1]. Multiple sclerosis is believed to consist of 1–2% of cases [5]. Symptomatic trigeminal neuralgia can be associated with sensory deficits and can present bilaterally and in younger patients [2]. Typical and atypical forms of trigeminal neuralgia are based on the constellation of symptoms rather than etiology [6].

Glossopharyngeal Neuralgia

Anatomical injury or compression along the ninth cranial nerve may result in glossopharyngeal neuralgia. Most common is compression by a mass or neurovascular compression. Compression by an elongated and calcified styloid process, known as Eagle's syndrome, is an infrequent cause. Up to 10% of cases of glossopharyngeal neuralgia can be associated with vagal symptoms manifesting as bradycardia, syncope, or cardiac arrest [7]. The incidence of this neuralgia is very low at 0.2–0.5 per 100,000 person per year [2, 8]. It is characterized by pain in the tonsillar pillars, angle of the jaw, ear, or base of the tongue. Sensory deficits may also be seen. Symptoms of hoarseness, coughing, and difficulty with swallowing have also been described [2]. Attacks are usually triggered by swallowing, mouth opening, coughing, or sneezing [9]. Palpation of the throat or ear canal or within the oropharynx may also trigger the pain. Painful episodes are typically transient but intense [1].

Auriculotemporal Neuralgia

Auriculotemporal neuralgia is a neuropathic condition resulting in pain in the distribution of the auriculotemporal nerve, which is a branch nerve stemming from the V3 division of the trigeminal nerve. It is characterized by pain near the temporomandibular joint, preauricular area, and parotid gland area and around the ear and temple. Episodes of pain are typically brief but intense. Symptoms are almost exclusively unilateral. The etiology usually involves entrapment of the auriculotemporal nerve or injury to the nerve such as with temporomandibular arthroscopy [10]. Mechanical compression to the nerve has also been described such as with synovial cysts, malformation or aneurysm of the middle meningeal artery, fracture of the mandibular condyle, or tumor spread along the course of the nerve [7].

Occipital Neuralgia

Occipital neuralgia is a headache variant involving pain in the distribution of the greater, lesser, or third occipital nerve. The greater occipital nerve originates from the dorsal ramus of C2, and lesser and third occipital nerves originate from C2 and C3 nerve roots [11]. Pain is typically felt in the upper cervical and posterior occipital region and can radiate upward to the apex of the scalp. It is characterized by paroxysmal attacks lasting seconds to minutes. Because of trigeminocervical interneuronal connections in the trigeminal spinal nuclei, pain can also be experienced in the orbital and frontal region. Pain is unilateral in 85% of patients and may be elicited by palpation over these nerves [2]. The incidence is thought to be approximately 3.2 per 100,000 [8]. Irritation of these nerves can be from mechanical compression by the suboccipital muscles of the scalp that these nerves traverse, tumors, vascular anomalies, and prior surgical scars. Other conditions known to cause inflammation of these nerves originate from cervical spine degenerative conditions, whiplash injury, vascular inflammation, and myelitis [7]. Recently, the role of ultrasound imaging was described as a diagnostic modality in identifying a potential source and location of occipital nerve entrapment and irritation [12].

Postherpetic Neuralgia

After remaining dormant for up to many decades, the varicella zoster virus can resurface from the trigeminal, autonomic, and dorsal root ganglia causing characteristic painful vesicles in the distribution of a single dermatome or cranial nerve. The vesicles can be preceded by pain for up to several days, but more commonly pain ensues after eruption of vesicles. Uncommonly, pain in a dermatomal or cranial nerve distribution can occur without vesicles, a condition known as zoster sine herpete [2]. The pain is neuropathic and characterized by burning, shooting, stabbing, and itching. Pain that persists beyond resolution of cutaneous vesicles beyond 4 months is termed postherpetic neuralgia [13]. Those who are immunocompromised and have age-related decline in immunity are at higher risk of developing the condition in which the lifetime risk is estimated to be 30% [14]. Most cases of herpes zoster erupting in the head occur in the ophthalmic division of the trigeminal nerve.

Other cranial nerve involvement such as geniculate zoster have been described in which eruption via cranial nerve VII manifests as painful vesicles in the external auditory canal, anterior two-thirds of the tongue, or hard palate. Ipsilateral facial palsy can also be a presenting sign [15]. There is no conclusive evidence that viral replication is the cause of postherpetic neuralgia. Studies do show reduced epidermal nerve fiber density measured from skin biopsy of patients with postherpetic neuralgia with preferential reduction in afferent unmyelinated fibers [7, 16, 17].

Superior Laryngeal Neuralgia

This uncommon disorder is characterized by pain along the lateral aspect of the neck. Pain may radiate to the angle of the mandible and to the ear. Pain can be evoked by swallowing, talking, mouth opening, coughing, or palpation along a focal point in the lateral neck where the nerve enters the larynx [7]. Hoarseness and persistent cough may also be presenting signs [18, 19]. The etiology is from trauma such as previous surgery, inflammation, laryngeal diverticulum, and displacement of the hyoid bone [20–22].

Optic Neuritis

Optic neuritis is caused by demyelination of the optic nerve from the optic chiasm and the bulb disc resulting in pain behind one or both eyes. The incidence is around 5 in 100,000 [23]. It is exacerbated by eye movements and gentle palpation of the eyes and accompanied by impaired vision. The disorder may be associated with other conditions such as multiple sclerosis or neuromyelitis optica or can be idiopathic [24–26]. More than 50% of patients who experience a first episode of autoimmune optic neuritis will develop multiple sclerosis. Demyelination may also occur from other autoimmune conditions such as Sjogren's syndrome, neurosarcoidosis, or vaccination. Infection can also result in demyelination, examples including syphilis, varicella zoster, and borreliosis among others [27].

Burning Mouth Syndrome

Burning mouth syndrome is characterized as chronic burning of the oral mucosa. It can also present with itching, dysesthesia, paresthesia, dry mouth, and altered sense of taste. Other associated findings include anxiety, depression, and nutritional deficiencies [28]. The syndrome affects over one million Americans with a greater incidence in women between the fifth and seventh decade of life [29]. Even though the prevalence is substantial, thorough understanding of the pathophysiology remains evasive. Proposed theories include neuropathic etiology related to the trigeminal complex or possibly a psychological phenomenon of an unknown mechanism. Recognition of the disorder can help some alleviate anxiety; however, lack of standard and effective therapy can be frustrating to the patient and physician [30].

Persistent Idiopathic Facial Pain

Persistent idiopathic facial pain is a debilitating condition of the face characterized as intense burning or a severe ache. It is often misdiagnosed as trigeminal neuralgia given the overlap in distribution of pain. However, unlike trigeminal neuralgia, it lacks autonomic features and is typically continuous rather than intermittent or episodic. Diminished sensation is not seen. Workup is unremarkable with more common causes of facial pain being ruled out [31, 32]. The incidence of persistent idiopathic facial pain is unclear, although it is estimated that 26% of the population will experience facial pain at some point in their life [33]. The pathophysiology of persistent idiopathic facial pain remains largely unclear. Quantitating sensory testing and functional brain imaging have shown sensory abnormalities such as hyperactive central neuronal activity [34–36]. Others propose that persistent idiopathic facial pain is on a continuum of trigeminal neuralgia given similarities [37]. There is a reported association with coexisting psychological disorders such as anxiety and depression; however, a causal relationship is not defined [38].

Conclusion

Pain in the head or face can usually be narrowed down to one specific nerve or a branch of a nerve. Often astute history taking and examination will confirm a correct diagnosis. The details of the nature of the pain and exacerbating factors assist the clinician in developing a differential diagnosis from the presenting symptoms.

References

1. Dorsch JN. Neurologic syndromes of the head and neck. Prim Care Clin Office Pract. 2014;41:133–49.
2. Chesire W. Cranial neuralgias. Continuum (Minneap Minn). 2015;21(4):1072–85.
3. Al-Quliti KW. Update on neuropathic pain treatment for trigeminal neuralgia. The pharmacological and surgical options. Neurosciences. 2015;20(2):107–14.
4. Hassan S, Khan NI, Sherwani OA, Bhatt W, Asif S. Trigeminal neuralgia: an overview of literature with emphasis on medical management. Int Res J Pharmcol. 2013;3:235–8.

5. De Santi L, Annunziata P. Symptomatic cranial neuralgias in multiple sclerosis: clinical features and treatment. Clin Neurol Neurosurg. 2012;114(2):101–7. https://doi.org/10.1016/j.clineuro.2011.10.044.
6. Cruccu G, Gronseth G, Alksne J, Argoff C, Brainin M, Burchiel K, Nurmikko T, Zakrzewska JM. AAN-EFNS guidelines on trigeminal neuralgia management. Eur J Neurol. 2008;15:1013–28.
7. O'Neil F, Nurmikko T, Sommer C. Other facial neuralgias. Cephalgia. 2017;37:1–12.
8. Koopman JS, Dieleman JP, Huygen FJ, et al. Incidence of facial pain in the general population. Pain. 2009;147(1–3):122–7. https://doi.org/10.1016/jpain200908.023.
9. Shephard MK, Macgregor EA, Zakrzewska JM. Orofacial pain: a guide for the headache physician. Headache. 2014;54(1):22–39. https://doi.org/10.1111/head.12272.
10. Fernández Sanromán J, Costas López A, Fernández Ferro M, de Sánchez AL, Stavaru B, Arenaz Bua J. Complications of temporomandibular joint arthroscopy using two-portal coblation technologies: a prospective study of 475 procedures. J Craniomaxillofac Surg. 2016;44(9):1221–5.
11. Cesmebasi A, Muhleman MA, Hulsberg P, et al. Occipital neuralgia: anatomic considerations. Clin Anat. 2014;28(1):101Y108. https://doi.org/10.1002/ca.22468.
12. Nourouze S. Occipital neuralgia diagnosis and treatment: the role of ultrasound. Headache. 2016;56(4):801–7.
13. Gadient PM, Smoth JH. The neuralgias: diagnosis and management. Curr Neurol Neurosci Rep. 2014;14:459. https://doi.org/10.1007/s11910-014-0459-3.
14. Yawn BP, Gilden D. The global epidemiology of herpes zoster. Neurology. 2013;81(10):928–30. https://doi.org/10.1212/WNL.0b013e3182a3516e.
15. Gilden D, Nagel MA, Cohrs RJ, Mahalingam R. The variegate neurological manifestations of Varicella Zoster virus infection. Curr Neurol Neurosci Rep. 2013;13(9):374. https://doi.org/10.1007/s11910-013-0374-z.
16. Oaklander AL, Romans K, Horasek S, et al. Unilateral post herpetic neuralgia is associated with bilateral sensory neuron damage. Ann Neurol. 1998;44:789–95.
17. Truini A, Haanpaa M, Provitera V, et al. Differential myelinated and unmyelinated sensory and autonomic skin nerve fiber involvement in patients with ophthalmic post herpetic neuralgia. Front Neuroanat. 2015;9:105.
18. O'Neill BP, Aronson AE, Pearson BW, et al. Superior laryngeal neuralgia. Headache. 1982;22:6–9.
19. Lee B, Woo P. Chronic cough as a sign of laryngeal sensory neuropathy: diagnosis and treatment. Ann Otol Rhinol Laryngol. 2005;114:253–7.
20. Baxter WF. Post-traumatic superior laryngeal neuralgia. Calif Med. 1958;88:235–9.
21. Aydin O, OzturkMand Anik Y. Superior laryngeal neuralgia after acute laryngitis and treatment with a single injection of a local anesthetic. Arch Otolaryngol Head Neck Surg. 2007;133:934–5.
22. Bagatzounis A, Geyer G. Lateral pharyngeal diverticulum causing superior laryngeal neuralgia. Laryngo Rhino-Otologie. 1994;73:219–21.
23. Pau D, Al Zubidi N, Yalamanchili S, et al. Optic neuritis. Eye. 2011;25:833–42.
24. Bradl M, Kanamori Y, Nakashima I, et al. Pain in neuromyelitis optica prevalence, pathogenesis and therapy. Nat Rev Neurol. 2014;10(9):529–36. https://doi.org/10.1038/nrneurol.2014.129.
25. Brownlee WJ, Miller DH. Clinically isolated syndromes and the relationship to multiple sclerosis. J Clin Neurosci. 2014;21(12):2065–71. https://doi.org/10.1016/j.jocn.2014.02.026.
26. Toosy AT, Mason DF, Miller DH. Optic neuritis. Lancet Neurol. 2014;13(1):83–99. https://doi.org/10.1016/S1474-4422(13)70259-X.
27. Evers S. Facial pain: Overlapping syndromes. Cephalgia. 2017;1–9. https://doi.org/10.1177/0333102417703761.
28. Klasser GD, Fischer DJ, Epstein JB. Burning mouth syndrome: recognition, understanding, and management. Oral Maxillofac Surg Clin North Am. 2008;20:255–71.
29. Thoppay JR, De Rossi SS, Ciarrocca RN. Burning mouth syndrome. Dent Clin N Am. 2013;57:497–512.

30. Liu YF, Kim Y, et al. Burning mouth syndrome: a systematic review of treatments. Oral Dis. 2017. https://doi.org/10.1111/odi.12660.
31. Obermann M, Holle D, Katsarava Z. Trigeminal neuralgia and persistent idiopathic facial pain. Expert Rev Neurother. 2011;11(11):1619–29.
32. Mueller D, Obermann M, Yoon MS, et al. Prevalence of trigeminal neuralgia and persistent idiopathic facial pain: a population-based study. Cephalalgia. 2011;31(15):1542–8.
33. Macfarlane TV, Blinkhorn AS, Davies RM, et al. Oro-facial pain in the community: prevalence and associated impact. Community Dent Oral Epidemiol. 2002;30(1):52–60.
34. Forssell H, Jaaskelainen S, List T, Svensson P, Baad-Hansen L. An update on pathophysiological mechanisms related to idiopathic orofacial pain conditions with implications for management. J Oral Rehabil. 2015;42(4):300–22.
35. Jääskeläinen SK, Forssell H, Tenovuo O. Electrophysiological testing of the trigeminofacial system: aid in the diagnosis of atypical facial pain. Pain. 1999;80(1):191–200.
36. Lang E, Kaltenhäuser M, Seidler S, Mattenklodt P, Neundörfer B. Persistent idiopathic facial pain exists independent of somatosensory input from the painful region: findings from quantitative sensory functions and somatotopy of the primary somatosensory cortex. Pain. 2005;118(1):80–91.
37. Vadivelu N, Vadivelu A, Kaye AD. Orofacial pain: a clinician's guide. Switzerland: Springer; 2014.
38. Weiss AL, Ehrhardt KP, Tolba R. Atypical facial pain: a comprehensive, evidence-based review. Curr Pain Headache Rep. 2017;21:8. https://doi.org/10.1007/s11916-017-0609-9.

Chapter 3
Pathophysiology of Head and Facial Pain

Matthew Helton and Erika A. Petersen

A variety of insults and mechanisms cause head and facial pain. Nociceptive pathways carrying the unpleasant physical and emotional perception of pain excite based on actual or impending tissue damage. Facial pain in particular possesses a large differential diagnosis that can be narrowed with historical facts pertinent to the patient. An understanding of the pathophysiology of facial pain will help the practitioner to the correct diagnosis and treatment for the patient. Causes of facial pain include acute insult, neurogenic, inflammatory, post-traumatic, and idiopathic.

Nociceptive Physiology of Head and Face

Afferents from the trigeminal nerve and from the C2 and C3 nerve roots innervate the head and face. The peripheral nerves contain axons originating from cell bodies of the trigeminal and dorsal root ganglia relaying sensation from the periphery. The largest diameter cells maintain the Aβ axons, which are large, myelinated fibers innervating the Pacinian corpuscle and detect innocuous stimuli such as vibration and pressure [1]. Nociceptive signals are received via transmission of two smaller fibers, the Aδ and C fibers. The Aδ fibers are lightly myelinated, of medium diameter, and considered the transmitters of "first" pain, associated with rapid, acute, and sharp sensations. The C fibers are smaller unmyelinated axons that have about one fifth the conduction velocity of Aδ fibers and present the sensations of diffuse, dull, and aching pain [2]. Transduction of pain begins via ligand-gated ion channels as

M. Helton · E. A. Petersen (✉)
Department of Neurosurgery,
University of Arkansas for Medical Sciences,
Little Rock, AR, USA
e-mail: mhelton2@uams.edu; eapetersen@uams.edu

J. Y. Suen, E. Petersen (eds.), *Diagnosis and Management of Head and Face Pain*, https://doi.org/10.1007/978-3-319-90999-8_3

well as G protein-coupled receptors, which are activated in response to inflammatory mediators released at sites of tissue of injury [1]. Action potentials transmit the noxious stimuli via Aδ and C fibers. In the C2 and C3 nerve root, the primary afferents pass the soma of the dorsal root ganglia and synapse in the dorsal horn, superficially, deep, or near the central canal. Two classes of second-order neurons exist, nociceptive-specific and wide-dynamic range. The latter receives input from non-nociceptive afferents as well, possibly providing avenue through which innocuous stimuli could be relayed as noxious. The second-order neurons decussate; join the spinoreticular, spinomesencephalic, spinoparabrachial, and spinothalamic tracts; and ascend in the anterolateral quadrant of the spinal cord and brainstem, where conscious, reflexive motor, and emotional responses to the pain signals are formed. The signals carried from trigeminal dermatomes differ initially because they are carried through a cranial rather than a peripheral nerve. The trigeminal afferents enter the brainstem in the pons and descend caudally to synapse in the trigeminal spinal nucleus in the rostral cervical cord and caudal medulla, where second-order neurons then decussate and join the anterolateral quadrant tracts.

Transition from Acute to Chronic Pain

Following the acute phase of pain from peripheral tissue injury, the tissue recovers, and inflammatory markers gradually decrease to a point where pain no longer exists, or unfortunately, the pain can persist long after the initial insult. In the acute phase of recovery, the normal nociceptive response is heightened in an evolutionary ploy to prevent further injury, referred to as peripheral sensitization [2]. Peripheral sensitization may lead to a chronic pain state via mechanisms that will be discussed further [3]. In the case of persistent damage to the somatosensory system, the pain can be classified as neuropathic [4]. In some individuals the acute onset of pain may not cease—even though local tissue has healed—instead evolving to a characteristically different pain. The resulting chronic pain from plasticity of the central nociceptive pathways is referred to as central sensitization [1, 5]. The key features of chronic pain include allodynia, pain in response to innocuous stimuli, and hyperalgesia, increased signal of pain in response to a noxious stimuli. Chronic pain can be due to effects of three general phenomena: peripheral sensitization, neuropathic pain, and central sensitization. These broad categories are not mutually exclusive in contributing to the pathophysiology of disease states of head and facial pain; however one particular disease may receive contributions to chronicity from all three of the categories.

Peripheral Sensitization

Acutely, peripheral sensitization refers to the upregulation of nociception immediately following tissue injury as a method to prevent further injury to the area. At the site of tissue injury, inflammatory mediators are released including neurotransmitters and peptides (serotonin, ATP, substance P, calcitonin gene-related peptide, bradykinin), prostaglandins (PGE2), leukotrienes, neurotrophins (NGF), cytokines, chemokines, extracellular proteases, and protons. This inflammatory, acidic soup bathes the peripheral nociceptor creating the transmission of painful stimuli and further decreases the threshold for nociceptive excitability through stimulation of protein kinase C (PKCε), adenylyl cyclases, G protein-coupled receptors, and voltage-gated ion channels [2]. Recent evidence suggests that the transient, local sensitization to pain may lead to symptoms of chronic pain locally such as allodynia and hyperalgesia. The transformation of acute to chronic pain peripherally is known as hyperalgesic priming. In a rat model of chronic pain, a local irritant is injected into a paw to begin hyperalgesic priming. When the acute inflammatory process has subsided, the paw has a more intense and longer nociceptive response to local prostaglandin injection than a control paw [6]. The researchers attributed the response to upregulation at the nociceptor to other isoforms of prostaglandin adenylyl cyclase receptors [3]. The change in expression of receptors at the periphery has been explained by neuronal modifications of mRNA enrichment and protein translation in the cell body [7]. Peripheral sensitization may not solely contribute to chronic pain states but may be a therapeutic target to limit hyperalgesia in chronic pain.

Neuropathic Pain

Neuropathic pain is inherently different from peripheral or central sensitization by definition. Treede et al. define neuropathic pain as "pain arising as a direct consequence of a lesion or disease affecting the somatosensory system" [4]. Several mechanisms explain neuropathic pain including inflammatory processes at the site of the damaged nerve and ephaptic transmission, where action potentials of axons "cross-talk" and excite adjacent neurons [8]. As with any tissue injury, axonal injury results in a release of pro-inflammatory mediators leading to complement activation, mast cell degranulation, neutrophil infiltration, macrophage recruitment, and infiltration of T lymphocytes. The inflammatory process furthers the initial allodynia and hyperalgesia. Unlike non-neuronal tissue, axonal damage leads to a process called Wallerian degeneration undertaken by Schwann cells and macrophages in an attempt to clear myelin and begin the process of axonal regeneration [5, 9]. Peripheral neuronal damage can lead to cross-excitation within the sensory ganglia via paracrine effects of inflammatory mediators. After sensing changes in the neuronal soma from peripheral injury, satellite glial cells release ATP, substance P, calcitonin gene-related peptide, and glial cell line-derived neurotrophic factor in the trigeminal sensory ganglion, which increase the excitability of small and medium diameter neurons [10]. Peripheral injury induces inflammatory changes in the central nervous system through microglia and astrocytes in a similar way as central sensitization, which will be discussed further [5, 11].

Not mutually exclusive of inflammatory-mediated neuropathy, Devor proposed a theory on neuropathic pain due to compression, specifically applied to trigeminal neuralgia, called the ignition hypothesis. Studies show that chronic nerve compression results in demyelination [12]. Peripheral innocuous stimuli create action potentials in the Aβ afferents. At the demyelinated site of compression, ephaptic coupling can occur, which is the transmission of action potentials from Aβ to adjacent axons that are lightly myelinated or have no myelin at all, the Aδ and C fibers. Therefore, the originally innocuous stimuli are perceived to be noxious by the central nervous system, explaining allodynia [12]. The ignition hypothesis was originally only applied to trigeminal neuralgia but may be extended to any neuropathic pain caused by compression or demyelination. Sites of damaged peripheral nerves not only cross-talk through ephaptic transmission but can spontaneously fire action potentials, known as ectopic activity. Several studies have shown spontaneous activity of C fibers in neuropathic pain [13–15]. Ectopic activity with ephaptic coupling and immunomodulation may all play a role in neuropathic pain.

Central Sensitization

Central sensitization is a theory based on brain plasticity of the nociceptive circuits past the primary afferents and explains dynamic tactile allodynia, secondary punctate/pressure hyperalgesia, temporal summation, and sensory aftereffects [16]. Central sensitization creates chronic pain states by increasing excitability and decreasing pain inhibition. In the spinal cord after peripheral injury, spinal microglia produce tumor necrosis factor and interleukin-1β and 6, which enhance transmission and suppress inhibitory signals in lamina II neurons [17]. Meanwhile, released brain-derived growth factor (BDNF) suppresses GABAergic inhibition in lamina I projections [18], which is consistent with the proposed gate control theory of pain [19]. The inhibitory and endogenous opioid neurons project to the dorsal horns from the periaqueductal gray and rostral ventral medulla; both are theorized to be influenced by central sensitization [20]. BDNF is also implicated in long-term potentiation in the hippocampus. Researchers propose that central sensitization is similar to memory formation or learning [21]. Unlike, neuropathic pain, central sensitization does not require neuronal injury [22]. Many patients experience pain in the absence of noxious stimuli or proven pathology. Central sensitization offers an explanation of how pain can be experienced without peripheral stimulation [16].

Neuralgias

The pathophysiology regarding trigeminal neuralgia continues to be debated. Originally, TN was attributed to abnormal central nervous system discharges similar to seizures as antiepileptic drugs were the first successful treatment [23]. Currently, the most commonly advanced mechanism of TN involves vascular compression of the nerve at the dorsal root entry zone to the pons, where central oligodendrocytes cede to Schwann cells for production of myelin [24, 25]. Evidence for the compression is provided by the curative benefit many patients experience with microvascular decompression of the trigeminal nerve. Biopsies from the trigeminal nerve dorsal root entry zone (DREZ) have shown compression of the nerve with loss of myelin [26, 27]. The loss of myelin at the DREZ allowed Devor to develop the ignition hypothesis discussed above. However, recent imaging studies demonstrate cases where patients have no compression of the nerve on MRI or intraoperatively [28]. Devor et al. (2002) explain these cases by hypothesizing patients must have compression of the trigeminal pathway elsewhere [27]. Other studies show small fiber (Aδ and C) dysfunction in TN patients suggesting symptoms of TN arise from compression of the smaller pain fibers resulting in ectopic discharges rather than the ephaptic coupling from demyelinated Aβ afferents [29, 30].

Trigeminal neuralgia must be distinguished into two subsets: typical or TN1, which is the more common form, involving intermittent intense lancinating pain for brief moments, and atypical or TN2, which shares symptoms with the typical form, but patients also develop a constant burning pain at baseline [25]. TN type 2 has been described as a chronic form of TN type 1, as a natural history study shows progression of intermittent pain to constant burning pain with intermittent eruptions [31]. Patients with TN2 were found to have increased central processing from stimulation than TN1 patients, likely representing overstimulation at the level of the medulla. This study implies central plasticity at wide-dynamic range second-order neurons or third-order neurons [30].

V2 and V3 dermatomes contain the most common trigger points and are the areas of greatest symptomology [26, 30], and superior cerebellar artery is the most likely culprit of compression at the dorsal root entry zone [26–28]. Anatomical studies demonstrate the rostral, superior projection of alpha fibers from V2 and V3 to the main trigeminal sensory nucleus in the pons, which would be the site of compression for superior cerebellar artery. The higher density of Aδ fibers at this location may explain the lancinating pain of typical TN. C fibers mostly project to the caudal medulla, which may be related to the increased central processing in atypical TN [32].

Other causes of trigeminal neuralgia exist beyond the idiopathic form discussed above such as cerebellopontine angle tumors and multiple sclerosis. TN caused by CPA tumors is thought to have a similar mechanism to neurovascular compression, as resection of tumor can provide relief of symptoms [33]. Multiple sclerosis is a demyelinating disease, so it causes TN via an axonopathy that is witnessed with chronic compression in vascular compression. MS plaques have been shown to involve the trigeminal nerve at the DREZ [34].

Glossopharyngeal neuralgia is a condition of hyperactivity of the glossopharyngeal nerve; therefore the same theories of pathophysiology apply here as in TN. It consists of intermittent, severe sharp pain affecting the sensory distribution of the ninth and tenth cranial nerve, particularly the throat, oropharynx, base of the tongue, ear canal, and areas inferior to the angle of the mandible [35]. Many cases of GPN are found to have vascular compression of the ninth nerve at the dorsal root entry zone to the medulla [36]. Other forms of neuronal damage and compression, including post-traumatic, Eagle's syndrome, postradiation, tumor compression, and multiple sclerosis, can produce symptoms of glossopharyngeal neuralgia [37].

Occipital neuralgia can present with strikingly similar symptoms to TN but covering the superior and inferior occipital nerves. Nerve dysfunction, mostly from compression, is the cardinal etiology of the disease process. Pathophysiology can include vascular compression from aberrant courses of the posterior inferior cerebellar artery or vertebral artery of the C1 and C2 nerve root, multiple sclerosis, C2 myelitis, tumor, or spondylosis of the C1/2 joint with tonic muscular contraction and compression [38].

Postherpetic neuralgia is continued pain after acute varicella zoster viral (VZV) infection and resolution of the rash. VZV can remain latent in the trigeminal ganglion of patients who have experienced chicken pox in the past. Postherpetic neuralgia exists in the same dermatome of the acute zoster infection and causes allodynia, hyperalgesia, constant burning, and intermittent lancinating common to other neuropathic diseases [39]. The inflammatory process of reactivation most likely creates peripheral and central sensitization resulting in unpleasant symptoms. Of cranial herpes zoster, 75% occur in the V1 (ophthalmic) division because of an unknown predilection for the latent VZV to settle in the ophthalmic portion of the gasserian ganglion [40]. The variety of symptoms may be explained best by the inconsistent proportional destruction of Aβ, Aδ, or C fibers [32].

Traumatic injuries to the afferent sensory nerves of the face and head can lead to neuropathic pain. After transection of peripheral sensory nerves, the transected axons begin Wallerian degeneration and form neuromas. Neuromas can also form after any damaging process including compression, stretch, postsurgical scar, and irritation [41]. Neuromas have been implicated in creating neuropathic pain. At the site of neuromas, the axons are highly disorganized in shape and myelinations. Several adjacent axons may not be myelinated by Schwann cells which can lead to ectopic discharge and ephaptic cross-talk, producing the symptoms of neuropathic pain [42]. Also, inflammatory results from traumatic nerve injuries can result in peripheral and central sensitization as discussed above [43].

Inflammatory

Inflammatory conditions such as infections or malignancy may have an entirely different pathophysiology than the syndromes previously discussed. Malignancy can cause a complex pain state involving neuropathic damage and compression, inflammatory signals, and ischemic mechanisms. Tumors can generate and secrete painful mediators like protons, bradykinin, endothelins, prostaglandins, proteases, and various growth factors [44]. Animal models show changes in centrally located microglia to enhance the synaptic transmission of pain signals [45]. Thus, peripheral and central sensitization play roles in cancer pain.

Many patients complain of facial pains from infectious bacteria, fungi, and viruses. Recent evidence suggests that some infectious elements may stimulate nociceptors through a novel mechanism. *Staphylococcus aureus* emits α-hemolysin which creates pores in the phospholipid bilayer of nociceptors causing loss of membrane potential and action potential firing. Other bacteria are known to emit ligands that directly bind receptors on nociceptors creating action potentials [46]. Lipopolysaccharides of bacterial cell walls peripherally sensitize nociceptors by binding a receptor and creating noxious hyperactivity [47].

Idiopathic

Some chronic pain disorders have no histopathological or instrumental evidence to explain the proportionality of symptoms. Temporomandibular disorder, persistent idiopathic facial pain, atypical odontalgia, and burning mouth syndrome have a high degree of comorbidity with other chronic pain states like fibromyalgia, headache, migraine, irritable bowel syndrome, and low back pain [20, 48, 49]. These neurophysiological disorders have been grouped into a category explained by their proposed pathophysiology, central sensitization syndromes. The mechanism behind central sensitization syndromes is in high likelihood multifactorial, and often these syndromes are diagnosed in patients with comorbid psychiatric disorder or autonomic dysfunction [20].

Temporomandibular disorder (TMD) is characterized as a clinical diagnose of generalized chronic pain of the stomatognathic system. In TMD, studies have shown functional and structural changes to prefrontal cortex and basal ganglia. Researchers suggest that patients suffer from decreased function of endogenous opioids of the periaqueductal gray and descending inhibitory pathways from the rostral ventral medulla [20]. Studies have shown that the central sensitization of TMD may begin with peripheral triggers like dental pain, oral surgery, or temporomandibular joint dysfunction [20]. Persistent idiopathic facial pain (PIFP) is a clinical diagnosis of chronic, nonspecific, and poorly localized pain without neurological deficit. Recent studies have shown some patients with PIFP have changes in blink reflex testing and thermal quantitative sensory testing, suggesting pathology of small fibers. However, the researchers were unable to localize the dysfunction to peripheral or central sensitization [50]. Atypical odontalgia is a clinical diagnosis defined as a chronic continuous pain symptom located in the dentoalveolar region, unexplainable by other disease processes. Many patients who experience atypical odontalgia recall onset after dental procedures, which is suggestive of a neuropathic pain syndrome rather than central sensitization [48]. However, 60% of patients in one study had a comorbid psychiatric condition, and antipsychotics were shown to be effective in treatment, suggesting a more central mechanism to the pain [51]. Burning mouth syndrome is characterized by a continuous burning sensation from the oral mucosa without a causative lesion. A relationship has been shown between oral pain and fibromyalgia, a central sensitization syndrome [52]. Histopathological studies have shown significantly lower density of epithelial and subepithelial nerve fibers in patients with burning mouth syndrome versus controls [48, 53]. In dry eye-like pain, patients suffer from the feeling of corneal irritation without a significantly decreased tear film; animal models have recently shown changes in the trigeminal brainstem nucleus after inducing reduced tear volume for 2 weeks, implying a central sensitization to the stimulus [54].

Like most syndromes proposed to be caused by central sensitizations, headaches are multifactorial in nature. Although different in symptomology, central sensitization may have a role in tension, cluster, and migraine headaches [55–59].

A variety of insults and mechanisms cause head and facial pain. Peripheral sensitization, neuropathic pain, and central sensitization phenomena—separately or combined—may result in chronic head and facial pain syndromes. A detailed understanding of the pathophysiology of each patient's facial pain will help the practitioner to arrive at the correct diagnosis and to assist in formulating optimal treatments.

References

1. Ingram SL. Molecular basis of nociception. In: Winn HR, editor. Youmans and Winn neurological surgery. Philadelphia: Elsevier; 2017. p. 1379.
2. Julius D, Basbaum AI. Molecular mechanisms of nociception. Nature. 2001;413(6852):203–10.
3. Reichling DB, Levine JD. Critical role of nociceptor plasticity in chronic pain. Trends Neurosci. 2009;32(12):611–8.
4. Treede RD, Jensen TS, Campbell JN, et al. Neuropathic pain: redefinition and a grading system for clinical and research purposes. Neurology. 2008;70(18):1630–5.
5. Austin PJ, Moalem-Taylor G. The neuro-immune balance in neuropathic pain: involvement of inflammatory immune cells, immune-like glial cells and cytokines. J Neuroimmunol. 2010;229(1–2):26–50.
6. Parada CA, Reichling DB, Levine JD. Chronic hyperalgesic priming in the rat involves a novel interaction between cAMP and PKCepsilon second messenger pathways. Pain. 2005;113(1–2):185–90.
7. Hirai T, Mulpuri Y, Cheng Y, et al. Aberrant plasticity of peripheral sensory axons in a painful neuropathy. Sci Rep. 2017;7(1):3407.
8. Cohen SP, Mao J. Neuropathic pain: mechanisms and their clinical implications. BMJ. 2014;348:f7656.
9. Conforti L, Gilley J, Coleman MP. Wallerian degeneration: an emerging axon death pathway linking injury and disease. Nat Rev Neurosci. 2014;15(6):394–409.
10. Takeda M, Takahashi M, Hara N, Matsumoto S. Glial cell line-derived neurotrophic factor modulates the excitability of nociceptive trigeminal ganglion neurons via a paracrine mechanism following inflammation. Brain Behav Immun. 2013;28:100–7.
11. Coull JA, Beggs S, Boudreau D, et al. BDNF from microglia causes the shift in neuronal anion gradient underlying neuropathic pain. Nature. 2005;438(7070):1017–21.
12. Devor M, Amir R, Rappaport ZH. Pathophysiology of trigeminal neuralgia: the ignition hypothesis. Clin J Pain. 2002;18(1):4–13.
13. Campero M, Bostock H, Baumann TK, Ochoa JL. A search for activation of C nociceptors by sympathetic fibers in complex regional pain syndrome. Clin Neurophysiol. 2010;121(7):1072–9.
14. Serra J, Solà R, Aleu J, Quiles C, Navarro X, Bostock H. Double and triple spikes in C-nociceptors in neuropathic pain states: an additional peripheral mechanism of hyperalgesia. Pain. 2011;152(2):343–53.
15. Kleggetveit IP, Namer B, Schmidt R, et al. High spontaneous activity of C-nociceptors in painful polyneuropathy. Pain. 2012;153(10):2040–7.

16. Woolf CJ. Central sensitization: implications for the diagnosis and treatment of pain. Pain. 2011;152(3 Suppl):S2–15.
17. Basbaum AI, Bautista DM, Scherrer G, Julius D. Cellular and molecular mechanisms of pain. Cell. 2009;139(2):267–84.
18. Ji RR, Chamessian A, Zhang YQ. Pain regulation by non-neuronal cells and inflammation. Science. 2016;354(6312):572–7.
19. Melzack R, Wall PD. Pain mechanisms: a new theory. Science. 1965;150(3699):971–9.
20. Monaco A, Cattaneo R, Marci MC, et al. Central sensitization-based classification for temporomandibular disorders: a pathogenetic hypothesis. Pain Res Manag. 2017;2017:5957076.
21. Kandasamy R, Price TJ. The pharmacology of nociceptor priming. Handb Exp Pharmacol. 2015;227:15–37.
22. Nijs J, Torres-Cueco R, Van Wilgen CP, et al. Applying modern pain neuroscience in clinical practice: criteria for the classification of central sensitization pain. Pain Physician. 2014;17(5):447–57.
23. Bergouignan M. Successful cure of essential facial neuralgia by sodium diphenylhydantoinate (in French). Rev Larygol Otol Rhinol (Bord). 1942;63:34–41.
24. Jannetta PJ. Arterial compression of the trigeminal nerve at the pons in patients with trigeminal neuralgia. J Neurosurg. 1967;26(1 Suppl):159–62.
25. Eller JL, Raslan AM, Burchiel KJ. Trigeminal neuralgia: definition and classification. Neurosurg Focus. 2005;18(5):E3.
26. Cheng J, Meng J, Liu W, et al. Nerve atrophy in trigeminal neuralgia due to neurovascular compression and its association with surgical outcomes after microvascular decompression. Acta Neurochir. 2017;159(9):1699 705.
27. Devor M, Govrin-lippmann R, Rappaport ZH. Mechanism of trigeminal neuralgia: an ultrastructural analysis of trigeminal root specimens obtained during microvascular decompression surgery. J Neurosurg. 2002;96(3):532–43.
28. Lee A, Mccartney S, Burbidge C, et al. Trigeminal neuralgia occurs and recurs in the absence of neurovascular compression. J Neurosurg. 2014;120(5):1048–54.
29. Liao MF, Lee M, Hsieh MJ, et al. Evaluation of the pathophysiology of classical trigeminal neuralgia by blink reflex study and current perception threshold testing. J Headache Pain. 2010;11(3):241–6.
30. Obermann M, Yoon MS, Ese D, et al. Impaired trigeminal nociceptive processing in patients with trigeminal neuralgia. Neurology. 2007;69(9):835–41.
31. Burchiel KJ, Slavin KV. On the natural history of trigeminal neuralgia. Neurosurgery. 2000;46(1):152–4.
32. Dasilva AF, Dossantos MF. The role of sensory fiber demography in trigeminal and postherpetic neuralgias. J Dent Res. 2012;91(1):17–24.
33. Shulev Y, Trashin A, Gordienko K. Secondary trigeminal neuralgia in cerebellopontine angle tumors. Skull Base. 2011;21(5):287–94.
34. Love S, Gradidge T, Coakham HB. Trigeminal neuralgia due to multiple sclerosis: ultrastructural findings in trigeminal rhizotomy specimens. Neuropathol Appl Neurobiol. 2001;27(3):238–44.
35. Minagar A, Sheremata WA. Glossopharyngeal neuralgia and MS. Neurology. 2000;54(6):1368–70.
36. Teixeira MJ, De Siqueira SR, Bor-Seng-Shu E. Glossopharyngeal neuralgia: neurosurgical treatment and differential diagnosis. Acta Neurochir. 2008;150(5):471–5.
37. Khan M, Nishi SE, Hassan SN, et al. Trigeminal neuralgia, glossopharyngeal neuralgia, and myofascial pain dysfunction syndrome: an update. Pain Res Manag. 2017;2017:7438326.
38. Choi I, Jeon SR. Neuralgias of the head: occipital neuralgia. J Korean Med Sci. 2016;31(4):479–88.
39. Mallick-Searle T, Snodgrass B, Brant JM. Postherpetic neuralgia: epidemiology, pathophysiology, and pain management pharmacology. J Multidiscip Healthc. 2016;9:447–54.

40. de Leeuw R, American Academy of Orofacial Pain. Orofacial pain: guideline or assessment, diagnosis, and management. Chicago: Quintessence; 2008.
41. Rajput K, Reddy S, Shankar H. Painful neuromas. Clin J Pain. 2012;28(7):639–45.
42. Fried K, Govrin-Lippmann R, Devor M. Close apposition among neighbouring axonal endings in a neuroma. J Neurocytol. 1993;22(8):663–81.
43. Benoliel R, Kahn J, Eliav E. Peripheral painful traumatic trigeminal neuropathies. Oral Dis. 2012;18(4):317–32.
44. Mantyh P. Bone cancer pain: causes, consequences, and therapeutic opportunities. Pain. 2013;154(Suppl 1):S54–62.
45. Yang Y, Li H, Li TT, et al. Delayed activation of spinal microglia contributes to the maintenance of bone cancer pain in female Wistar rats via P2X7 receptor and IL-18. J Neurosci. 2015;35(20):7950–63.
46. Chiu IM, Heesters BA, Ghasemlou N, et al. Bacteria activate sensory neurons that modulate pain and inflammation. Nature. 2013;501(7465):52–7.
47. Diogenes A, Ferraz CC, Akopian AN, et al. LPS sensitizes TRPV1 via activation of TLR4 in trigeminal sensory neurons. J Dent Res. 2011;90(6):759–64.
48. Forssell H, Jääskeläinen S, List T, et al. An update on pathophysiological mechanisms related to idiopathic oro-facial pain conditions with implications for management. J Oral Rehabil. 2015;42(4):300–22.
49. Seccia TM, Rossitto G, Calò LA, Rossi GP. Oral burning with dysphagia and weight loss. Medicine (Baltimore). 2015;94(31):e1163.
50. Lang E, Kaltenhäuser M, Seidler S, et al. Persistent idiopathic facial pain exists independent of somatosensory input from the painful region: findings from quantitative sensory functions and somatotopy of the primary somatosensory cortex. Pain. 2005;118(1-2):80–91.
51. Takenoshita M, Miura A, Shinohara Y, et al. Clinical features of atypical odontalgia; three cases and literature reviews. Biopsychosoc Med. 2017;11:21.
52. Rhodus NL, Fricton J, Carlson P, Messner R. Oral symptoms associated with fibromyalgia syndrome. J Rheumatol. 2003;30(8):1841–5.
53. Lauria G, Majorana A, Borgna M, et al. Trigeminal small-fiber sensory neuropathy causes burning mouth syndrome. Pain. 2005;115(3):332–7.
54. Rahman M, Okamoto K, Thompson R, et al. Sensitization of trigeminal brainstem pathways in a model for tear deficient dry eye. Pain. 2015;156(5):942–50.
55. Bendtsen L. Central sensitization in tension-type headache–possible pathophysiological mechanisms. Cephalalgia. 2000;20(5):486–508.
56. Buchgreitz L, Lyngberg AC, Bendtsen L, Jensen R. Frequency of headache is related to sensitization: a population study. Pain. 2006;123(1-2):19–27.
57. Fernández-de-las-Peñas C, Cuadrado ML, Arendt-Nielsen L, et al. Myofascial trigger points and sensitization: an updated pain model for tension-type headache. Cephalalgia. 2007;27(5):383–93.
58. Sandrini G, Proietti Cecchini A, Milanov I, et al. Electrophysiological evidence for trigeminal neuron sensitization in patients with migraine. Neurosci Lett. 2002;317(3):135–8.
59. Fernández-de-las-Peñas C, Ortega-Santiago R, Cuadrado ML, et al. Bilateral widespread mechanical pain hypersensitivity as sign of central sensitization in patients with cluster headache. Headache. 2011;51(3):384–91.

Chapter 4
Nomenclature and Differential Diagnosis

Rabia Tari and Konstantin V. Slavin

Introduction

Facial pain is a debilitating pain condition which can affect at one point or another up to 26% of the general population [1]. As a matter of fact, it may be safe to assume that every living person has experienced facial pain at some point of her/his life due to dental issues, sinus problems, diseases, and injuries of the eyes, face, etc. In general, the facial pain may be a sign of various pathologies of facial structures, central nervous system (i.e., brain stem, thalamus, etc.) lesions, and cranial nerves or, in many of the cases, originate from an unknown source.

The general category of facial pain disorders includes diverse number of pathological conditions; these may be divided into neuropathic and nociceptive, odontogenic and non-odontogenic, neurogenic and non-neurogenic, etc. The differentiation and subcategorization vary among the disciplines and with different grouping strategies.

Neuropathic facial pain is a common term used for facial pain associated with nerve lesions or injuries [2]. The sensory innervation of the face is provided by both spinal nerves (C2–C4) and cranial nerves (V, VII, IX, X), and the trigeminal nerve is the source of the facial pain in the majority of the anatomically obvious neuralgias and neuropathies. Trigeminal neuralgia (TN) is worth particular attention as a distinct subtype of the facial pain as this potentially devastating condition can be successfully managed with multiple well-established interventions. While its diagnosis is quite straightforward, the exact terminology of its variants remains a common issue in publications.

According to a recent systematic review, the prevalence of trigeminal neuralgia (TN) ranges from 0.03 to 0.3% [3]. This tenfold discrepancy may be explained by a relatively small number of studies that fulfill the commonly accepted criteria of

R. Tari · K. V. Slavin (✉)
Department of Neurosurgery, University of Illinois at Chicago, Chicago, IL, USA
e-mail: kslavin@uic.edu

J. Y. Suen, E. Petersen (eds.), *Diagnosis and Management of Head and Face Pain*, https://doi.org/10.1007/978-3-319-90999-8_4

quality but also by heterogeneity of TN characteristics and subtypes [4–6]. The situation with confusing terminology gets even more complicated when it comes to more general facial pain epidemiology studies. There are only few meta-analyses in this field as multiple studies that use different classification strategies and criteria get discarded.

The general understanding of common facial pain terminology and differential diagnosis is the purpose of this chapter. Emphasis is placed on neuropathic facial pain.

Nomenclature

The terms used in this field are based on classifications and taxonomies proposed by study groups, author-based consensus, and individual expert opinions. In some classification systems, facial pain is grouped separately or together with the headache and orofacial pain. Five current major classifications that are used worldwide include facial pain disorders:

1. International Classification of Headache Disorders (ICHD), by the International Headache Society (IHS)
2. Classification of Chronic Pain, by the International Association for the Study of Pain (IASP)
3. International Classification of Diseases (ICD) coding, by the World Health Organization (WHO)
4. Classification from the American Association of Orofacial Pain (AAOP)
5. Burchiel classification

Among these, only IASP, ICHD, and Burchiel classifications contain descriptive information and diagnostic criteria for neuropathic facial pain [7–9].

Nonetheless, there are many publications do not follow the terms used in these classifications. The need for a terminological clearout for the confusing pool of interpretations is therefore quite evident [10]. The misinterpretations of pain conditions create a burden for decision-making, prescribing of treatments, evaluation of treatment efficacy, and planning of research and communication [11].

The attempt of Nixdorf et al. for orofacial pain taxonomy was promising. They have used persistent dentoalveolar pain disorder as an example to show how ontological principles can be used to improve related taxonomy [10]. However, the problem is not always the terms. Different stages of disease progression or overlapping conditions may have an impact on confusing nomenclature in literature [12, 13]. One example is the term "atypical odontalgia" which can also refer to phantom tooth pain, deafferentation pain, trigeminal neuropathy, or atypical facial pain [10, 13]. Although it was advised not to group these disorders for the aim of improving treatment selections, the confusing terms are still being used [14, 15].

Table 4.1 Comparative table of facial pain classifications

Facial pain classifications	Year	Extent of classification	Structure	Comments
The International Classification of Diseases (ICD) coding-ICD 10	2015	All diseases	Coding system Not diagnostic, not categorized Etiologically based	ICD-11 will be integrated with ICHD
International Headache Society (IHS) International Classification of Headache Disorders (ICHD-3 beta)	2013	Headache and facial pain	Diagnostic, theoretical, etiological, unidimensional Consensus of experts Criteria for each disorder	Validation problem for atypical pain Insufficient evidence
International Society for the Study of Pain (IASP)-Classification of Chronic Pain	1994	Pain disorders	Multiaxial, descriptive theoretical No criteria	Validation problem for atypical pain
American Association of Orofacial Pain (AAOP)	2005	Orofacial pain	Based on symptomatology Multiaxial No criteria	Two axes (physical and psycho); first axis: six subgroups

Despite the recent attempts to combine and integrate some of them, current terminology remains problematic and will be mentioned in context of relevant classifications under the section of differential diagnosis.

Diagnostic Classifications (Table 4.1)

The first consensus on the classification of headache disorders was pursued by an ad hoc committee formed by the US National Institutes of Health in 1962 [16] . In 1986, it was followed by IASP task force classification which was revised in 1994 and updated twice since then [17]. Recently, it was announced that ICD-11 will be integrated with new classification of IASP task force [18]. One out of seven main chronic pain topics, the "chronic headache and orofacial pain," contains four subgroups, and chronic orofacial pain is among them:

1. Chronic primary headaches
2. Chronic secondary headaches
3. Chronic orofacial pains
4. Headache and orofacial pain not otherwise specified

ICHD is another general diagnostic classification that is used in most epidemiological studies; it was first published in 1988. Two revisions later, its latest version, so-called beta-edition, was published to collect evidence and provide field testing opportunities [19, 20] (Table 4.2). All physicians working in the related fields were

Table 4.2 ICHD-3 beta classification with brief descriptions

Painful cranial neuropathies and other facial pains
1. Trigeminal neuralgia
A. *Classical trigeminal neuralgia*
(a) Classical TN, purely paroxysmal
(b) Classical TN with concomitant persistent facial pain
B. Painful trigeminal neuropathy
(a) Painful trigeminal neuropathy attributed to acute herpes zoster
(b) Postherpetic trigeminal neuropathy
(c) Painful post-traumatic trigeminal neuropathy
(d) Painful trigeminal neuropathy attributed to multiple sclerosis (MS) plaque
(e) Painful trigeminal neuropathy attributed to other disorder
2. Glossopharyngeal neuralgia
3. Nervus intermedius (facial nerve) neuralgia
A. Classical nervus intermedius neuralgia
B. Nervus intermedius neuropathy attributed to herpes zoster
4. Occipital neuralgia
5. Optic neuritis
6. Headache attributed to ischemic ocular motor nerve palsy
7. Tolosa-Hunt syndrome
8. Paratrigeminal oculosympathetic (Raeder's) syndrome
9. Recurrent painful ophthalmoplegic neuropathy
10. Burning mouth syndrome (BMS)
11. Persistent idiopathic facial pain (PIFP)
12. Central neuropathic pain
A. Central neuropathic pain attributed to MS
B. Central poststroke pain (CPSP)

invited to submit evidence to the chair persons of the relevant chapter for the next ICHD revision [19, 20]. ICHD-3 is expected to be published in 2018.

Neuropathic pain is classified in most pertinent fashion by Burchiel in 2003 with partial subsequent revision in 2005 (Table 4.3) [8, 21]. Here, we use Burchiel classification as a diagnostic guide (Table 4.4).

Questionnaires

While clinically based differential diagnosis is achieved by the classifications' diagnostic criteria and physicians' clinical assessments, instrument-based differential diagnosis was tested by various authors as well (Table 4.5).

Table 4.3 Trigeminal neuralgia types in different classifications

Classification, year	# of sub-categories for TN	TN type							Other
Burchiel classification, 2005	7	TN1 Idiopathic sharp, shooting, electric shock-like episode pain	TN2 Idiopathic aching, throbbing burning, >50% constant pain	TNP Unintentional trigeminal injury	Trigeminal deafferentation pain Intentional trigeminal injury	Resulting from herpes outbreak	ATN Somatoform pain disorder	Associated with MS	
International Classification of Diseases (ICD), 2015	6	G50.0 TN: syndrome of paroxysmal facial pain	–	–	S04.3 Injury of trigeminal nerve	B02.22 Postherpetic TN	G50.1 Atypical facial pain	–	G.50.8 Other disorders of TN G50.9 Disorders of TN, unspecified
IASP, 1994 (updated 2011, 2012)	5	TN	–	–	Secondary trigeminal neuralgia from facial trauma	Acute HZV (trigeminal) Postherpetic neuralgia	–	Secondary TN from CNS lesions	
ICHD, 2013	8	Classical TN	Classical TN with concomitant persistent facial pain (previously ATN/TN2)	–	Painful post-traumatic trigeminal neuropathy (previously anesthesia dolorosa)	Painful trigeminal neuropathy attributed to acute herpes zoster Postherpetic trigeminal neuropathy	Persistent idiopathic facial pain (PIFP)	–	

(continued)

Table 4.3 (continued)

Classification, year	# of sub-categories for TN	TN type							Other
AAN-EFNS guidelines, 2016	4	Classical TN (MR proved)	TN with continuous pain	–	–	–	–	Secondary TN from lesions including MS	Idiopathic TN when no etiology found Grading system added

Table 4.4 Burchiel TN classification (2003)

1. Trigeminal neuralgia type 1 (TN1): Idiopathic, sharp shooting, electrical shock-like, episodic pain
2. Trigeminal neuralgia type 2 (TN2): Idiopathic, aching, throbbing, burning, >50% constant pain
3. Trigeminal neuropathic pain (TNP): It is caused by unintentional injury to the trigeminal system from trauma; oral surgery, root injury from posterior fossa, or cranial base surgery, stroke, etc. can be causes of this type of pain
4. Trigeminal deafferentation pain: The presence of numbness as a result of intentional injury from denervating pain procedures
5. Symptomatic trigeminal neuralgia: Associated with multiple sclerosis
6. Facial postherpetic neuralgia: Resulting from outbreak of facial herpes zoster
7. Atypical trigeminal neuralgia: Somatoform disorder

Table 4.5 Diagnostic questionnaires

Author/s	Year	Topic	Predictability rate (%)	# of groups, subgroups
Hapak et al.	1994	Craniofacial pain	74.3	Three groups and nine subgroups
Limonadi et al.	2006	Trigeminal neuralgia	95	Seven groups
Aggarwal et al.	2007	Orofacial pain	94	Three groups
McCartney et al.	2014	Facial pain	87.1	10
MacFarlane et al.	2004	Orofacial pain	71, 71, 57	Three groups; 23 subgroups

In 1975, Melzack first published a pain questionnaire that can measure pain and provide quantitative information at the same time [22]. It has been found that McGill's questionnaire may help differentiate between TN and atypical facial pain with 90% correct prediction [23].

In 1994, a self-administered questionnaire based on diagnostic classification was proposed by Hapak et al. [24]. Three categories were obtained: musculoligamentous, neurologic, and dentoalveolar. Neurologically based conditions included atypical facial pain, TN, migraine, cluster headache, and muscular contraction headache. The findings indicated that the sensitivity and specificity of this diagnostic questionnaire were 78.7%, 78.9%, and 37.5% and 81.5%, 78.2%, and 97% for the musculoligamentous, neurologic, and dentoalveolar groups, respectively. They used questionnaire and digital pain scales for undiagnosed patients and then classified them according to the most probable diagnosis.

In 2004, Macfarlane et al. presented a new classification questionnaire for orofacial pain and classified a total of 125 patients into three groups: musculoligamentous with 71%, dentoalveolar with 71%, and neurological/vascular with 57% good prediction [25].

Another questionnaire-based tool for classifying self-reported orofacial pain was developed and validated in population-based studies by Aggarwal et al. [26].

However, this tool grouped together the orofacial pain conditions that were likely to have an underlying pathology and those likely to be idiopathic. In a second study, these authors aimed to develop and validate a questionnaire-based tool that would enable classification of idiopathic orofacial pain in the general population [27]. They classified three categories, idiopathic, dentoalveolar, and musculoligamentous, based on distinct characteristics reported in a self-administered questionnaire. Ninety-four percent of the cases were successfully classified.

In 2006, Limonadi et al. presented the artificial neural network (ANN) which provided a tool for self-diagnosis based on a computerized questionnaire for TN patients [28]. Patients were classified according to Burchiel classifications. Predictability rates were higher than 95%. However, the study population was skewed due to a high percentage of typical TN patients. In 2014, an update was published by the same group [29]. They added four more questions and turned the questionnaire into a web-based diagnostic tool for ten different facial pain diagnoses. The sensitivity and specificity of new ANN were reported to be 92.4% and 87.8% for TN1, respectively, which was an improvement compared to the previous results of 84 and 83% of the earlier version. The ANN was still less sensitive at determining an accurate TN2 diagnosis (62.5% sensitive) but also better than the previous version. They mentioned that in forthcoming data sets, they are determined to improve temporomandibular joint disorders, nervus intermedius neuralgia, and glossopharyngeal neuralgia diagnoses as well.

Pain is a uniquely personal experience, and measuring it is highly perceptional. The controversy in the literature about the validation of the pain questionnaires is therefore almost inevitable.

Differential Diagnosis

Diagnostic criteria offered in classifications and/or extensive clinical experience draw the path to an accurate diagnosis. The first step is the clinical data gathering. History-taking stands as a gold standard method for facial pain diagnostic process. It should be integrated with the physical examination and imaging, with particular emphasis on the relevant differential diagnosis. The differential diagnosis of facial pain is detailed in (Table 4.2).

Neuralgia

The term neuralgia generally refers to a painful condition of a named nerve; it is considered a true example of painful mononeuropathy. When it comes to classification of neuralgias, the terminology varies, but in general, they are divided into primary and secondary, typical, or classic and atypical, central and peripheral, idiopathic, or unknown, and these terms are used freely in multiple publications making nomenclature definition very complex.

Use of the term "secondary" is expected to be limited to those cases where the painful nerve is affected by a known distinct pathological process such as tumor, vascular malformation, trauma, infection, or demyelination. Such straightforward distinction becomes somewhat controversial when IHS classification suggests naming neuralgia "secondary" if a vascular compression is identified during surgical intervention and "primary" if surgical intervention never took place. In surgeon's mind, however, the neuralgia that occurs in the absence of conditions listed above (tumor, etc.) is considered "primary" whether or not there is a documented vascular compression.

Trigeminal Neuralgia/Trigeminal Pain

Trigeminal neuralgia is a heterogeneous group of disorders presenting with neuropathic pain in one or more branches of the trigeminal nerve.

Pre-trigeminal Neuralgia

This term refers to a continuous dull pain in the upper or lower jaw that later develops into classic TN [30].

Idiopathic Trigeminal Neuralgia. Type I

(ICD: G50.0 trigeminal neuralgia, syndrome of paroxysmal facial pain, tic douloureux; ICHD, 13.1.1.1 classical TN, purely paroxysmal; IASP, 006.X8a trigeminal neuralgia, tic douloureux) (Table 4.6)

Table 4.6 ICHD-3 beta diagnostic criteria for classical TN

A. At least three attacks unilateral facial pain fulfilling criteria B and C
B. Occurring in one or more divisions of the trigeminal nerve, with no radiation beyond the trigeminal distribution
C. Pain has at least three of the following four characteristics:
1. Recurring in paroxysmal attacks lasting from a fraction of a second to 2 min
2. Severe intensity
3. Electric shock-like, shooting, stabbing, or sharp in quality
4. Precipitated by innocuous stimuli to the affected side
D. No clinically evident neurologic deficit
E. Not better accounted for by another ICHD-3 diagnosis

Idiopathic TN, previously known as classical or typical TN, is characterized by unilateral severe brief sharp pain attacks in one or more branches of the trigeminal nerve with spontaneous onset or triggered by non-painful stimuli. In between these electric shock-like pain attacks, there are refractory periods when triggering no longer produces pain. It may be bilateral in some cases.

It has been hypothesized that this condition may further advance to the type of TN formerly known as atypical, characterized by more than 50% constant pain [31]. The vascular compression of the trigeminal nerve root has been accepted as an etiopathogenetic factor for TN1 as the surgical decompression may cure this condition. However, multiple anatomical and radiological studies showed that vascular compression does not always result in TN symptoms [31–33]. As a matter of fact, up to 32% of people without pain have been found to have neurovascular compromise on high resolution imaging [31].

Idiopathic Trigeminal Neuralgia: Type II

(ICD: G50.0 syndrome of TN with concomitant persistent pain; IASP, 006.X8a trigeminal neuralgia, tic douloureux)

This type of facial pain is characterized by an aching, throbbing, or burning constant pain that is present at least 50% of the time. Sharp/episodic pain may accompany TN2 but is not required for diagnosis. Both ICHD-2 and ICHD-3 beta describe a new term of "TN with concomitant persistent pain" [34, 35]. In Burchiel classification, this condition is referred to as TN2 [8].

Postherpetic Neuralgia

(ICD, B02.22 postherpetic trigeminal neuralgia; ICHD, 13.1.2.2 postherpetic trigeminal neuropathy; and 13.1.2.1 painful trigeminal neuropathy attributed to acute herpes zoster; IASP, 003.X2b postherpetic neuralgia [trigeminal])

Pain in the trigeminal nerve territory that developed after a herpetic infection in the same area is considered postherpetic neuralgia. There are theories that pain in acute and late periods of viral infection with herpes zoster is caused by different mechanisms. The pain is burning and dysesthetic and may be associated with sensory loss and some degree of allodynia; trophic changes may also occur.

Trigeminal Deafferentation Pain

This condition is characterized by burning crawling itching tearing pain and is seen after intentional injury of the trigeminal system, usually as a result of neuroablative intervention (neurectomy, gangliolysis, rhizotomy, nucleotomy, tractotomy, etc.) Anesthesia dolorosa is an advanced form of this kind of pain; in addition to neurodestructive procedures, it may also be seen in brainstem and mesencephalic infarctions.

Post-traumatic Trigeminal Neuropathy

(ICHD: 13.1.2.3 painful post-traumatic trigeminal neuropathy)

This type of neuralgia develops as a result of unintentional direct insult of to the trigeminal system, such as trauma, maxillofacial surgery, skull base surgical procedures, and posterior fossa surgery.

Constant, dull, throbbing, or burning pain with or without sharp pain paroxysms may be observed in the affected area. Nerve involvement in post-traumatic pain is distal to the trigeminal root and ganglion, and the character of pain differs from deafferentation pain and idiopathic types of TN.

Symptomatic Trigeminal Neuralgia

(ICHD: 13.1.2.4 painful trigeminal neuropathy attributed to multiple sclerosis (MS) plaque)

The term *symptomatic* is not present in the latest versions of HIS and IASP classifications. The neurosurgeons and neurologists continue using this term [8, 36, 37]. TN is seen in up to 10% of MS patients. The associated neuropathic pain can be either constant or episodic.

Secondary Trigeminal Neuralgia

(ICHD: 13.1.2.5–13.1.2.6 painful trigeminal neuropathy attributed to space-occupying lesion or other disorder)

Secondary TN is caused by other primary conditions that are summarized in Box 2. The underlying condition should be treated first to relieve this type of pain. According to the American Academy of Neurology—European Federation of Neurological Societies (AAN-EFNS) guidelines, "secondary" TN is caused by a major neurological disease such as tumor of the cerebellopontine angle or multiple sclerosis [38]; these guidelines group secondary and symptomatic TN into one category.

Geniculate Neuralgia

(ICD, G51.1 geniculate ganglionitis, disorder of geniculate ganglion; ICHD, 13.3 geniculate (facial nerve) neuralgia; IASP, 006.X2 geniculate neuralgia (VII cranial nerve), Ramsay Hunt syndrome)

Geniculate neuralgia presents with sharp and lancinating unilateral pain that is localized to an area behind the ear and/or the external auditory canal. It may be accompanied by other symptoms such as salivation, tinnitus, and bitter taste. ICHD-3 beta criteria require at least three attacks of brief paroxysms of pain felt deeply in the auditory canal, sometimes radiating to the parieto-occipital region. The term "geniculate neuralgia" is frequently used interchangeably with "neuralgia of nervus intermedius" (see below).

Glossopharyngeal Neuralgia

(ICD, G52.1 disorders of glossopharyngeal nerve, glossopharyngeal neuralgia; ICHD, 13.2 glossopharyngeal neuralgia; IASP, 006.X8b glossopharyngeal neuralgia)

Glossopharyngeal neuralgia is also called vagoglossopharyngeal neuralgia. It presents with sharp shooting pain in the posterior part of the tongue, pharynx, tonsils, and ear, sometimes with trigger zones located in the ipsilateral half of the tongue and throat. The pain can be provoked by chewing, swallowing, and talking. Vascular compromise can be seen on imaging and during surgery. ICHD criteria require the number of attacks to be three or more.

Sphenopalatine Neuralgia (Sluder)

Sluder neuralgia is a rare condition that presents with infraorbital or retro-orbital pain radiating toward the neck. It may be accompanied by lacrimation and conjunctival injection.

Superior Laryngeal Neuralgia

(ICD, G52.2 disorders of vagus nerve, superior laryngeal neuralgia; IASP, 006.X8e neuralgia of superior laryngeal nerve [vagus nerve neuralgia])

Superior laryngeal neuralgia presents with severe paroxysmal pain felt in the throat, in the mandibular region, or under the ear. Pain is triggered by swallowing, head turning, and straining the voice.

Paratrigeminal Neuralgia (Raeder)

(ICHD, 13.8 paratrigeminal oculosympathetic (Raeder's) syndrome; IASP, 002.X4 [tumor]/002.X1a [trauma]/002.X3b [inflammatory, etc.]/002X8 [unknown] Raeder's syndrome (Raeder's paratrigeminal syndrome) Type I–Type II)

Paratrigeminal neuropathic pain presents in the frontotemporal region with associated partial Horner syndrome.

Occipital Neuralgia (Arnold)

(ICD, M53.82 other specified dorsopathies in cervical region, occipital neuralgia; ICHD, 13.4 occipital neuralgia; IASP: 004.X8–004.X1 [trauma] occipital neuralgia)

Occipital neuralgia is localized primarily in the occipital area and radiates to ear and retromandibular region.

Nervus Intermedius Neuralgia

(ICD, G52.9 disorders of other cranial nerves; ICHD, 13.3 nervus intermedius [facial nerve] neuralgia, [13.3.1 classical; 13.3.2 attributed to herpes zoster]; IASP, 006.X8c neuralgia of the nervus intermedius)

Nervus intermedius neuralgia presents with unilateral paroxysmal attacks deep in the ear. This term is used interchangeably with geniculate neuralgia, and this commonality is reflected in ICHD but not clear in other classifications.

Atypical Facial Pain

Frazier and Russell first used the term "atypical" in 1924 for facial pain that did not respond to surgical therapy [39]. Since that time terms "atypical facial pain" and "atypical trigeminal neuralgia" have often been used interchangeably even though these two terms describe very different conditions. In general, atypical facial pain refers to a poorly localized, vaguely described facial pain, nonanatomical in distribution, and with no evidence of a defined organic cause [3, 16]. Atypical trigeminal neuralgia, on the other hand, refers to condition that stems from trigeminal dysfunction but differs from "typical" TN by the presence of constant pain in addition to the classical electric shock-like attacks (typical TN is expected to be episodic only), by the presence of sensory deficits (typical TN patients have normal neurological examination), by the absence of trigger zones, by lack of response to anticonvulsants primarily carbamazepine (response to carbamazepine is considered pathognomonic for typical TN), etc. The pain in atypical TN, however, remains very anatomically defined and does not cross midline. To avoid this confusion, it is now recommended to stop using the term "atypical TN" and instead refer to it as TN type 2, or TN2, based on Burchiel classification.

According to one published concept, the main difference in symptomatology of "typical" TN and "atypical" TN is the severity and/or duration of the vascular compression of the trigeminal nerve root [12]. This concept is supported by clinical experience; it postulates that typical TN, atypical TN, and trigeminal neuropathic pain may not be separate conditions but just different degrees (or successive stages) of progressive injury of the trigeminal nerve. Well-known observations of vascular compression by nearby arterial or venous vessels in patients with atypical TN support this theory. As a further proof of this concept, Miller et al. in 2009 reported six patients with TN1 who subsequently progressed to TN2 [31]. They suggested that TN type at the onset is more meaningful than its ultimate presentation at the time of clinical evaluation.

With this, the term "atypical facial pain" (AFP) is currently reserved for patients with unequivocal evidence of a somatoform pain disorder that can be objectively diagnosed by psychological testing [21]. This term should not be used for those patients who are refractory to treatment or those "not-completely-typical" pain conditions that may be included in any other diagnostic category. Similarly, the other terms that were used to describe the atypical facial pain, such as dental causalgia, atypical facial neuralgia, and phantom orofacial pain, are no longer recommended for use [40].

Although both IASP and IHS excluded the term "atypical facial pain" from their lists and suggested the terms "other and unspecified pain in the jaws" or "facial pain not fulfilling other criteria," this term remains widely used by various authors [41]. A recent survey of UK clinicians from all specialties who treat facial pain showed that 89% of them still use the term [41]. One hundred forty-three randomly selected specialists (oral and maxillofacial surgeons, oral medical experts, ear nose and throat surgeons, anesthetists, psychiatrists, and neurologists) completed questionnaires; 127 of them used the term atypical facial pain, and the rest used various other terms.

Persistent Idiopathic Facial Pain (PIFP)

In general, "idiopathic" refers to conditions with no identifiable cause. In case of trigeminal neuralgia, "idiopathic" is usually the same as "primary" TN, but in case of the persistent idiopathic facial pain (PIFP), idiopathic refers to the absence of identifiable organic disease and serves as substitute to the term "psychogenic" [11].

In ICHD PIFP, formerly known as atypical facial pain, describes chronic facial pain without evidence of structural or other specific causes of pain [9, 42]. Alternatively, PIFP is defined as a pain along the territory of the trigeminal nerve, which does not fit criteria for other cranial neuralgias [2, 43, 44]. ICHD suggests that "atypical odontalgia," based on the history, can either be PIFP or a painful post-traumatic trigeminal neuropathy.

Headache Disorders

Trigeminal autonomic cephalgias (TACs) and migraine have been linked to the ophthalmic division of the trigeminal nerve. Based on a study of prevalence of facial pain in the migraine population, only 9% out of 517 migraine patients were found to experience pain in the lower half of the face [45]. This was attributed to the anatomical overlap of the trigeminal and cervical afferents throughout the trigeminocervical complex causing a referral of pain with otherwise typical clinical symptoms of a migraine attack. TACs are normally perceived in the upper part of the person's face but every now and then radiate to the face and teeth, and in turn, orofacial structures may give rise to headaches [46]. These conditions are characterized by short-lasting pain, some in the facial region and some in the head, and are accompanied by different autonomic features. As a matter of fact, there was a suggestion that short-lasting unilateral neuralgiform headache with cranial autonomic features (SUNA), short-lasting unilateral neuralgiform headaches occurring with conjunctival injection and tearing (SUNCT), TN may represent different stages of a single continuum [47].

In general, most causes of headache and craniofacial pain, including SUNCT, cluster-tic syndrome, paroxysmal hemicrania, and primary stabbing headache, should be considered in the differential diagnosis of TN.

Non-neurogenic Orofacial Pain and Temporomandibular Causes

Classic TN or secondary TN may sometimes be confused with dental causes of pain. Dental pain is usually continuous, intraoral pain that is dull or throbbing, whereas classic TN is typically intermittent and sharp pain. Furthermore, some patients describe a phase of "pre-trigeminal neuralgia" characterized by atypical (for TN) symptoms (e.g., jaw or tooth pain) that might mimic dental pain [30].

Non-neurogenic oral cavity diseases can present with stimulus-evoked, sharp, throbbing, or continuous pain; they may be easily confused with neurogenic pain, but oral examination and radiographs would help in establishing correct diagnosis.

Differential Diagnosis Algorithm

Our facial pain diagnosis and management algorithm was published in 2007 [48] (Table 4.7). Determination of anatomical distribution of pain and its correlation with representation of neurological structure(s) is the first step. Then, to differentiate secondary and primary causes, radiological evaluation—usually brain MRI with contrast—is performed. Pain nature and significant history information (previous surgery, infection, trauma, vascular formation, etc.) help to establish correct diagnosis and chose proper medical and surgical management.

If the pain does not follow anatomical distribution, a psychological evaluation may be in order to establish diagnosis of AFP/PIFP.

Table 4.7 Differential diagnosis of facial pain

Trigeminal neuralgia
Trigeminal neuralgia Type I: Idiopathic typical trigeminal neuralgia
Trigeminal neuralgia Type II: Idiopathic atypical trigeminal neuralgia
Symptomatic/secondary trigeminal neuralgia
Trigeminal neuropathic pain
Post-traumatic trigeminal pain
Trigeminal deafferentation pain
Anesthesia dolorosa
Central deafferentation syndrome
Postherpetic neuralgia
Glossopharyngeal neuralgia
Geniculate neuralgia
Sphenopalatine (Sluder) neuralgia
Paratrigeminal (Raeder) syndrome
Pain ophthalmoplegia (Tolosa-Hunt syndrome)
Petrous apex syndrome (Gradenigo syndrome)
Cancer-related pain
Atypical facial pain
Non-neurogenic orofacial pain and temporomandibular joint-related pain
Headache and other conditions

Table 4.8 Comparison of IASP and IHS classification

IASP	IHS	
Central pain (if confined to the head and face)	12.7.2	Thalamic pain
Trigeminal neuralgia (tic douloureux)	12.2.1	Trigeminal neuralgia
Secondary neuralgia (trigeminal) from central nervous system lesions (tumor or aneurysm)	12.2.2.2	Symptomatic trigeminal neuralgia
Acute herpes zoster (trigeminal)	12.1.4.1	Herpes zoster
Postherpetic neuralgia (trigeminal)	12.1.4.2	Chronic postherpetic neuralgia
Geniculate neuralgia (seventh cranial nerve): Ramsay Hunt syndrome	12.1.4.1	Herpes zoster
Glossopharyngeal neuralgia (ninth cranial nerve)	12.3.1 12.3.2	Idiopathic glossopharyngeal neuralgia Symptomatic glossopharyngeal neuralgia
Neuralgia of the superior laryngeal nerve (vagus nerve neuralgia)	12.5	Superior laryngeal neuralgia
Occipital neuralgia	12.6	Occipital neuralgia
Hypoglossal neuralgia	12.1.7	Other causes of persistent pain of cranial nerve origin
Glossopharyngeal pain from trauma	12.3.2	Symptomatic glossopharyngeal neuralgia
Hypoglossal pain from trauma	12.1.7	Other causes of persistent pain of cranial nerve origin
Tolosa-Hunt syndrome (painful ophthalmoplegia)	12.1.5	Tolosa-Hunt syndrome

Conclusion

Since the time of Hippocrates (circa 400 BC), there are some challenges related to diagnosis and treatment of facial pain [49]. Both surgical and nonsurgical approaches are used in facial pain patients; the choice of approach is generally guided by practical treatment algorithms.

Most challenge remains with so-called atypical pain patients, as their diagnosis and management require advanced multidisciplinary expertise. Meanwhile, the lack of universally accepted classification makes therapeutic decisions more difficult [27]. This is further complicated by a fact that somewhere between 7 and 44% of cases may be unclassifiable in view multiple diagnostic classifications [20] (Table 4.8). Even when symptoms point toward involvement of a specific nerve(s), there is a general lack of imaging tools that may help in establishing clinical diagnosis. The key to a proper diagnostic approach is to evaluate the symptoms as a whole and present the patient with treatment options in a goal-oriented manner. Since the duration of chronic pain may affect the treatment results, a timely and accurate diagnosis remains a cornerstone of efficient management.

The use of a grading system such as "definite," "probable," or "possible" has been suggested for use in case of diagnosing neuropathic pain. It has been suggested that this type of grading may be extended to various orofacial pain diagnoses as a means of managing the uncertainty in providing diagnoses for conditions that have varied clinical presentations [37].

Although the head and face are closely related, diagnostic classifications of headache and orofacial pain are not properly integrated. It does appear, however, that chronic orofacial pain and headaches can be classified together as they may be sharing similar underlying pathophysiology, clinical characteristics, and neurovascular issues. To test this concept, the headache definitions have been applied in a cohort of chronic orofacial pain patients. The researchers concluded that both headaches and OFP should own their own subclassifications.

In general, the use of comprehensive classification systems does not guarantee better outcomes. But discrepancy in terminology and existence of conflicting classification systems may delay diagnosis, negatively affect interprofessional communication, or result in inaccurate labeling. In addition to this, use of different classifications may make meta-analyses difficult if not impossible.

Summary

Chronic facial pain often requires multidisciplinary and multi-interventional therapy. Pain medicine, neurology, neurosurgery, otolaryngology, ophthalmology, dentistry, and maxillofacial surgery are those disciplines that deal with diagnosis and treatment of facial pain.

Major classification guidelines lack the common language for diagnosis. It is therefore not surprising that most studies and publications include unclassified, overlapping, and mixed (combined) cases making it problematic for further analysis. The approach to gather evidence as used in the last version of ICHD and publish a beta version for field testing is a promising step in creating a unified and comprehensive classification. Inclusion of orofacial pain groups in this collaboration is expected to strengthen the future versions of classifications.

The unfortunate part of classifications that are not validated or supported by evidence/validation is that they not only result in the wrong selection of patients for treatment but also facilitate collection of uncategorizable data that cannot be properly analyzed, making it all but impossible to create the evidence-based approach that is desperately needed for management of this complicated group of patients.

References

1. Macfarlane TV, Blinkhorn AS, Davies RM, Kincey J, Worthington HV. Oro-facial pain in the community: prevalence and associated impact. Community Dent Oral Epidemiol. 2002;30(1):52–60.
2. Weiss AL, Ehrhardt KP, Tolba R. Atypical facial pain: a comprehensive, evidence-based review. Curr Pain Headache Rep. 2017;21(2):9.
3. De Toledo IP, Conti Réus J, Fernandes M, Porporatti AL, Peres MA, Takaschima A, et al. Prevalence of trigeminal neuralgia: a systematic review. J Am Dent Assoc. 2016;147(7):576.e2.
4. Koopman JSHA, Dieleman JP, Huygen FJ, de Mos M, Martin CGM, Sturkenboom MCJM. Incidence of facial pain in the general population. Pain. 2009;147(1):122–7.
5. Rasmussen P. Facial pain. II. A prospective survey of 1052 patients with a view of: character of the attacks, onset, course, and character of pain. Acta Neurochir. 1990;107(3-4):121–8.
6. Tjakkes GHE, De Bont LGM, van Wijhe M, Stegenga B. Classification of chronic orofacial pain using an intravenous diagnostic test. J Oral Rehabil. 2009;36(7):469–75.
7. Merskey H, Bogduk N. Classification of chronic pain: descriptions of chronic pain syndromes and definitions of pain terms. 2nd ed. Seattle: IASP Press; 1994.
8. Burchiel KJ. A new classification for facial pain. Neurosurgery. 2003;53(5):1164–7.
9. International Headache Society. The International Classification of Headache Disorders: 2nd edition. Cephalalgia. 2004;24(Suppl 1):9–160.
10. Nixdorf DR, Drangsholt MT, Ettlin DA, Gaul C, De Leeuw R, Svensson P, et al. Classifying orofacial pains: a new proposal of taxonomy based on ontology. J Oral Rehabil. 2012;39(3):161–9.
11. Aghabeigi B. Background: neurobiology of pain. In: Zakrzewska JM, Harrison SD, editors. Assessment and management of orofacial pain. Amsterdam: Elsevier; 2002. p. 17–34.
12. Burchiel KJ, Slavin KV. On the natural history of trigeminal neuralgia. Neurosurgery. 2000;46(1):152–5.
13. Melis M, Lobo SL, Ceneviz C, Zawawi K, Al-Badawi E, Maloney G, et al. Atypical odontalgia: a review of the literature. Headache. 2003;43(10):1060–74.
14. Agostoni E, Frigerio R, Santoro P. Atypical facial pain: clinical considerations and differential diagnosis. Neurol Sci. 2005;26(S2):s71–4.
15. Leeuw RD, Klasser GD, American Academy of Orofacial Pain. Orofacial pain: guidelines for assessment, diagnosis, and management. Chicago: Quintessence Publishing; 2013.
16. Ad Hoc Committee on Classification of Headache of the National Institute of Health. Classification of headache. JAMA. 1962;179(9):717–8.
17. International Association of the Study of Pain. Scheme for coding chronic pain diagnoses. Pain. 1986;24:S10–2.
18. Treede RD, Rief W, Barke A, Aziz Q, Bennett MI, Benoliel R, et al. A classification of chronic pain for ICD-11. Pain. 2015;156(6):1003–7.

19. Olesen J. From ICHD-3 beta to ICHD-3. Cephalalgia. 2016;36(5):401–2.
20. Renton T, Kahwaja N. Pain part 5a: chronic (neuropathic) orofacial pain. Dent Update. 2015;42(8):744–60.
21. Eller JL, Raslan AM, Burchiel KJ. Trigeminal neuralgia: definition and classification. Neurosurg Focus. 2005;18(5):1–3.
22. Melzack R. The McGill Pain Questionnaire: major properties and scoring methods. Pain. 1975;1(3):277–99.
23. Dubuisson D, Melzack R. Classification of clinical pain descriptions by multiple group discriminant analysis. Exp Neurol. 1976;51(2):480–7.
24. Hapak L, Gordon A, Locker D, Shandling M, Mock D, Tenenbaum HC. Differentiation between musculoligamentous, dentoalveolar, and neurologically based craniofacial pain with a diagnostic questionnaire. J Orofac Pain. 1994;8(4):357–68.
25. Macfarlane GJ, Macfarlane TV, Blinkhorn AS, Craven R, Zakrzewska JM, Atkin P, et al. Can one predict the likely specific orofacial pain syndrome from a self-completed questionnaire? Pain. 2004;111(3):270–7.
26. Aggarwal VR, Lunt M, Zakrzewska JM, Macfarlane GJ, Macfarlane TV. Development and validation of the Manchester orofacial pain disability scale. Community Dent Oral Epidemiol. 2005;33:141–9.
27. Aggarwal VR, McBeth J, Lunt M, Zakrzewska JM, Macfarlane GJ. Development and validation of classification criteria for idiopathic orofacial pain for use in population-based studies. J Orofac Pain. 2007;21(3):203–15.
28. Limonadi FM, McCartney S, Burchiel KJ. Design of an artificial neural network for diagnosis of facial pain syndromes. Stereotact Funct Neurosurg. 2006;84(5-6):212–20.
29. McCartney S, Weltin M, Burchiel KJ. Use of an artificial neural network for diagnosis of facial pain syndromes: an update. Stereotact Funct Neurosurg. 2014;92(1):44–52.
30. Evans RW, Graff-Radford SB, Bassiur JP. Pretrigeminal neuralgia. Headache. 2005;45(3):242–4.
31. Miller JP, Acar F, Hamilton BE, Burchiel KJ. Radiographic evaluation of trigeminal neurovascular compression in patients with and without trigeminal neuralgia. J Neurosurg. 2009;110(4):627–32.
32. Hardy DG, Rhoton AL Jr. Microsurgical relationships of the superior cerebellar artery and the trigeminal nerve. J Neurosurg. 1978;49(5):669–78.
33. Klun B, Prestor B. Microvascular relations of the trigeminal nerve: an anatomical study. Neurosurgery. 1986;19(4):535–9.
34. Maarbjerg S, Gozalov A, Olesen J, Bendtsen L. Concomitant persistent pain in classical trigeminal neuralgia–evidence for different subtypes. Headache. 2014;54(7):1173–83.
35. Maarbjerg S, Sørensen MT, Gozalov A, Bendtsen L, Olesen J. Field-testing of the ICHD-3 beta diagnostic criteria for classical trigeminal neuralgia. Cephalalgia. 2015;35(4):291–300.
36. Gronseth G. Practice parameter: the diagnostic evaluation and treatment of trigeminal neuralgia (an evidence-based review): report of the Quality Standards Subcommittee of AAN abd EFNS. Neurology. 2008;71(15):1183–90.
37. Cruccu G, Finnerup NB, Jensen TS, Scholz J, Sindou M, Svensson P, et al. Trigeminal neuralgia: new classification and diagnostic grading for practice and research. Neurology. 2016;87(2):220–8.
38. Cruccu G, Gronseth G, Alksne J, Argoff C, Brainin M, Burchiel K, et al. AAN-EFNS guidelines on trigeminal neuralgia management. Eur J Neurol. 2008;15(10):1013–28.
39. Frazier C, Russell E. Neuralgia of the face: an analysis of 754 cases with relation to pain and other sensory phenomena before and after operation. Arch Neurol Psychiatry. 1924;11:557–63.
40. Woda A, Tubert-Jeannin S, Bouhassira D, Attal N, Fleiter B, Goulet J-P, et al. Towards a new taxonomy of idiopathic orofacial pain. Pain. 2005;116(3):396–406.
41. Elrasheed AA, Worthington HV, Ariyaratnam S, Duxbury AJ. Opinions of UK specialists about terminology, diagnosis, and treatment of atypical facial pain: a survey. Br J Oral Maxillofac Surg. 2004;42(6):566–71.

42. International Headache Society. The International Classification of Headache Disorders, 3rd edition (beta version). Cephalalgia. 2013;33(9):629–808.
43. Zakrzewska JM. Classification issues related to neuropathic trigeminal pain. J Orofac Pain. 2004;18(4):325–31.
44. Zebenholzer K, Wober C, Vigl M, Wessely P, Wober-Bingol C. Facial pain in a neurological tertiary care centre–evaluation of the International Classification of Headache Disorders. Cephalalgia. 2005;25(9):689–99.
45. Yoon MS, Mueller D, Hansen N, Poitz F, Slomke M, Dommes P, et al. Prevalence of facial pain in migraine: a population-based study. Cephalalgia. 2010;30(1):92–6.
46. Benoliel R, Birman N, Eliav E, Sharav Y. The International Classification of Headache Disorders: accurate diagnosis of orofacial pain? Cephalalgia. 2008;28(7):752–62.
47. Lambru G, Matharu MS. SUNCT, SUNA and trigeminal neuralgia: different disorders or variants of the same disorder? Curr Opin Neurol. 2014;27(3):325–31.
48. Slavin KV, Nersesyan H, Colpan ME, Munawar N. Current algorithm for the surgical treatment of facial pain. Head Face Med. 2007;3(1):30.
49. Eboli P, Stone JL, Aydin S, Slavin KV. Historical characterization of trigeminal neuralgia. Neurosurgery. 2009;64(6):1183–7.

Part II
Evaluation and Diagnosis

Chapter 5
History and Physical Examination

James Y. Suen

Introduction

Headaches and facial pain are very common and are a major medical problem in this country and the world [1]. It is critical to obtain an accurate history and physical exam to determine the etiology of facial and head pain. If the head pain is severe and abrupt in onset, one must rule out a ruptured aneurysm or intracranial hemorrhage because time is critical to treat that problem.

We feel that pain in the face and head is commonly related to a peripheral trigeminal neuritis secondary to multiple factors, such as herpes zoster, trauma, nerve compression from accompanying blood vessels similar to the classic trigeminal neuritis, and many other causes, as well as idiopathic [2].

The nerve supply to the face and head is easy to learn. Knowing the nerve anatomy and with an accurate history can lead to an accurate diagnosis and lead to successful treatment. Most facial and head pain will be recurrent, chronic, and severe, leading to many physician visits.

History

Facial Pain

The face is primarily supplied by the trigeminal nerve, except for the earlobes and along the jaw line, which are innervated by the upper cervical plexus nerves (Fig. 5.1).

J. Y. Suen
Department of Otolaryngology—Head and Neck Surgery, University of Arkansas for Medical Sciences, Little Rock, AR, USA
e-mail: suenjamesy@uams.edu

J. Y. Suen, E. Petersen (eds.), *Diagnosis and Management of Head and Face Pain*, https://doi.org/10.1007/978-3-319-90999-8_5

Obtaining an accurate and good history can lead to identifying the nerves involved. It is important to ask if there was a precipitating event, how long the pain has been present, the characteristics of the pain, and if it is intermittent or chronic. Also it is important to know what treatment has been tried, how successful it was, and whether any medications caused side effects. Other history would include previous trauma requiring surgery with reconstruction metal plates, herpes zoster infection, sinus problems, dental pain, and dental treatment. Previous neck surgery or trauma must be known because it can cause lower facial pain or occipital headaches.

The classic trigeminal neuritis, type I is important to differentiate from the peripheral type trigeminal neuritis. Type I is secondary to a vascular compression of the trigeminal nerve at the root entry zone in the brain stem. It has the potential for cure with surgical decompression or radiosurgery. Patients with Type I pain will usually describe severe, sharp, electrical shock-like pain which can be intermittent and debilitating. Most often it involves the third division of the trigeminal nerve which will cause jaw and face pain on one side. If the patient describes this type of pain, it is important to rule out a vascular compression of the nerve with a specific MRI scan focusing on cisternal segment of the trigeminal nerve.

Once Type I trigeminal neuritis is ruled out, the history should focus on identifying "trigger points" which are where the facial pain usually begins. Patients commonly point to half of their face or head and even both sides, but when questioned carefully, they usually can identify a "starting point." As this history is obtained, the clinician should begin to think about the trigeminal nerve innervation to that area (Fig. 5.1). These trigger points are important, because we have found that nerve blocks to one or more of the peripheral trigeminal nerves can abort the facial pain and headaches [3].

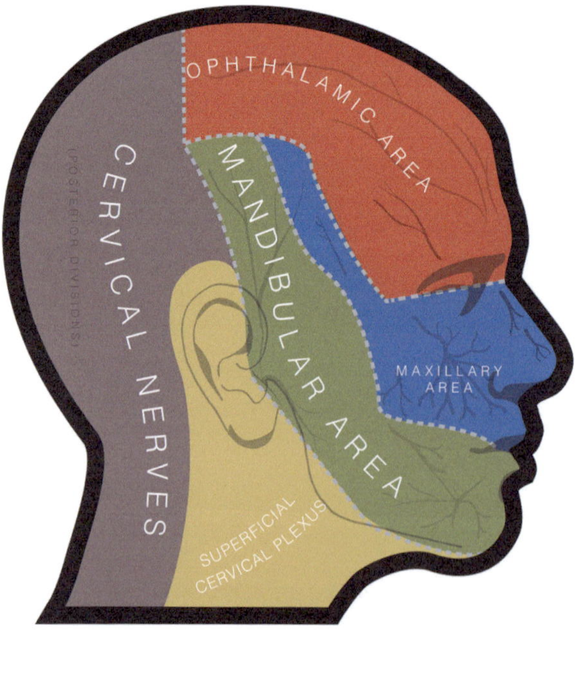

Fig. 5.1 Nerve supply to the face, head, and upper neck. Dermatomes supplied by the three divisions of the trigeminal nerve and the upper cervical nerves—C2, 3

Headache Pain

Most headaches are called "migraine" or "tension" headaches. It is important to understand that a lot of facial pain or occipital pain will provoke headaches or head pain, so the history must ascertain where the pain started. If it does start in the face or in the back of the head, the same history as above should be obtained. Other history should include if the patient has been evaluated by a neurologist, whether the patient has nausea and vomiting with the headache, and what, if anything, will relieve the pain. Also it is important to know if scans have been done to rule out brain tumors, subdural hematomas, or sinus or ear infections.

The following case is an example of how important the history can be:

A 43-year-old white female had a history of severe pain behind and around the right lower ear for over 6 years. After failing to respond to medications, she underwent a vascular decompression procedure performed, and it helped the pain for about 2 months. The severe, sharp pain returned in the "right occipital area" and was so severe that she would cry and almost pass out. She was referred to a neurologist, who tried a greater occipital nerve block with minimum improvement. She was tried on anticonvulsants, amitriptyline, and baclofen with no improvement. The pain started involving her right temple and forehead area. She was seen by a neurosurgeon who recommended re-exploration of the trigeminal nerve for concern for persistent compression, so she underwent another vascular decompression surgery. It was noted during that surgery that there was not an artery compressing the trigeminal nerve. She again experienced a period of postoperative pain relief which lasted 2 months, and then her severe pain recurred. When we saw her, she stated the pain would start over the right mastoid area near the lower end of her craniotomy scar and then the facial pain would start. When examined, she pointed to the trigger points: at the lower end of her craniotomy incision line and around the earlobe and angle of her jaw, which is innervated by the lesser occipital and greater auricular nerves (Fig. 5.1). When questioned closely about her original pain, she said it was in the same area of the mastoid and earlobe at the beginning and was still the main trigger point (Fig. 5.2). I recommended a nerve block of her right lesser occipital and greater auricular nerves with xylocaine. Within 5 min after the nerve block, she had over 50% pain relief but still had some pain over her right temple and forehead. I then did a block of her right zygomaticotemporal (Fig. 5.3) and supraorbital nerves and her pain resolved. The nerves were also blocked with bupivacaine.

She returned 1 week later, and she said she had 3 days of complete pain relief and that her severe pain episodes decreased from over 50 a day to about 10–15 per day. The pain was starting to recur in the lesser occipital nerve area, but the temple and forehead pain had not recurred. Another block of her lesser occipital nerve helped significantly. We offered to resect the upper cervical plexus, and this was performed. She has been pain free for over 6 months, and the numbness does not bother her.

In talking with her neurosurgeon who performed the second surgery, it was noted that the patient did not have arterial compression of her main trigeminal nerve. It is likely that this patient's original pain was from her lesser occipital and greater auricular nerves and that if a good history and exam had been performed initially, the proper diagnosis would have been made.

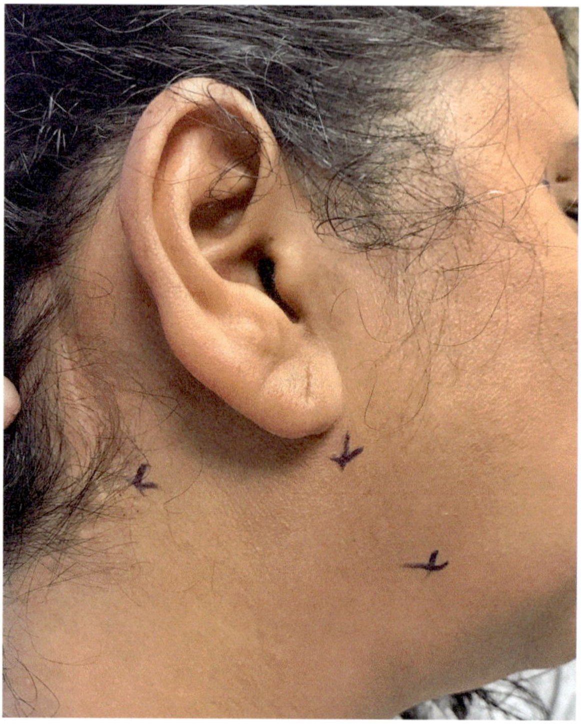

Fig. 5.2 Photo of the original and recurrent pain areas. Note the craniotomy incision over the mastoid area. The "X" at the bottom of the incision is where the lesser occipital nerve is located. The "X" near the earlobe is the greater auricular nerve distribution. The "X" at the angle of the jaw is the transverse cervical nerve innervation. All of these are part of the upper cervical plexus nerves from C2, 3

Physical Exam

This is where the knowledge of the nerves supplying the face and head is crucial. As the patient describes where the pain originates and what areas are involved, the examiner's mind should be thinking which nerves innervate that area.

During the physical exam, it is important to determine where the pain or headache began and if there is a "trigger point." Most patients will say, it hurts everywhere, but if pinned down, they frequently will point to one area where it starts. Having the patient *point specifically* to where the pain starts is critical. If this trigger point can be ascertained, nerve blocks are helpful to diagnose and treat the pain or headaches.

We have found that many patients who complain of bilateral face or head pain will have a trigger point only on one side and if that area or nerve is treated, it commonly will prevent the opposite side from hurting.

If the patient can give you a trigger point, this is where your anatomy knowledge is crucial. It is common to have even two or more trigger points. That is important to know also, because several nerves may need to be blocked.

The physical exam should also look for scars from previous skin cancer excisions and titanium plates from previous trauma surgery or craniotomies. Palpation of the face and head for sensitive areas should be performed. Many nerves that cause facial pain and headaches may be sensitive to pressure from palpation.

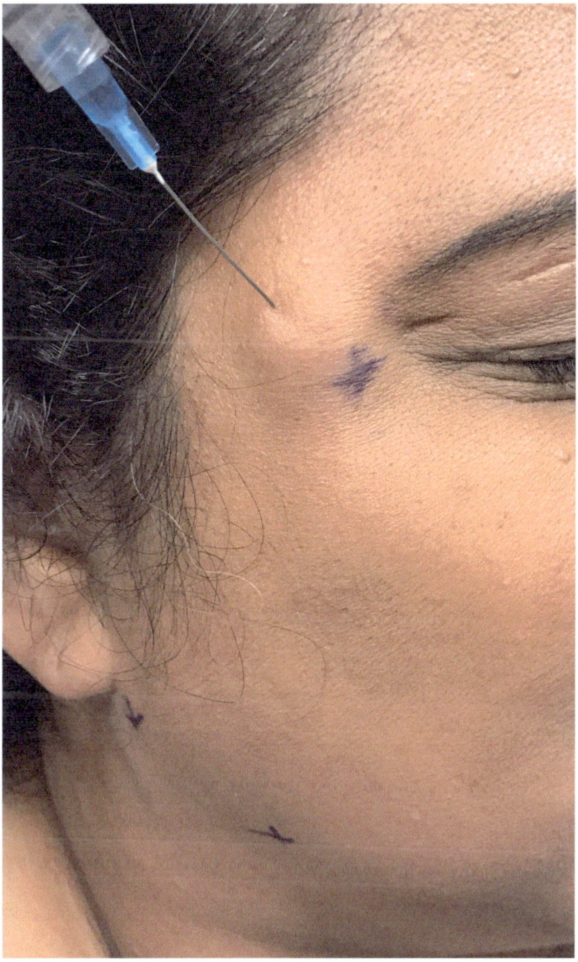

Fig. 5.3 "X" indicates the location of the zygomatico-temporal nerve which can hurt when the cervical plexus nerves hurt

The nose should also be examined to look for septal spurs which can impinge on the adjacent middle turbinate which can trigger pain in the V1 or V2 distribution [4].

Summary

It cannot be emphasized enough that an accurate history and physical exam are crucial to help diagnose the origin of pain in the face and head. *Ask where does the pain seem to start and find the trigger points!*

Also learn the nerve innervation to the face and head—it is the *key* to proper diagnosis and effective treatment.

References

1. Goldberg LD. The cost of migraine and its treatment. Am J Manag Care. 2005; 11(2 Suppl):S62–7.
2. Brisman. Trigeminal neuralgia: diagnosis and treatment. World Neurosurg. 2011;76(6):533–4.
3. Janis JE, Dhanik A, Howard JH. Validation of the peripheral trigger point theory of migraine headaches: single-surgeon experience using botulinum toxin and surgical decompression. Plast Reconstr Surg. 2011;128:123–31.
4. Ahamed SH, Jones NS. What is Sluder's neuralgia. J Laryngol Otol. 2003;117(6):437–43.

Chapter 6
Imaging Approach for the Diagnosis of Head and Face Pain

Ryan T. Fitzgerald and Vikas Agarwal

Headache

Indications for Imaging

Headache is a common complaint constituting 1–3% of all emergency room presentations and an estimated 18 million outpatient visits annually in the USA alone [1]. Whether or not imaging is a necessary component of the workup, and if so what imaging strategy is best suited for a particular patient, depends on a variety of clinical factors. Evidence suggests that routine use of neuroimaging is not warranted in pediatric or adult patients with a primary headache syndrome in the absence of a recent change in headache onset pattern, development of seizures, pain that is exacerbated by exertion or Valsalva, or focal neurological signs or symptoms [2]. The American College of Radiology provides guidance and recommendations through its Appropriateness Criteria, a free online resource that was developed to assist clinicians choose the most appropriate study, if any is indeed indicated, for a given indication (https://www.acr.org/Quality-Safety/Appropriateness-Criteria). Within the ACR guidelines, headache is divided into 16 variants based on presenting signs/symptoms and comorbidities. For each headache variety, each imaging modality (CT, MRI, catheter angiography, etc.) is assigned a numeric rating reflecting its appropriateness to the specific presentation based on factors such as study efficacy, safety, and cost.

R. T. Fitzgerald (✉)
Department of Radiology, University of Arkansas for Medical Sciences, Little Rock, AR, USA

V. Agarwal
Department of Radiology, University of Pittsburgh Medical Center, Pittsburgh, PA, USA
e-mail: agarwalv@upmc.edu

J. Y. Suen, E. Petersen (eds.), *Diagnosis and Management of Head and Face Pain*, https://doi.org/10.1007/978-3-319-90999-8_6

For example, a sudden onset severe headache is most appropriately imaged using non-enhanced CT of the head (ACR appropriateness score 8/9), whereas a new headache in a cancer patient is most appropriately imaged by brain MRI with and without contrast (ACR appropriateness score 9/9). For a chronic headache with no new features and a normal neurologic examination, no imaging modality received a score higher than a 4, indicating that imaging may not be necessary. The ACR has estimated the yield of positive imaging studies in patients referred with isolated, non-traumatic headache to be less than 0.5% [3]. As such, based on an estimated cost to the patient of $400 for CT of the head and $900 for MRI brain, the cost to detect an actionable finding with CT is $100,000 and $225,000 with MRI. Such costs must be weighed against the emotional and psychological value to the patient of a negative scan.

Modalities and Techniques

For headache of rapid onset, extreme severity, or headache accompanied by neurologic deficits or altered mental status, non-enhanced computed tomography (NECT) serves as the preferred initial imaging technique [1]. NECT is highly accessible, expedient, and facilitates stratification of headaches into two broad categories: primary and secondary headache disorders. The rapidity with which NECT can be obtained and interpreted, particularly in an emergency room setting, is crucial given that secondary headache disorders requiring prompt clinical attention, such as intracranial hemorrhage and herniation, are readily detected by NECT. Further, a negative NECT, in the absence of "red flag" signs and symptoms, provides both clinicians and patients assurance that any subsequent workup can be undertaken on a non-emergent basis. Contrast-enhanced head CT (CECT) has little utility with the exception of patients for whom MRI is contraindicated (e.g., due to ferromagnetic implants) given that any indication for which contrast would be advantageous (suspected neoplasm, meningitis, etc.) would be more appropriately imaged by MRI rather than CECT. CT angiography (CTA) has a limited role in the workup of headache in the absence of positive findings on the initial NECT such as subarachnoid hemorrhage, headache in the setting of suspected injury of the vertebral or carotid arteries, or headache accompanied by Horner's syndrome [1].

Outside of the acute setting, most headache variants are most appropriately imaged by MR rather than CT owing to its superior tissue characterization and spatial resolution. Additional benefits of MR are the absence of ionizing radiation entailed by CT, the ability to obtain high-quality angiographic imaging without contrast administration, and the option to obtain physiologic information such as cerebrospinal fluid (CSF) dynamics that may be relevant to some types of headache, such as headache in the setting of Chiari I malformation. Thus, the overall efficacy of MR for the exclusion of secondary headache etiologies such as primary or metastatic neoplasm, infection, and intracranial hypertension/hypotension is superior to that of CT.

Trigeminal Neuralgia

Trigeminal neuralgia (TN), characterized by rapid onset of severe, unilateral, and paroxysmal pain in one or more of the trigeminal nerve distributions (second or third divisions in 95% of cases), is the most common facial neuralgia with a prevalence of 3–6 cases per 100,000 population [4]. Neurovascular compression was recognized as a source of TN symptomatology as early as 1934 [5]. Imaging plays a crucial role in treatment planning of suspected vascular compression of the trigeminal nerve through its ability to provide detailed anatomic depiction of the relationship of the nerve to adjacent arterial and venous vasculature (Fig. 6.1). Because not all neurovascular contacts elicit symptomatology, high-resolution MR imaging is of particular value due to its ability to distinguish between arterial and venous contact and also to clearly define the anatomic location of neurovascular contact [6]. Further, imaging in patients with trigeminal nerve pain serves to exclude a variety of additional etiologies that could potentially impact the nerve along its course including neoplasm (either arising from the nerve itself [e.g., trigeminal schwannoma] or extra-neural neoplasms that compress or infiltrate the trigeminal nerve [e.g., meningioma]), nonneoplastic masses such as arachnoid or epidermoid cysts, autoimmune or idiopathic neural inflammation, and demyelination.

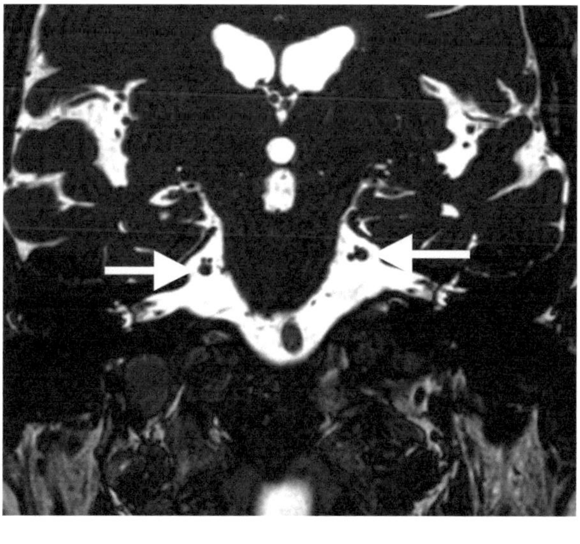

Fig. 6.1 Coronal T2-weighted SSFP image depicts the cisternal segments of each trigeminal nerve (arrows). Both nerves are bordered by pairs of vessels (hypointense foci along the superior border of the right CN V and medial and superior-medial borders of the left CN V

Modalities and Techniques

At most centers, MRI serves as the first-line modality for detection and characterization of trigeminal neurovascular compression in patients being considered for surgical or interventional treatment. Thin-section (1 mm or less), heavily T2-weighted, multi-planar steady-state free procession (SSFP) acquisition serves as the backbone of the MR evaluation due to its exceptional contrast between cisternal CSF and adjacent soft tissue/vascular structures (Fig. 6.2). Further, owing to the volumetric acquisition of the SSFP technique, images can be reformatted at any obliquity in order to best delineate and display relevant anatomy and neurovascular relationships. Specific protocols will of course vary according to variations in the technical capabilities of various hardware and software packages and institutional preferences; however, a typical TN protocol MR exam would include routine whole-brain sagittal T1-weighted, axial FLAIR, and thin-section SSFP images through the cisterns and brainstem in three planes. Recommended SSFP acquisition parameters adapted from Hughes et al. [7] are as follows: TR/TE = default to minimum; flip angle = 65°; slice thickness = 1 mm; matrix = 384 × 256; number of excitations, 2; and FOV, 18–20 cm.

Many institutions also obtain an MR angiogram (MRA) as part of the TN protocol. Due to the flow velocity-dependent nature of signal on a 3D time-of-flight MRA, this study can assist in distinguishing between high velocity flow arteries and relatively slow-flow venous vasculature. Further, MRA can provide an overview of

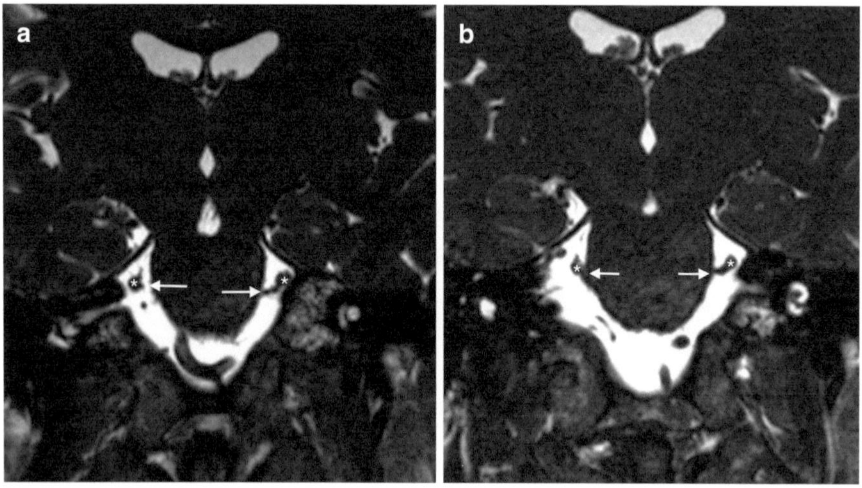

Fig. 6.2 Coronal T2-weighted SSFP images show the trigeminal nerves at their mid-cisternal segments (**a**) and more posteriorly near the root entry zones (**b**). A single branch of the right superior cerebellar artery (SCA) borders the medial aspect of the right CN V along its cisternal segment (right arrow, **a**) and persists at this location at the root entry zone (left arrow, **b**). Similarly, paired SCA branches medial and inferior to the left CN V along its cisternal segment (left arrow, **a**) also track along the root entry zone (left arrow, **b**)

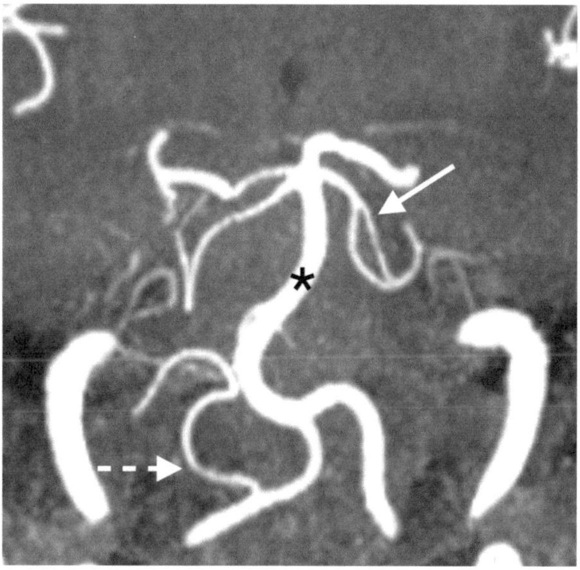

Fig. 6.3 Maximal intensity projection (MIP) reconstruction from a 3D time-of-flight, non-enhanced MRA data set readily depicts posterior circulation vasculature; dashed arrow = right PICA, asterisk = basilar artery, arrow = early bifurcating left SCA with dual distal branches

an individual's vascular anatomy that can aid in interpretation of cross-sectional imaging (Fig. 6.3). Depending on institutional and practice preferences, protocols may also include additional routine sequences through the brain such as diffusion-weighted imaging and T2*-weighted or susceptibility-weighted sequences. Contrast-enhanced T1-weighted MR imaging also readily depicts vasculature but depending on acquisition parameters may not reliably differentiate small arteries from veins (Fig. 6.4).

In the setting of TN, the primary goal of imaging is to depict the anatomy of the trigeminal nerve and detect any sites of vascular contact and/or compression. Neurovascular conflict is recognized as the most common etiologic factor in cases of idiopathic trigeminal neuralgia and was confirmed surgically in over 96% of TN cases in a series published by Sindou et al. [8]. Sites of contact should be reported based on their position along the course of the trigeminal nerve through its cisternal segment from the portis trigeminus to the root entry point. Given that not all trigeminal neurovascular contacts elicit symptoms, the greater prevalence of symptomatology with contact at the root entry site or along the posterior oligodendrocyte-myelinated segment versus contact of the anterior segment lends salience to the finding of posterior contact sites in symptomatic patients prior to surgery or other interventions [7]. In fact, contact along the anterior one third of the cisternal segment has been reported in less than 10% of surgically treated TN patients ($n = 579$) [8].

Beyond mere neurovascular contact, Leal et al. showed that high-resolution MRI is able to accurately characterize vessel-associated compression, displacement, and/

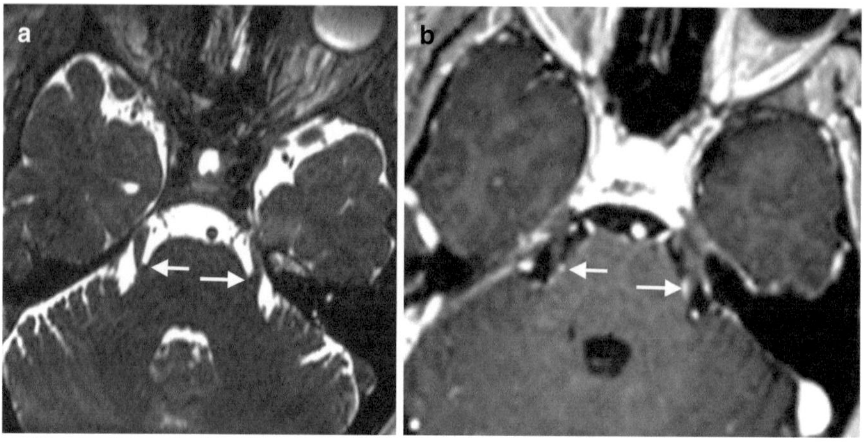

Fig. 6.4 Axial T2-weighted SSFP image (**a**) and a contrast-enhanced T1-weighted turbo field echo (TFE) acquisition (**b**) reveal bilateral neurovascular contact at the trigeminal root entry zones (arrows)

or distortion of the trigeminal nerve relative to subsequent operative findings [9]. Such information has the potential to greatly impact the preoperative prognosis as the mid- and long-term outcome after surgery is strongly related to the degree of neural compression, as shown by Sindou et al. in their study of 350 TN patient with arterial contact and/or compression [10]. Cure rates following MVD at year 1 and year 15 were 83.3% and 58.3% in those subjects with contact but no compression versus 96.6% and 88.1% is patients with severe neurovascular compression [10].

Gamma Knife surgery (GKS), a stereotactic radiosurgical technique directly facilitated by MR imaging guidance, has proven utility in treatment-refractory trigeminal neuralgia (Fig. 6.5). Studies exploring the efficacy of GKS have shown initial resolution of symptoms in greater than 90% of subjects and decreased morbidity relative to surgical decompression [11, 12]. As reported after MVD, the return of symptoms over time is not uncommon following GKS ablation. In a large cohort of 497 GKS-treated patients, the actuarial probabilities of remaining pain free without medication at 3, 5, 7, and 10 years were 71.8%, 64.9%, 59.7%, and 45.3% [12].

Beyond initial diagnosis and treatment planning in patients with trigeminal neuralgia, imaging plays a role for patients whose symptoms persist following MVD, either due to failure to identify the true culprit vessel or failure to successfully alleviate neurovascular contact. In their study of patients with recurrent or persistent hemifacial spasm after MVD, Hughes et al. found that in most cases, decompression, as determined by position of the surgical pledget, had been performed beyond the most clinically salient centrally myelinated zone of the facial nerve [13]. By analogy considering the overlapping pathophysiologic basis of trigeminal neuralgia and hemifacial spasm attributable to neurovascular compression, careful attention to the location of surgical material along the long axis of the trigeminal nerve and its relationship to the most likely site of relevance (adjacent to the root entry zone)

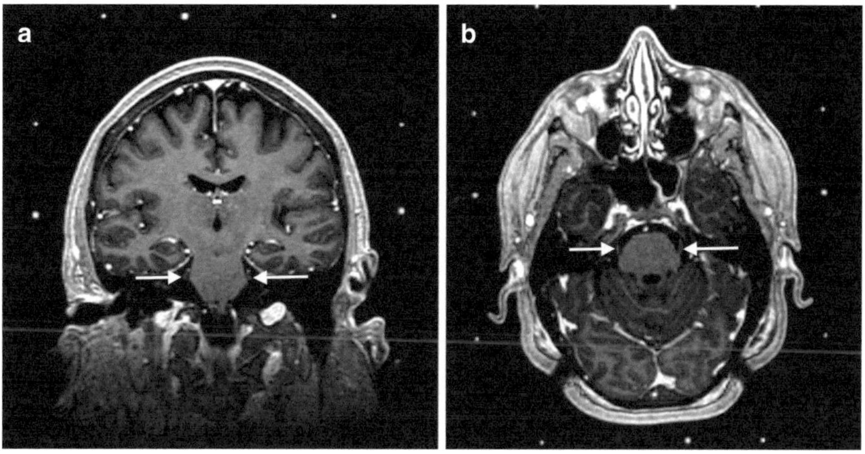

Fig. 6.5 Coronal (**a**) and axial (**b**) images from a contrast-enhanced T1-weighted turbo field echo (TFE) data set performed for purposed of stereotactic guidance precisely depict each trigeminal nerve (arrows). Note the dots around the periphery of the field of view that serve as fiducial markers facilitating operative planning for Gamma Knife surgery

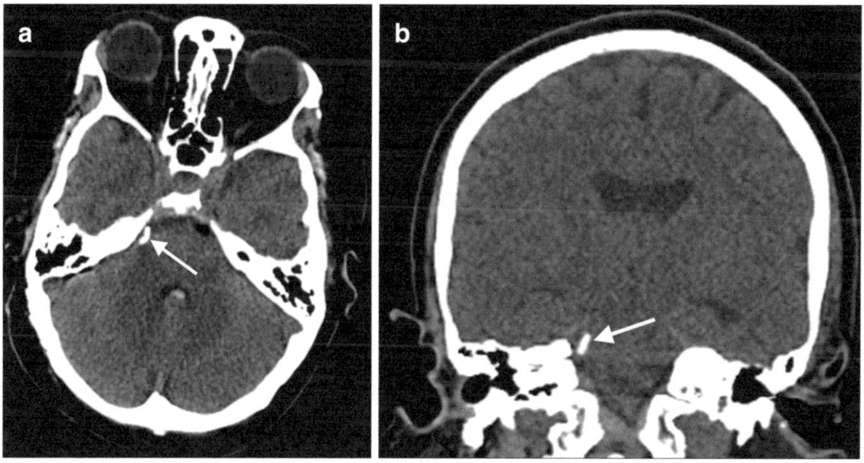

Fig. 6.6 Axial (**a**) and coronal reformatted (**b**) CT images show the expected hyperdense cylindrical appearance of a surgical pledget along the lateral aspected of the right CN V root entry zone. Pledgets may be straight or curved, as in this case

can help guide efficacious revision surgery in select patients. CT can depict the general position of surgical material following MVD (Fig. 6.6), but MRI is the preferred modality for assessment of the etiology of persistent or recurrent trigeminal neuralgia symptoms following treatment.

Imaging may also play a role, albeit limited, in patients with trigeminal neuralgia treated with implantable peripheral nerve stimulators, particularly in the assessment

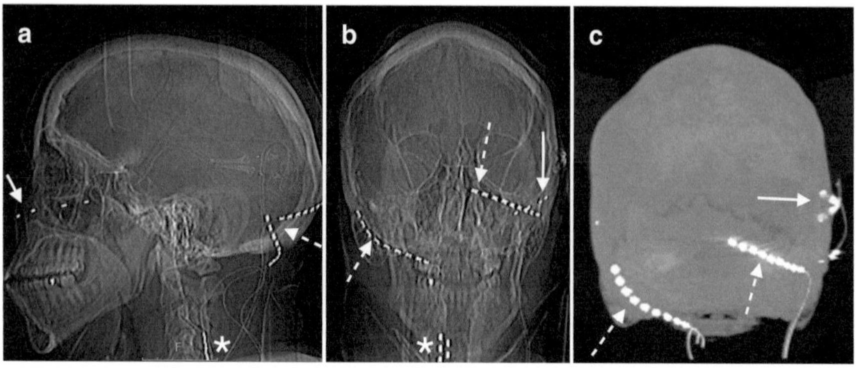

Fig. 6.7 Sagittal (**a**) and frontal (**b**) scout images from a CT scan and a maximal intensity projection (MIP) reconstruction (**c**) reveal multiple implantable devices including a left V2 division stimulator device (solid arrow), bilateral occipital nerve stimulators (dashed arrows), and a cervical spinal stimulator within the dorsal epidural space at C4 (asterisk)

of potential placode dislodgment, lead dehiscence, or implant infection. As many devices may not be MRI compatible, CT is the primary imaging modality employed for implant assessment (Fig. 6.7).

Glossopharyngeal Neuralgia

Glossopharyngeal neuralgia manifests as severe, unilateral, paroxysmal pain in the sensory distribution of the ninth cranial nerve (CNIX), similar to trigeminal neuralgia in terms of pathophysiology but much rarer. Pain localizes to the oropharynx, oral tongue or base of the tongue, tonsillar fossa, or ears and may be accompanied by palatal myoclonus, bradycardia, or even syncope and cardiac arrest [4, 14]. Cases of glossopharyngeal neuralgia have been attributed to a variety of etiologies including tumor, infection, Chiari I malformation, and neurovascular compression. Along its course from the upper medulla to the pars nervosa portion of the jugular foramen, CNIX may be impacted by the posterior inferior cerebellar artery (PICA), vertebral artery, or the anterior inferior cerebellar artery (AICA) in decreasing order of reported frequency, or a combination thereof [14, 15]. In 47 subjects who underwent microvascular decompression of CNIX for glossopharyngeal neuralgia, the PICA was the most commonly encountered offending vessel (68%) [15]. The authors found compression of the root entry zone by multiple arteries in 17% of subjects and attributed glossopharyngeal symptomatology to vein contact in 6% of subjects. The efficacy of microvascular decompression for glossopharyngeal neuralgia is robust, as demonstrated by complete resolution of symptoms in 46 of 47 subjects in this study [15].

MRI serves as the primary imaging modality for the exclusion of secondary causes of glossopharyngeal symptomatology, delineation of CNIX anatomy and

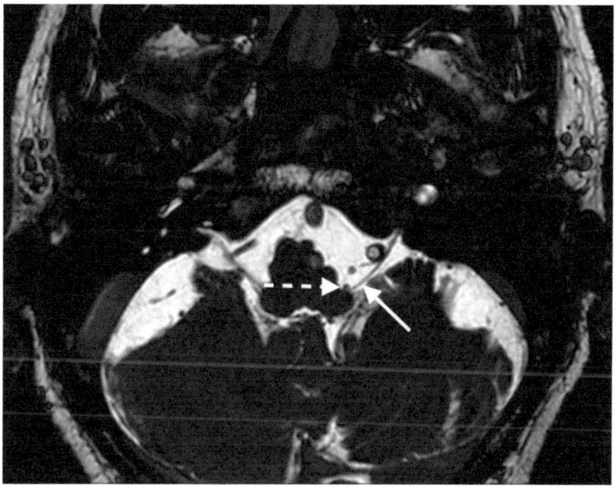

Fig. 6.8 Axial T2-weighted SSFP image shows the left glossopharyngeal nerve (solid arrow) as it approaches its root entry zone in the supra-olivary fossette being compressed by the ipsilateral posterior inferior cerebellar artery (dashed arrow)

course, and assessment for potential neurovascular conflict, all of which are readily accomplished by the addition of thin-section (1 mm or less) SSFP imaging to a routine brain MRI protocol. As in the assessment of trigeminal neuralgia, MRA may provide additional information regarding flow velocity within vessels in proximity to or contacting the glossopharyngeal nerve. Anatomically, the supra-olivary fossette, the most medial portion of the cerebello-pontomedullary angle, serves as an important radiologic and surgical landmark given its proximity to the root entry zone of CNIX [14]. In their cohort of ten patients with glossopharyngeal neuralgia, Hiwatashi et al. found arterial contact of the CNIX root entry zone in all ten subjects [14]. Thus, similar to the anatomic considerations in trigeminal neuralgia, the site of vascular contact relative to the root entry zone is a critical factor in determining the salience of CNIX neurovascular contact.

Figure 6.8 is an axial T2-weighted SSFP image showing the left glossopharyngeal nerve as it approaches its root entry zone in the supra-olivary fossette being compressed by the ipsilateral posterior inferior cerebellar artery.

Conclusion

Facial and head pain can be a feature of a wide array of disease entities across several medical domains. Several potentially life-threatening conditions such as intracranial hematoma or aneurysmal hemorrhage should be eliminated as part of the workup of new onset head pain. Clinicians should avail themselves of the American College of Radiology Appropriateness Criteria for guidance on optimal imaging techniques for patient evaluation. Imaging evaluation can play a crucial role in diagnosis and treatment planning.

References

1. Kuruvilla DE, Lipton RB. Appropriate use of neuroimaging in headache. Curr Pain Headache Rep. 2015;19(6):17.
2. May A. New insights into headache: an update on functional and structural imaging findings. Nat Rev Neurol. 2009;5(4):199–209.
3. Douglas A, et al.. American College of Radiology ACR Appropriateness Criteria® Headache. Available at: https://acsearch.acr.org/docs/69482/Narrative/. Accessed 4 April 2017.
4. Siccoli MM, Bassetti CL, Sándor PS. Facial pain: clinical differential diagnosis. Lancet Neurol. 2006;5(3):257–67.
5. Dandy WE. Concerning the cause of trigeminal neuralgia. Am J Surg. 1934;24(2):447–55.
6. Haller S, et al. Imaging of neurovascular compression syndromes: trigeminal neuralgia, hemifacial spasm, vestibular paroxysmia, and glossopharyngeal neuralgia. Am J Neuroradiol. 2016;37(8):1384–92.
7. Hughes MA, et al. MRI of the trigeminal nerve in patients with trigeminal neuralgia secondary to vascular compression. Am J Roentgenol. 2016;206(3):595–600.
8. Sindou M, Howeidy T, Acevedo G. Anatomical observations during microvascular decompression for idiopathic trigeminal neuralgia. Acta Neurochir (Wien). 2002;144(1):1–12.
9. Leal PRL, et al. Visualization of vascular compression of the trigeminal nerve with high-resolution 3T MRI: a prospective study comparing preoperative imaging analysis to surgical findings in 40 consecutive patients who underwent microvascular decompression for trigeminal neuralgia. Neurosurgery. 2011;69(1):15–25, discussion 26.
10. Sindou M, et al. Microvascular decompression for primary trigeminal neuralgia: long-term effectiveness and prognostic factors in a series of 362 consecutive patients with clear-cut neurovascular conflicts who underwent pure decompression. J Neurosurg. 2007;107(6):1144–53.
11. Régis J, et al. Prospective controlled trial of gamma knife surgery for essential trigeminal neuralgia. J Neurosurg. 2006;104(6):913–24.
12. Régis J, et al. Long-term safety and efficacy of Gamma Knife surgery in classical trigeminal neuralgia: a 497-patient historical cohort study. J Neurosurg. 2016;124(4):1079–87.
13. Hughes MA, et al. MRI findings in patients with a history of failed prior microvascular decompression for hemifacial spasm: how to image and where to look. Am J Neuroradiol. 2015;36(4):768–73.
14. Hiwatashi A, et al. MRI of glossopharyngeal neuralgia caused by neurovascular compression. Am J Roentgenol. 2008;191(2):578–81.
15. Sampson JH, et al. Microvascular decompression for glossopharyngeal neuralgia: long-term effectiveness and complication avoidance. Neurosurgery. 2004;54(4):884–90.

Chapter 7
Psychological Assessment in the Context of Head and Facial Pain

Leanne R. Cianfrini and Daniel M. Doleys

Introduction

Let's play "one of these things is not like the other": diabetes, cardiovascular disease, cancer, and chronic pain. In three of these conditions, a health-care provider is able to run diagnostic tests—a comprehensive metabolic blood panel, cardiac catheterization, X-ray/CT imaging—and "prove" the patient has the suspected disease. In three of these conditions, a clinician can track quantitative physiological outcomes of their chosen treatment—Does insulin bring A1C and blood glucose back within the reference ranges? Does the cardiac stent improve blood flow? Is the tumor shrinking? In contrast, the disease of chronic pain stands apart. Although testing can provide some evidence of pathology in certain cases of acute pain, there is no definitive medical test that correlates well to the patient's personal, subjective experience of the phenomenon of "pain." Although medical imaging techniques can lead to objective diagnoses (e.g., cervical facet arthropathy, osteoarthritis of the right temporomandibular joint), they are not designed to assess pain-related emotions or to predict individual behavior. Furthermore, in the face of being challenged to blindly trust the patient in front of us to be able to realistically evaluate and effectively verbalize their pain, we are often asked to provide invasive treatments and potent analgesics.

The disease of chronic pain is like no other medical condition in requiring a leap of faith in the face of frankly incomplete data. In the mental health profession, where there is likewise no blood test or diagnostic scan to "prove" mood disorders, anxiety, or a personality disorder, methods of comprehensive assessment have been developed to translate a patient's subjective experience into one that can be better understood and tracked over time. One must heed the advice shared by Hippocrates and Sir William Osler: "It is more important to know what sort of person has a

L. R. Cianfrini (✉) · D. M. Doleys
The Doleys Clinic, Birmingham, AL, USA

J. Y. Suen, E. Petersen (eds.), *Diagnosis and Management of Head and Face Pain*, https://doi.org/10.1007/978-3-319-90999-8_7

disease than to know what sort of disease the person has." One must become as dogged and thorough as an investigative journalist to delve into a complex, dynamic experience that has deep-seated and costly individual, familial, and societal ramifications. One must think through the analysis in a systematic way, asking "Why, Where, How, When, What?" to get the complete picture. This chapter will ask and answer these questions in the context of psychological assessment for head and facial pain, highlighting the rationale and domains of relevance for a biopsychosocial pain assessment, providing examples of assessment instruments in each domain, and offering practical approaches for implementing screening and/or comprehensive assessment into various types of clinical practices.

Why?

The tongue-in-cheek answer to "*Why* conduct psychological assessment of the pain patient?" is "Why wouldn't you?" We'll ask some additional questions to help frame our answer further:

- Would you like to know in advance if your patient is likely to benefit from your proposed interventions? Is the person before you likely to be one with persistent pain and a strong degree of pathophysiology who seems to function well, or is he one with minimal pathology that will become so overwhelmed by pain that it becomes the primary focus of his reduced quality of life?
  - Hint: It's not the degree of physical damage alone that dictates outcomes but also complex individual genetic and psychosocial factors.
- Would you like to improve the chance of success for your patient to reach appropriate and individualized treatment goals?
  - Hint: Psychological variables can represent significant potential impediments to optimal response and ability to benefit from physical or pharmacological treatment programs, including surgical interventions and other invasive procedures. Early therapeutic interventions can mitigate potential for poor outcomes.
- Would you like to identify any "red flags" for patient safety?
  - Hint: Risk stratification models based on evidence-based psychosocial risk factors are readily accessible and can be a medicolegal safeguard for your practice.

A better response to "Why?" warrants a discussion of the biopsychosocial model of chronic pain. The scope of the role of psychological assessment has evolved in parallel with our expanding understanding of the pain experience. In the early days when pain and other diseases were approached solely from a reductionistic and dualistic biomedical conceptualization, the realm of the "mind" was considered irrelevant. Explanations for health and disease were offered primarily in terms of discrete, measurable biological variables. Although the concept of a direct correlation between specific organic pathology and pain report tended to explain adaptive and acute pain fairly well, using purely physiological evidence failed to predict the experience of chronic pain. Clinical observations also indicated that many patients complained of persistent pain refractory to medical and surgical treatments and that functional disability often appeared in excess of what might be expected based on physical pathology alone. Specifically, the biomedical model was inadequate in situations when a patient complained of pain which was not commensurate with the degree of observable pathology. This "disconnect" is common in chronic pain conditions as headache, fibromyalgia, and temporomandibular disorders. It became obvious that other factors—likely psychological and social factors—must contribute to the pain experience and to treatment outcomes.

The evolution of comprehensive pain models incorporating a biopsychosocial approach has developed over decades, and a thorough description of the systematic attempts to produce these models is beyond the scope of this chapter. It is sufficient to note that more recent pain models have been constructed to incorporate multiple dimensions of the pain experience, acknowledging that pain does not exist in a social vacuum and that nonphysiological factors such as personality, cognitions, beliefs, sociocultural variables, learning, and emotional reactivity all contribute significantly to a patient's perception of pain. One enduring model [1] characterizes pain along three distinct, interrelated dimensions: (a) sensory/discriminative, which acknowledges underlying physical pathology and incorporates nervous system pathways; (b) affective-motivational, which reflects emotional responses to pain; and (c) cognitive-evaluative, which takes into account individual beliefs and ascribes meaning to the pain experience. The integration of each of these factors is required for the conscious experience of pain. When pain becomes chronic, sensory input plays a diminished role, while affective and cognitive pathways play a more prominent role in the creation of painful perceptions.

The International Association for the Study of Pain [2] nods to the dual nature of pain in their oft-cited definition: "an unpleasant sensory and emotional experience associated with actual or potential tissue damage or described in terms of such damage." As the sophistication of brain imaging techniques evolved, a clearer picture of the brain regions involved in pain processing was formed, with dynamic overlap in pain and limbic structures, such as the anterior cingulate cortex, amygdala, and insular cortex, among others [3, 4]. The 2011 Institute of Medicine (IOM) report [5] concluded that pain has biological, psychological, and social components, and effective treatments for pain must address all three areas. The IOM report also acknowledged that the risk of acute and chronic pain, as well as the risk for "chronification" of pain, is affected by an interplay between demographic and cultural factors, modifiable psychological factors, and disease-related factors. Figure 7.1 summarizes these factors using a life-span approach.

Thus, chronic pain—a separate clinical entity with underlying mechanisms that distinguish it from simply prolonged acute pain [6]—requires accurate assessment of not only the medical aspects of pain but the psychosocial factors as well. Most chronic pain guidelines (VA/DoD, CDC, state medical boards) recommend a psychological evaluation as an integral part of the diagnostic workup, and such assessments are required by insurance carriers prior to certain surgical/implantable device interventions.

From Birth	Childhood	Adolescence	Adulthood
Genetics, female sex, minority race or ethnicity, congenital disorders, prematurity Parental anxiety, irregular feeding and sleeping Parents' pain exposure and reactions Temperament and personality			
	Physical/sexual abuse and other traumatic events (e.g., death of a parent, witness to violence) Low socioeconomic status Emotional, conduct, and peer problems Hyperactivity Serious illness or injury, hospitalization Separation from mother Acute or recurrent pain experience		
		Changes of puberty, gender roles Education level, learning (behavioral reactions to pain) Injuries Obesity Low levels of fitness	
			Vivid recall of childhood trauma Lack of social support, accumulated stress ("allostatic load") Surgery Overuse of joints and muscles Occupational exposures, job dissatisfaction, low work status Development of chronic disease Aging

Fig. 7.1 Life-span factors associated with the development of chronic pain. Reprinted with permission from Relieving Pain in America: A Blueprint for Transforming Prevention, Care, Education, and Research (2011) by the National Academy of Sciences, Courtesy of the National Academies Press, Washington, D.C. [5]

Beyond an inclination to accept and adhere to the biopsychological model in theory or to follow consensus recommendations, it is simply helpful in actual practice to know and be able to address psychosocial factors that predispose a patient to pain, that may precipitate flares, or that may prolong their pain. For example, individuals with temporomandibular disorders (TMD) show a higher prevalence of stress, anxiety, posttraumatic stress disorder, depression, somatic awareness, pain catastrophizing, suicidal ideation, and kinesiophobia (fear of movement and reinjury) compared with controls [7–13]. Beyond prevalence or correlational studies, one well-done prospective cohort study (The Orofacial Pain: Prospective Evaluation and Risk Assessment, or OPPERA study) demonstrated that several psychological variables predicted *first onset* of TMD pain, but the strongest predictors were perceived stress, previous stressful life events, and negative affect at a 3-year follow-up [14]. Studies have also demonstrated that psychological comorbidities such as depression contribute to the *persistence or chronicity* of TMD pain, regardless of the presence of painful comorbidities [15–18].

Patients with migraine are more likely to develop depression than those without migraine. In a review of the literature, the prevalence of depression varied from 8.6 to 47.9% in patients with migraine [19], with the overall risk of developing depression 2.2 times higher in patients with migraine. There is also a high degree of comorbidity between bipolar disorder II and migraine, with further research required to better understand the relationships between the two conditions [20]. Disability and quality of life are impacted when migraines or other headache pain conditions are associated with depression or anxiety [21, 22]. Studies also have found high utilization of health resources when migraine is comorbid with psychiatric disorders [23]. Depression and anxiety also seem to play relative roles in the transformation from acute to chronic migraine [24] and in the development of migraine overuse headache separate from factors that are typically associated with substance abuse [25].

In summary, an approach that ignores the complex and dynamic interactions among medical, cognitive, and affective variables is incomplete and likely to be ineffective. Clearly, psychological assessment has a role in identifying nonphysiological factors contributing to a patient's pain complaints, quality of life, persistence of pain and dysfunction, and treatment outcomes. This perspective suggests a role for psychological assessment earlier rather than later in the treatment process, as well as at various points along the treatment process.

When?

The psychological evaluation can prove helpful during several critical points within a comprehensive pain management program, with timing chosen depending on the provider's needs and those of the particular patient. There have been lists of indications published for psychological evaluation, such as those developed by a multidisciplinary occupational medicine panel [26]. However, these recommendations often seem reactionary, in that patients would be sent for evaluation only after all treatments fail, if there are aberrant prescription medication behaviors, if there is lack of adherence to medical treatment, or once cognitive impairment or suicidality is suspected. We recommend earlier involvement to identify and mitigate future problems; in other words, the psychological evaluation does not have to be limited to a role of last resort.

If the patient is only sent for psychological interaction after they already violate the terms of a medical agreement, e.g., seeking prescriptions from multiple providers or having an abnormal drug screen, the visit with the mental health professional is seen as a punishment. If the patient is sent only once they exhibit emotional reactions in the office or if they express frustration with the failures of several medication or treatment trials, the psychological referral seems like a dismissal of the patient's valid physical concerns. Conversely, if the evaluation occurs early on in the process of the pain experience, encouraged and supported by the physician, it is better received as part of the interdisciplinary care program.

At our outpatient chronic pain management clinic, the psychological evaluation is the first step in patient care. An opioid risk stratification analysis is done, which guides the frequency of follow-up visits and determines the plan for compliance monitoring throughout the treatment program. This serves as medicolegal safeguard for the prescribing physician. The evaluation also suggests appropriate outcome measures for the particular patient. For example, for a patient who continues to work full time but exhibits anxiety and avoidance of recreational and social activities, return-to-work or physical therapy quotas may not be the ideal post-intervention outcome measurements. Instead, one might consider administering measures of anxiety, quality of life, social support, or pain beliefs at various points during treatment to assess change in these domains important for this particular individual.

In our tertiary care setting, the pretreatment interview and testing are followed by an educational program led by the behavioral medicine specialist to teach the patient risks and benefits of treatment, how the brain processes pain and emotion (a biopsychosocial explanation tailored to the patient level), how to manage mood, how to improve sleep and make dietary choices to calm inflammation, and about the clinic expectations for safety, adherence, and the patient's own role in the team care. The psychologist stays involved periodically for therapeutic interventions and for compliance monitoring. We have found that this method of early assessment and intervention enhances compliance, helps with patient retention, makes it easier to advocate and communicate if future issues do arise, and has improved patient involvement in their own care.

Where and How (To Frame It)?

Individuals with chronic pain seldom spontaneously seek assistance from psychologists; the encounters nearly always involve consultation with third-party referral sources. Referring clinicians may understand that collaboration with a psychologist or a screening in office can be a valuable part of comprehensive pain management, but may not be comfortable explaining the recommendation for testing or the psychology referral to the patient.

It is critical for the patient to be adequately prepared for the assessment. It is evident from concern expressed by patients that the role of psychological assessment in pain management is not always well understood. There is evidence that patients are more receptive to referral when it is introduced by the physician as part of an essential routine for treatment results. Anxious patients express concern that their physician suspects the pain is "not real," or is insinuating that they are "faking it" or "crazy" [27]. Clearly, these assumptions or perceptions of dismissiveness can lead to patient resistance [28]. When possible, referring health professionals can assist the process by (a) explaining the reason for the evaluation, (b) emphasizing the importance of understanding how pain affects the person's quality of life, and (c) indicating that the intention is to derive information that will maximize treatment effectiveness. The patient should be given the opportunity to ask questions and provide consent. At our outpatient pain management clinic, we typically use a variation of the following language included on our website and in our patient scheduling letter and presented verbally during the interview introduction:

> "We understand that chronic pain can impact mood, activities, sleep, and social functioning, among other things. The purpose of the psychological evaluation is to help us understand how your pain is impacting your life and how the stresses of life, in turn, might be affecting your pain. This will help guide your comprehensive treatment plan and can increase the effectiveness of your medical treatments."

Full evaluations can be conducted in office or at bedside during a hospital inpatient consultation. In office assessments can last up to 60–90 min face-to-face and are often covered by behavioral medicine or psychological codes under most insurance plans.

The question often arises as to how to find a local pain psychologist. There are at least three avenues. First, obtain the membership rosters from the American Pain Society and the International Association for the Study of Pain; members are listed by location and specialty. Second, contact the nearest institution that grants a doctoral degree in psychology. The department of psychology often is aware of graduates in the area and their specialty interests. Third, contact your state board of examiners in psychology. Once a person is identified, there may be some practical and financial advantages to having them as an employee of the practice vs. using them as an outside consultant. For those psychologists interested, but requiring some additional training, there are many such opportunities through workshops offered by the various local, regional, and national pain societies. Darnall and colleagues recently issued a national call to action to improve pain education and training of psychologists; the goal is to reduce reported barriers for medical providers to access qualified pain psychologists and facilitate biopsychosocial treatment [29].

A growing trend is also to incorporate a psychological *screening* assessment in the setting of the busy medical practice. This is often done through an electronic assessment, in which a battery of brief questionnaires is delivered by iPad or other computerized software that can interface with your electronic health record system. Several companies have predetermined batteries that might take 5–10 min for the patient to complete to give a sense of psychological risk factors such as depression, medication compliance risk, and perceived functional impairment. We discourage use of these batteries as a stand-alone or final step—results should be used to guide referral onto appropriate mental health providers to address underlying concerns raised by the screening score profile.

What?

There are three major components to a thorough psychological assessment, in addition to medical record review: (a) the interview, (b) behavioral observations, and (c) standardized testing. Although the "what" of testing in the context of pain management is not universally agreed upon and can vary with treatment setting, medical condition, and referral question, most recommendations fall within the context of a multidisciplinary and biopsychosocial paradigm.

Interview and Behavioral Observations

The usual first step and main event in any comprehensive psychological evaluation is the interview. This may be conducted in a structured or unstructured format but essentially is the opportunity to "get to know the person behind the pain." A thorough interviewer trained in pain or health psychology will gather a rich and detailed portrait of the patient from information spanning several domains, including (a) pain description and history, (b) contributing psychosocial factors, and (c) issues like cognitive or behavioral barriers to appropriate treatment adherence.

The psychologist is also trained to make specific behavioral observations throughout the interview about the patient's obvious or subtle pain behaviors, affect, cognitive limitations, mental status, communication style, and pathological personality indicators. Patients often communicate their private experience of pain through overt pain behaviors such as postures (e.g., bracing, guarding), nonverbal groans, or facial expressions or through verbal communication [30]. An escalation of such behaviors in medical settings can be witnessed when the patient feels their message is inaccurately received or is not being acknowledged. Situations like the frustrating "12 out of 10" pain rating arise and can cloud the clinical picture. For example, how can you tell whether a patient who winces and grimaces to the slightest stimulus is intentionally exaggerating, is experiencing a true neuropathic pain state with allodynia, or is simply an unsophisticated communicator? Interviews will routinely involve caretakers, spouses, significant others, and/or relevant family members to gather information about possible secondary gain/reinforcement issues and communication patterns and to secure the most accurate and complete historical information. Solicitous partners may unintentionally encourage patients to increase pain behaviors by offering more support in the presence of such behaviors, rather than reinforcing more adaptive behavior [31].

The specific information collected during the interview is flexible and may vary depending on the patient, the psychologist, and the needs of the referring physician (e.g., a presurgical screening vs. diagnostic interview vs. assessment of compliance risk factors). Typical interview topics and behavioral observations are summarized in Table 7.1.

Table 7.1 Possible psychological interview topics

Pain-related information	Psychosocial information	Medication/adherence issues	Behavioral observations
Pain location, intensity ratings, descriptors	Brief social history (e.g., educational attainment, work history, family background, living situation)	Medication management (e.g., list of medications, doses, dose timing, prescribing physician, side effects, etc.)	Good/poor historian
Pain treatment history and outcomes	Job satisfaction/ dissatisfaction	Personal and family substance use/abuse history	Cognitive status (performance on brief mental status test)
Exacerbating factors	Family reactions to pain	Adherence to medications (e.g., missed doses, running out ahead of time)	Alertness, affect
Helpful self-management interventions	Current mood status (e.g., depression, anxiety, anger, frustration, presence of affective disorders)	Side effects	Interaction with family members (supportive, solicitous, adversarial)
Impact of pain on activity and quality of life	Psychological diagnosis and mental health treatment history	Signs of tolerance	Personality indicators, rapport with interviewer and staff
Activity pacing efficacy	Suicidal ideation and intent for self-harm	Illicit behaviors surrounding obtaining medication (e.g., borrowing from family, purchasing off street)	Overt pain behaviors (e.g., wincing, guarding)
Understanding of diagnosis and prognosis	Legal or social reinforcements/secondary gain	Irrational fears of addiction	Barriers to medication compliance (e.g., poor judgment, impulsivity, poor memory)
Expectations for treatment gains	Current coping skills and confidence in their use	Adherence to other medical treatments (e.g., diabetic diet, sleep hygiene or CPAP use, exercise program)	Consistency between verbal complaint and behavior
	Availability and quality of social support		
	Cognitive styles: presence of pain catastrophizing, somatic hypervigilance		
	History of developmental trauma (e.g., sexual abuse)		
	Readiness for change/ chronic pain acceptance		

Psychological Testing

Assessments relying solely on interview data are often considered incomplete if not inadequate. Paper-and-pencil or computerized tests are recommended to examine consistency of patient self-report and to provide quantitative data for repeat comparison. This is presently the closest answer we can give to the call from third-party payors for "objective" outcome tracking. Tests should ideally be well-standardized, validated using appropriate normative samples (e.g., for comparison with other pain patients), and psychometrically sound.

Indeed, there is growing evidence of the utility of psychological tests for patients with pain. A review of 125 meta-analyses and 800 samples concluded that psychological tests provide information beyond what can be obtained in an interview and are scientifically comparable to medical test validity [32]. Furthermore, baseline psychological testing can sometimes exceed the ability of medical tests to predict the outcome of medical treatments for certain pain conditions like low back pain [33, 34].

Numerous questionnaire and psychological assessment instruments are available for clinical use which allow for evaluation of multiple domains at once or specific domains allowing the clinic to tailor a battery to their needs. The recently published revised Diagnostic Criteria for TMD (DC/TMD; [35]), which is based on multi-center clinical studies and international consensus conferences, includes recommendations for an "Axis II" protocol beyond a medical assessment. This involves a psychosocial evaluation, either through brief assessment that can be conducted by a general practitioner or through a comprehensive set of instruments for expanded assessment by an orofacial pain specialist. The recommended questionnaires cover the domains of pain location, physical function, functional limitations, distress, depression, anxiety, physical symptoms, and orofacial parafunctions.

We'll begin with a discussion of instruments within specific recommended domains and then identify a few of the available comprehensive batteries for pain assessment.

Specific Testing Domains

Pain Intensity and Descriptive Measures: Pain perception is a personal, covert process, and as mentioned earlier, there is no fail-safe mechanical means of measuring an individual's pain experience. Many of our patients have lamented the lack of such an instrument of empathy: "I wish my doctor or my wife could feel what I feel for just 20 seconds so they'd know what I'm going through." Imagine that sense of isolation, knowing that traditional verbal communication is inadequate to share what you feel, why the pain seems like an insurmountable barrier to accomplishing your goals, and why you're so desperate for compassionate and immediate care. In chronic pain especially, signs of overt autonomic arousal (e.g., increased blood pressure, perspiration) do not always correspond directly to pain intensity, so one must be cautioned against "judging a book by its cover" during an office consultation. Quantitative sensory testing has been developed for use in experimental pain research settings (e.g., responses to thermal, mechanical, ischemic stimulation) and can illuminate some psychophysiological parameters in neuropathic pain states like an individual's pain threshold, tolerance, or degree of central sensitization/allodynia/hyperalgesia [36] but is still dependent on patient self-report.

That leaves us with quantified subjective measures to identify pain intensity at its worst, least, current, and average. The Numerical Rating Scale (NRS) is the widely used 0–10 or 0–100 scale with endpoints usually defined as "no pain" to "most intense pain imaginable." Visual analogue scales (VAS), in which a patient marks a vertical line along a 10 cm horizontal line, is often used in research to detect subtle changes across time.

There are some clinical issues to note with such scales. For example, if a patient has multiple sites of pain (e.g., tension-type headache, TMD pain, and low back pain), for which site are they providing that single numerical rating? Should multiple intensity ratings be generated for each pain site, or can pain intensity be accurately aggregated into a single number? How are scale anchors defined—is a patient's 10/10 the same as ours? Is their scale the same across time or are their anchors dynamic and situationally dependent? Experienced clinicians are well aware of the discrepancy between subjective pain ratings and objective measures of function [37–39]. Patients who give similar pain intensity ratings may exhibit a very different degree of psychological and physical impairment. There is also a disconnect between changes in numerical ratings and patient satisfaction with treatment [40]. Prominent researchers in the field [41, 42] have strongly questioned the use of the NRS as the primary metric for chronic pain.

The DC/TMD also encourages the use of a pain drawing or body map to capture a sense of pain location. We encourage use of both a whole body map and a head diagram, since many patients have multiple pain complaints concurrent with a head or facial pain complaint (e.g., coexisting functional somatic syndromes like migraine, irritable bowel syndrome, fibromyalgia [43]). In a recent study of 135 patients referred to tertiary care for TMD pain, only 21% reported localized TMD pain, 20% reported regional pain such as headaches and neck pain, and the majority reported widespread pain at multiple body sites [44]. A verbal explanation may be warranted to help patients explore all sites of pain [45].

As conceptualized eloquently by D.A. Williams [46], "if you are listening to music, knowing only the volume setting tells you little about instrumentation, quality, key or tempo of the piece that is being played." In other words, we need to go *beyond the 0–10* and consider additional aspects of the patient's experience, such as the unpleasantness or "suffering" component. The McGill Pain Questionnaire (MPQ; [47]) can be used for evaluating pain intensity or the sensory component but also captures qualities of the affective-motivational dimension of pain. The measure presents several groups of adjectives ranked in terms of severity and can be administered as a paper-and-pencil test or by an evaluator reading each subclass of words. Studies have shown that the MPQ is able to discriminate among discrete pain conditions, such as between migraine and tension-type headache [48] or between trigeminal neuralgia and atypical facial pain [49]. A clinician can use the information from the MPQ to guide interventions. For example, a patient who endorses several affective pain descriptors of high intensity (i.e., "terrifying," "unbearable," "vicious") may respond to treatment that targets pain anxiety, maladaptive pain beliefs, unrealistic expectations, or coping mechanisms. This plan may differ from a behavioral treatment program designed for a patient that primarily endorses sensory descriptors such as "aching," "tender," and "cramping," in which techniques such as muscle relaxation may be better suited.

Quality of Life (QoL)/Functional Impact of Pain: A reduction in pain intensity ratings may continue to be a principal outcome, but only in the context of the patient's overall QoL/function. This is consistent with the recommendations for outcome domains in chronic pain studies and clinical trials presented in the recent IMMPACT guidelines [50]. In this category of testing, the patient's perceived functional limitations due to their pain are delineated, and areas of behavioral intervention are identified. Validity of such measures can be questionable because of the self-report nature (e.g., we have had patients rate a sitting tolerance of only 10 min but proceed to sit through an hour interview or class), and daily activity diaries for improved short-term recall are not always feasible. General QoL measures allow for broad comparisons between illness conditions and are useful in health research (e.g., the Short Form Health Survey [51], Sickness Impact Profile [52]), but administration can be lengthy, and these measures are often unresponsive to change in specific pain conditions. The Pain Disability Index [53] is shorter and widely used and produces ratings of general pain limitations on obligatory and discretionary activities across seven functional content areas (e.g., family/home responsibilities, recreation, social life).

Disease-specific QoL instruments better reflect the impact associated with single disease states. For example, we use the Oswestry Disability Index [54] quite a bit in our practice, but these items (e.g., impact on lifting, sitting) were designed to measure disability in patients with low back pain and would not translate well to assess the unique functional and parafunctional interference possible with head and facial pain (e.g., impact on chewing, yawning, creating facial expressions of emotion). Several of the most widely used headache- and facial pain-specific QoL instruments with adequate psychometric properties are listed in Table 7.2.

The clinician can use this information about the extent of pain interference, the domains of functioning most affected by the pain, and the activities the patient can still perform to guide appropriate medical intervention, to improve functional ability, and to assess the outcome of treatment.

Mood Symptoms: Psychiatric illnesses such as major depressive disorder, bipolar disorder, and anxiety disorders commonly occur in individuals with head and facial pain. Such mental disorders are best diagnosed with interview based on Diagnostic and Statistical Manual criteria [63], but screeners exist to signal whether fuller evaluation is warranted. The three most commonly assessed moods in chronic pain studies have been depressed mood, anxiety, and anger. It is also important clinically to make the distinction between clinical/psychiatric diagnoses and normal pain-related mood changes. The most common phrase we hear during our psychological evalua-

Table 7.2 Relevant disease-specific quality of life instruments

Questionnaire	Reference	Brief description
Headache specific		
Migraine Disability Assessment Scale (MIDAS)	[55]	5-item questionnaire designed to evaluate headache impact/disability within previous 3 months in domains of work/school, household work, family/social activities
Headache Impact Test (HIT-6)	[56]	6-item survey that measures headache-induced burden in domains of pain, social and role functioning, vitality, cognitive function, and psychological distress
Migraine-Specific Quality of Life Questionnaire (MSQoL), most recent version MSQ 2.1	[57, 58]	14-item questionnaire to assess impact of migraine on health-related QoL over the past 4 weeks across three dimensions: role function-restrictive, role function-preventive, and emotional function
Jaw/facial pain specific		
Jaw Functional Limitation Scale (JFLS)	[59]	Measures global functional limitation of the jaw along 3 constructs: mastication, vertical jaw mobility (e.g., open wide), and emotional and verbal expression (e.g., ability to frown, put on a happy face); available in 20- and 8-item versions
Mandibular Function Impairment Questionnaire (MFIQ)	[60]	11-item assessment of perceived difficulty with particular mandibular movements or tasks (e.g., speaking, yawning), with 6 additional questions about mastication impairment for various foods
Oral Health Impact Profile, most recent version OHIP-14	[61, 62]	14-item measure of impact of oral disorders on well-being: functional limitation, physical pain, psychological discomfort, social disability, etc.

tions is, "I'm sad/frustrated/upset because I can't do the things I used to do." Often, a patient would not necessarily meet criteria for premorbid clinical depression but is simply confronting a natural grieving process over their pain-related losses. Similarly, a patient presenting with panic disorder with agoraphobia would require a different course of therapy than a patient who is withdrawing and isolating from social activities due to fear of exacerbating pain. For excellent reviews of psychological risk factors in headache and facial pain, see [64] and the OPPERA study [14], respectively.

Depression Screening Tools: There are some older scales that are widely used to evaluate depression in a variety of settings (e.g., Beck Depression Inventory [65]; Center for Epidemiological Studies—Depression Scale [66]). Although it has been postulated that these may be prone to artificial score inflation and false positives for depression in patients with pain-related somatic complaints [67], others have found that both the BDI and CES-D significantly discriminated between patients with chronic pain who did and did not have major depression [68].

More recent recommendations are moving toward use of various versions of the Patient Health Questionnaire [69], which was designed for use in primary care patients and is easily accessible for Internet download. The PHQ 4-, 9-, and 15-item versions are all mentioned as part of the DC/TMD Axis 2 psychosocial assessment [35].

The PHQ-9 is a valuable 9-item screening instrument for detecting MDD based on DSM-IV criteria, and the PHQ-2 includes the first 2 items critical for the diagnosis: (a) anhedonia, or loss of pleasure/interest, and (b) depressed, sad, or hopeless mood. These instruments are easily comprehended and quickly completed by patients and have been validated for use in migraine patients [70]. It is important to note, however, that these instruments provide only a probable diagnosis of major depressive disorder that should be investigated by further psychological diagnostic evaluation.

Anxiety Screening Tools: Anxiety assessments can include the generalized anxiety disorder-7 (GAD-7, [71]) as recommended by the DC/TMD. The shorter version (GAD-2) has also been widely used and validated as a screening tool in patients with migraines [72]. The Pain Anxiety Symptoms Scale (PASS-20) measures fear avoidance and anxiety responses specific to pain [73]. A construct called "cogniphobia" has emerged out of the kinesiophobia (fear and avoidance of movement) literature. Cogniphobia refers to the fear, and subsequent avoidance, of cognitive exertion in patients with migraine headaches out of concern for triggering a migraine episode. It was initially discussed in context of a posttraumatic headache disorder population but has been observed in primary headache disorder patients as well [74], and a new scale is under development for use in headache disorders in general [75]. There is also an adaptation of a kinesiophobia scale for use in TMD patients [13].

Anger Assessment: Anger, anywhere along a spectrum from frustration to fury, has long been recognized as common among individuals with chronic pain [76]. Anger may also be an expression of unresolved grief secondary to losses suffered in response to chronic pain. There is robust relationship between anger expression style and adverse pain outcomes above and beyond that of general negative affect, and this relationship may even be modulated by endogenous opioids [77]. Trost and colleagues [78] explored various cognitive dimensions of anger in chronic pain, such as goal frustration and perceived injustice. The authors also proposed pathways through which anger may undermine outcome, e.g., anger expression impairing the patient-physician therapeutic alliance. The State-Trait Anger Expression Inventory (STAXI; [79]) is the most widely used questionnaire in this domain.

By first assessing mood and then intervening through medications or behavioral lifestyle interventions, clinicians can modify how pain is processed and modulated via descending affective pathways. Reduction of the mood impact on disability and quality of life—whether from a primary mood diagnosis or from pain-related mood changes—is critical for outcomes regardless of the medical treatment selected.

Pain Beliefs and Attitudes: Thoughts, beliefs, attitudes, and appraisals about the pain experience, as well as patient expectations about treatments and their own role in the process, are powerful predictors of health-care utilization [80, 81] and treatment adherence/response [82]. One study showed that 41% of variance in physical functioning outcomes in patients entering a multidisciplinary pain treatment program was attributable simply to what patients think about their pain and how they cope with pain, even after controlling for effects of age, sex, and pain intensity [28]. You can imagine a different outcome for a patient who believes, "My pain is curable, but my doctor doesn't understand it, and they're the one responsible for fixing it!" vs. one who appraises, "My pain may be lifelong, but I can learn to manage my own lifestyle and follow appropriate medical treatments." Thus, assessment of locus of control (belief in who is responsible for symptom relief), coping resources, confidence/self-efficacy for the use of those resources, and pain acceptance gives the clinician a sense of which patients already have a viable armamentarium of self-management skills and those who may need additional pain coping training. Recent studies are elucidating the complex interplay of modifiable psychological factors, health beliefs, and disability in patients with head and facial pain (e.g., [83]). Examples of psychometrically sound questionnaires in this domain are highlighted in Table 7.3.

One cognitive process in particular has emerged as a defining predictor of pain-related disability and warrants special mention: pain catastrophizing [93]. You have met patients with this negative evaluation style if you've heard phrases like "This pain is killing me," "I can't think of anything except the pain," and "I feel helpless to ease the pain." This triad of beliefs has a strong impact on the sufferer. Catastrophizing is considered an important predictive factor for the transition from an acute pain state to one that is chronic—predicting up to 47% of the variance in this transition [94].

Table 7.3 Common questionnaires for pain beliefs and attitudes

Questionnaire	Reference	Brief description
Survey of Pain Attitudes (SOPA)	[84]	57 items to assess adaptive (control, emotion) and maladaptive (disability, harm, medication, solicitude, medical cure) beliefs
Chronic Pain Coping Inventory-42 (CPCI-42)	[85]	42-item abbreviated version to assess illness-focused coping (e.g., guarding, resting, asking for assistance) vs. wellness-focused coping (e.g., pacing, exercise, seeking social support)
Coping Strategies Questionnaire (CSQ)	[86]	6 cognitive (diverting attention, reinterpreting pain sensations, coping self-statements, ignoring pain sensations, praying or hoping, and catastrophizing) and 1 behavioral (increasing activity level) pain coping scales
Pain Self-Efficacy Questionnaire (PSEQ)	[87]	10-item measure of confidence in one's ability to engage in activities despite pain; 2-item version also validated [88]
Chronic Pain Acceptance Questionnaire-Revised (CPAQ-R)	[89]	20 items designed to measure acceptance of pain across 2 factors: activity engagement and pain willingness
Belief in Pain Control Questionnaire (BPCQ)	[90]	13 items to measure the power of individual beliefs regarding pain management across 3 subscales: internal or personal control of pain, beliefs that powerful others (doctors) control pain, and beliefs that pain is controlled by chance events
Headache-Specific Locus of Control	[91]	33-item scale to measure individual perceptions that headache problems and headache relief are determined primarily by internal factors, health-care professionals, or chance factors
Pain Catastrophizing Scale (PCS)	[92]	13-item instrument assessing pain catastrophizing across 3 subscales: rumination, magnification, and helplessness

Comprehensive Pain Inventories

There are several clinical testing instruments that can be used by trained and licensed psychologists for assessing a variety of psychological variables at once. The Minnesota Multiphasic Personality Inventory (MMPI-2) is a 567-item true/false measure of personality function and emotional status that has predictive ability based on more than 50 years of collection and analysis [95]. In its various formats, including a major recent revision (MMPI-2 RF [96]), a picture of psychological states, traits, and styles can emerge through the profile of results on clinical scales (e.g., excessive anxiety, hostility, somatization/somatic focus, sociopathy, social withdrawal). The profile can also provide a sense of the patient's reporting style (e.g., openness, defensiveness, "faking good," or "faking bad") through responses on validity scales. Although designed for assessment of psychiatric patients, it is commonly used in chronic pain and presurgical assessment, with certain profile patterns identified among independent samples of patients with diverse chronic pain syndromes. In a sample of headache patients, for example, significant elevations on the hypochondriasis, depression, hysteria, psychasthenia, and social introversion scales distinguished treatment-seeking headache patients from non-treatment-seeking controls [97]. Recently, Manfredini and colleagues demonstrated that chronic TMD pain patients without MRI-detected temporomandibular joint effusion have a different personality profile than patients with TMJ effusion and pain-free individuals [98]. Psychologists can use information from this measure to guide treatment plans and to suggest "red flag" personality characteristics to referring physicians. For example, a patient with an MMPI profile suggesting high levels of hostility, resistance to authority, and an elevated energy level may tend to test limits and may exhibit medication compliance issues down the line.

The Millon Behavioral Medicine Diagnostic (MBMD; [99]) has been normed on pain patients and can screen for a broad range of psychiatric diagnoses. The Battery for Health Improvement-2nd edition (BHI-2) and the brief version (BBHI-2) intended for use as a screener in medical offices are excellent inventories designed specifically to address biopsychosocial factors in patients with chronic pain [100].

Neurocognitive Testing

Testing can also include structured measures designed to examine neurocognitive functioning. Many patients involved in pharmacological management wish to or are expected to maintain their daily activities, including work, operating machinery/automobiles, maintaining their household, and/or managing finances. However, cognitive and neurological processes such as attention, concentration, planning, reaction time, and memory may be impaired in patients with pain [101, 102]. Cognitive deficits may result from head injuries or concussions, other organic processes, interference from pain itself or pain-related depression, or medication effects. In older patients, cognitive impairment may also occur as a result of dementia or increased susceptibility to side effects of sedating medications.

Brief screening tools such as the Repeatable Battery for the Assessment of Neuropsychological Status (RBANS, [103]) are easy to administer, can be sensitive to cognitive changes over time, and give some basic information about the cognitive processes listed above. As a most basic screener, inclusion of the Mini Mental Status Exam (MMSE, [104]) can be administered in 5–10 min for a gross assessment of orientation, attention, immediate recall, and language. Patients can also be asked to complete a self-appraisal of cognitive impairment using a tool such as the Multiple Ability Self-Report Questionnaire (MASQ, [105]) for perception of abilities in five cognitive domains: language, visuo-perceptual, verbal memory, visual memory, and attention. Psychologists trained for administration and interpretation of neuropsychological tests can also conduct formal batteries to examine suspected cognitive deficits in a more comprehensive and thorough manner. Patients can be released to function and work within the confines of the test parameters (e.g., minimizing competing stimuli, with stability of the current medication regimen). In addition, the results of testing can also guide the development of cognitive rehabilitation therapies for cognitively impaired patients.

Other Testing Domains

Sleep Quality: Testing can also be selected for comorbid issues affected by pain. For example, sleep disorders, including insomnia, obstructive sleep apnea, and sleep-related bruxism, are common comorbidities in both headache and TMD patients [106] and have a bidirectional relationship with pain [107]. The two most frequently used sleep questionnaires with good psychometric properties in orofacial pain populations [108] are the Epworth Sleepiness Scale [109] and the Pittsburgh Sleep Quality Index [110]. Psychological interventions such as biofeedback-assisted relaxation, sleep hygiene training, and graded exposure to tolerate CPAP therapy can be employed to improve sleep quality and may indirectly raise pain threshold and tolerance [111].

Autonomic Nervous System Activity: Analysis of autonomic nervous system activity in headache or facial pain patients can also prove helpful to guidAe biofeedback-assisted relaxation interventions. For example, measurements of heart rate variability and skin conductance have been used successfully to elucidate elevated sympathetic nervous system activity in patients with migraine and tension-type headaches [112], and the use of electromyographic (EMG) biofeedback assessment and treatment has been supported for use in patients with TMD [113]. For use in a typical medical practice, Autonomic Nervous System Testing machines are available for noninvasive testing under reimbursable testing codes; results can suggest which patients could benefit from referral to a psychologist trained in biofeedback interventions.

Risk for Aberrant Drug Behaviors: If your practice involves prescriptions for controlled substances, current clinical guidelines make a strong recommendation based on weak evidence to assess for current substance abuse, misuse, or addiction and risk for aberrant drug behaviors prior to initiation of opioid therapy for chronic pain [114]. Indeed, many state medical boards require/mandate such an initial risk stratification for controlled substances as well as ongoing compliance monitoring. Risk assessments help determine the amount of treatment structure and risk mitigation strategies needed for an individual patient (e.g., frequency of urine drug testing, pill counts, follow-up visits). The diagnostic interview is still considered to have clearest sensitivity and specificity, and no one risk tool has been shown to be better than another [115]. Some brief, validated, and nonconfrontational risk assessment tools in the public domain include:

- Substance Abuse Assessment
  - CAGE-AID [116] assesses likelihood and severity of alcohol and drug abuse, suited for use in primary care facilities but not specific for pain patients.
  - Drug Abuse Screening Test (DAST) [117] assesses problems and consequences related to drug (including prescription) misuse.
- Opioid Risk Assessment
  - Opioid Risk Tool [118] assesses the risk of aberrant behaviors in patient's prescribed opioid medications for chronic pain.
  - Screener and Opioid Assessment for Patients with Pain-Revised (SOAPP-R) [119] predicts possible opioid abuse in chronic pain patients and includes a companion measure for ongoing reassessment of opioid risk, the Current Opioid Misuse Measure [120].

Response Bias

In some cases, patient credibility may be questioned, especially in instances in which significant financial incentives are involved, e.g., worker's compensation, ongoing litigation, or disability applications. Factitious disorder and malingering are rare in clinical practice [121] and as such may be missed in the pain medicine setting. These nonorganic syndromes may present as pain or neurological complaints, with intentional fabrication or feigning of physical symptoms, or exaggerated expression of physical conditions in order to adopt a sick role. However, confirming these diagnoses requires difficult exclusions, including (a) conversion disorder, expression of a psychiatric disorder as head or facial pain as a symbolic transformation; (b) somatoform disorders, in which the preoccupation with physical symptoms exceeds organic pathology; and (c) hypochondriasis, conviction that pain is part of a malignant disease process. Inferences must also be based upon external data as well as clinician judgments about patient's motives and motivation. Unnecessary and invasive medical interventions, especially implanted devices which the patient may refuse to have removed, may cause further complications. On the other end of the spectrum, some patients may present with denial and unawareness of symptoms or minimize symptoms in a consciously motivated desire to continue activities that might otherwise be restricted (e.g., driving).

Rather than jumping to conclusions or judgment about the motives of a patient, it is recommended to make an attempt through assessment methods to screen for symptom validity and level of effort/motivation to identify the multiple driving forces behind patient motivation for symptom report. The MMPI-2 mentioned earlier has a set of validity scales for such purposes. The Modified Somatic Perception Questionnaire (MSPQ) and Pain Disability Index (PDI) are also used in pain populations to differentiate between malingered pain-related disability and non-malingering patients [122].

Conclusion

So, back to some questions: Do you want to implant an occipital stimulator in a migraine patient or perform neurosurgery on a trigeminal neuralgia patient with a strong degree of catastrophizing and anxiety? Do you want to perform that second or third jaw surgery for complaints of pain on a patient striving for disability? Do you want to give controlled substances to a person with an undiagnosed addiction? If not, consider a psychological assessment early on in your treatment algorithm. There may be times that surgical intervention may be required despite the psychological status of the patient to preserve neurological integrity and minimize further compromise. Even in such cases, understanding the patient will help to set proper expectations and establish a long-term care plan.

Do not be put off by the breadth of psychological constructs highlighted in this chapter or the volume of tests available. In a screening situation in a medical office, one can make the burden of testing as minimal as possible for the patient by using shorter, electronic versions of the tests mentioned above validated for use in clinical settings. For example, in just 17 items, a physician could screen for pain intensity, migraine-related disability, depression, anxiety, pain self-efficacy, and opioid risk with use of a NRS, the MIDAS, PHQ-2, GAD-2, PSEQ-2, and ORT. The trend toward more comprehensive assessment conveys an interest in the person as a whole rather than as a mere receptacle of treatment.

In summary, psychological assessment can (a) create a picture of the "person behind the pain"; (b) flag warning signs for potential patient noncompliance; (c) provide an estimated prognosis based on psychosocial barriers or boons to recovery; (d) establish whether psychological counseling for emotional distress might improve chances of treatment success; (e) guide the health-care team in creating appropriate and realistic treatment goals and algorithms; (f) indicate whether pretreatment education (e.g., about surgical risks/possible benefits, about safety with opioids or triptans), addiction recovery, behavior change (e.g., smoking cessation, weight management), or counseling is warranted; (g) help you meet the recommended or required practice guidelines for your medical specialty; and (h) practice within the accepted biopsychosocial model of pain care.

References

1. Melzack R, Casey KL. Sensory, motivational, and central control determinants of pain: a new conceptual model. In: Kenshalo D, editor. The skin senses. Springfield: Chas. C. Thomas; 1968. p. 423–39.
2. International Association for the Study of Pain. Pain terms: a list with definitions and notes on usage recommended by the IASP Subcommittee on Taxonomy. Pain. 1979;6:249–52.
3. Apkarian AV, Bushnell MC, Treede RD, Zubieta JK. Human brain mechanisms of pain perception and regulation in health and disease. Eur J Pain. 2005;9(4):463–84.
4. Wager TD, Atlas LY, Lindquist MA, Roy M, Woo CW, Kross E. An fMRI-based neurologic signature of physical pain. N Engl J Med. 2013;368(15):1388–97.
5. Institute of Medicine. Relieving pain in America: a blueprint for transforming prevention, care, education, and research. Washington, DC: The National Academies Press; 2011.
6. Bonica JJ, Loeser JD, Chapman CR, Fordyce WE. History of pain concepts and theories. In: Bonica JJ, editor. The management of pain. 2nd ed. Philadelphia: Lea & Febiger; 1990.
7. De Leeuw R, Bertoli E, Schmidt JE, Carlson CR. Prevalence of traumatic stressors in patients with temporomandibular disorders. J Oral Maxillofac Surg. 2005;63:42–50.
8. De Leeuw R, Bertoli E, Schmidt JE, Carlson CR. Prevalence of post-traumatic stress disorder symptoms in orofacial pain patients. Oral Surg Oral Med Oral Pathol Oral Radiol Endod. 2005;99(5):558–68.
9. Bertoli E, De Leeuw R. Prevalence of suicidal ideation, depression, and anxiety in chronic temporomandibular disorder patients. J Oral Facial Pain Headache. 2016;30(4):296–301.
10. Manfredini D, Landi N, Bandettini Di Poggio A, Dell'Osso L, Bosco M. A critical review on the importance of psychological factors in temporomandibular disorders. Minerva Stomatol. 2003;52:321–6.
11. Quartana PJ, Buenaver LF, Edwards RR, Klick B, Haythornthwaite JA, Smith MT. Pain catastrophizing and salivary cortisol responses to laboratory pain testing in temporomandibular disorder and healthy participants. J Pain. 2010;11:186–94.
12. Pompili M, Serafini G, Di Cosimo D, Dominici G, Innamorati M, Lester D, et al. Psychiatric comorbidity and suicide risk in patients with chronic migraine. Neuropsychiatr Dis Treat. 2010;6:81–91.
13. Visscher CM, Ohrbach R, van Wijk AJ, Wilkosz M, Naeije M. The Tampa Scale for Kinesiophobia for temporomandibular disorders (TSK-TMD). Pain. 2010;150:492–500.
14. Fillingim RB, Ohrbach R, Greenspan JD, Knott C, Diatchenko L, Dubner R, et al. Psychological factors associated with development of TMD: the OPPERA prospective cohort study. J Pain. 2013;14(12 Suppl):T75–90.
15. Velly AM, Look JO, Carlson C, Lenton PA, Kang W, Holcroft CA, et al. The effect of catastrophizing and depression on chronic pain—a prospective cohort study of temporomandibular muscle and joint pain disorders. Pain. 2011;152:2377–83.
16. Epker J, Gatchel RJ. Coping profile differences in the biopsychosocial functioning of patients with temporomandibular disorder. Psychosom Med. 2000;62:69–75.
17. Garofalo JP, Gatchel RJ, Wesley AL, Ellis E. Predicting chronicity in acute temporomandibular joint disorders using the research diagnostic criteria. J Am Dent Assoc. 1998;129:438–47.
18. Ohrbach R, Dworkin SF. Five-year outcomes in TMD: relationship of changes in pain to changes in physical and psychological variables. Pain. 1998;74:315–26.
19. Antonaci F, Nappi G, Galli F, Manzoni GC, Calabresi P, Costa A. Migraine and psychiatric comorbidity: a review of clinical findings. J Headache Pain. 2011;12:115–25.
20. Fornaro M, Stubbs B. A meta-analysis investigating the prevalence of moderators of migraines among people with bipolar disorder. J Affect Disord. 2015;178:88–97.
21. Lanteri-Minet M, Radat F, Chautard MH, Lucas C. Anxiety and depression associated with migraine: influence on migraine subjects' disability and quality of life, and acute migraine management. Pain. 2005;118:219–26.

22. Kim S, Park SP. The role of headache chronicity among predictors contributing to quality of life in patients with migraine: a hospital-based study. J Headache Pain. 2014;15:68.
23. Wu J, Davis-Ajami ML, Kevin Lu Z. Impact of depression on health and medical care utilization and expenses in US adults with migraine: a retrospective cross sectional study. Headache. 2016;56(7):1147–60.
24. Lipton RB. Tracing transformation: chronic migraine classification, progression, and epidemiology. Neurology. 2009;72(Suppl 5):53–7.
25. Galli R, Pozzi G, Frustaci A, Allena M, Anastasi S, Chirumbolo A, et al. Differences in the personality profile of medication-overuse headache sufferers and drug addict patients: a comparative study using MMPI-2. Headache. 2011;51(8):1212–27.
26. American College of Occupational and Environmental Medicine. Chronic pain treatment guidelines. In: Hegmann K, editor. Occupational medicine practice guidelines. 2nd ed. Beverly Farms: OEM Press; 2008.
27. White KS. Assessment and treatment of psychological causes of chest pain. Med Clin North Am. 2010,94(2):291–318.
28. Turner JA, Jensen MP, Romano JM. Do beliefs, coping, and catastrophizing independently predict functioning in patients with chronic pain? Pain. 2000;85(1–2):115–25.
29. Darnall BD, Scheman J, Davin S, Burns JW, Murphy JL, Wilson AC, et al. Pain psychology: a global needs assessment and national call to action. Pain Med. 2016;17:250–63.
30. Fordyce WE. Behavioral methods for chronic pain and illness. St. Louis: Mosby; 1976. p. 236.
31. Keefe FJ, Somers TJ, Williams DA, Smith SJ. Assessment of pain behaviors. In: Turk DC, Melzack R, editors. Handbook of pain assessment. 3rd ed. New York: Guilford Press; 2011. p. 134–50.
32. Meyer GJ, Finn SE, Eyde LD, Kay GG, Moreland KL, Dies RR, et al. Psychological testing and psychological assessment. A review of evidence and issues. Am Psychol. 2001;56(2):128–65.
33. Carragee EJ, Alamin TF, Miller JL, Carragee JM. Discographic, MRI and psychosocial determinants of low back pain disability and remission: a prospective study in subjects with benign persistent back pain. Spine J. 2005;5(1):24–35.
34. Carragee EJ, Barcohana B, Alamin T, van den Haak E. Prospective controlled study of the development of lower back pain in previously asymptomatic subjects undergoing experimental discography. Spine. 2004;29(10):1112–7.
35. Schiffman E, Ohrbach R, Truelove E, Look J, Anderson G, Goulet J-P, et al. Diagnostic criteria for temporomandibular disorders (DC/TMD) for clinical and research applications: recommendations of the International RDC/TMD Consortium Network and Orofacial Pain Special Interest Group. J Oral Facial Pain Headache. 2014;28(10):6–27.
36. Walk D, Sehgal N, Moeller-Bertram T, Edwards RR, Wasan A, Wallace M, et al. Quantitative sensory testing and mapping: a review of nonautomated quantitative methods for examination of the patient with neuropathic pain. Clin J Pain. 2009;25(7):632–40.
37. McCracken LM, Evon D, Karapas ET. Satisfaction with treatment for chronic pain in a specialty service: preliminary prospective results. Eur J Pain. 2002;6(5):387–93.
38. Jensen MP, Mendoza T, Hanna DB, Chen C, Cleeland CS. The analgesic effects that underlie patient satisfaction with treatment. Pain. 2004;110:480–7.
39. Shaw WS, Means-Christensen AJ, Slater MA, Webster JS, Patterson TL, Grant I, et al. Psychiatric disorders and risk of transition to chronicity in men with first onset low back pain. Pain Med. 2010;11:1391–400.
40. Comley AL, DeMeyer E. Assessing patient satisfaction with pain management through a continuous quality improvement effort. J Pain Symptom Manage. 2001;21(1):27–40.
41. Sullivan MD, Ballantyne JC. Must we reduce pain intensity to treat chronic pain? Pain. 2016;157(1):65–9.
42. Ballantyne JC, Sullivan MD. Intensity of chronic pain—the wrong metric? N Engl J Med. 2015;373:2098–9.

43. Warren JW, Langenberg P, Clauw DJ. The number of existing functional somatic syndromes (FSSs) is an important risk factor for new, different FSSs. J Psychosom Res. 2013;74(1):12–7.
44. Suvinen TI, Kemppainen P, Le Bell Y, Kauko T, Forssell H. Assessment of pain drawings and self-reported comorbid pains as part of the biopsychosocial profiling of temporomandibular disorder pain patients. J Oral Facial Pain Headache. 2016;30(4):287–95.
45. Hawkins JM, Schmidt JE, Hargitai IA, Johnson JF, Howard RS, Bertrand PM. Multimodal assessment of body pain in orofacial pain patients. Pain Med. 2016;17(5):961–9.
46. Williams DA. The importance of psychological assessment in chronic pain. Curr Opin Urol. 2013;23(6):554–9.
47. Melzack R. The McGill pain questionnaire: major properties and scoring methods. Pain. 1975;1:277–99.
48. Mongini F, Deregibus A, Raviola F, Mongini T. Confirmation of the distinction between chronic migraine and chronic tension-type headache by the McGill pain questionnaire. Headache. 2003;43(8):867–77.
49. Melzack R, Terrence C, Fromm G, Amsel R. Trigeminal neuralgia and atypical facial pain: use of the McGill Pain Questionnaire for discrimination and diagnosis. Pain. 1986;27:297–302.
50. Turk DC, Dworkin RH, McDermott MP, Bellamy N, Burke LB, Chandler JM, et al. Analyzing multiple endpoints in clinical trials of pain treatments: IMMPACT recommendations. Pain. 2008;139:485–93.
51. Ware JE Jr, Sherbourne CD. The MOS 36-item short-form health survey (SF-36). I. Conceptual framework and item selection. Med Care. 1992;30(6):473–83.
52. Bergner M, Bobbitt RA, Carter WB, Gilson BS. The sickness impact profile: development and final revision of a health status measure. Med Care. 1981;19:787–805.
53. Pollard CA. Preliminary validity study of the pain disability index. Percept Mot Skills. 1984;59:974.
54. Fairbank JC, Pynsent PB. The Oswestry disability index. Spine. 2000;25(22):2940–52.
55. Stewart WF, Lipton RB, Dowson AJ, Sawyer J. Development and testing of the migraine disability assessment (MIDAS) questionnaire to assess headache-related disability. Neurology. 2001;56(6 Suppl 1):S20–8.
56. Kosinski M, Bayliss MS, Bjorner JB, Ware JE Jr, Garber WH, Batenhorst A, et al. A six-item short-form survey for measuring headache impact: the HIT-6. Qual Life Res. 2003;12:963–74.
57. Jhingran P, Osterhaus JT, Miller DW, Lee JT, Kirchdoerfer L. Development and validation of the migraine-specific quality of life questionnaire. Headache. 1998;38:295–302.
58. Martin BC, Pathak DS, Sharfman MI, Adelman JU, Taylor F, Kwong WJ, et al. Validity and reliability of the migraine-specific quality of life questionnaire (MSQ Version 2.1). Headache. 2000;40:204–15.
59. Ohrbach R, Larsson P, List T. The jaw functional limitation scale: development, reliability, and validity of 8-item and 20-item versions. J Orofac Pain. 2008;22(3):219–30.
60. Stegenga B, de Bont LGM, de Leeuw R, Boering G. Assessment of mandibular function impairment associated with temporomandibular joint osteoarthrosis and internal derangement. J Orofac Pain. 1993;7:183–95.
61. Slade GD, Spencer AJ. Development and evaluation of the Oral Health Impact Profile. Community Dent Health. 1994;11(1):3–11.
62. Slade GD. Derivation and validation of a short-form oral health impact profile. Community Dent Oral Epidemiol. 1997;25:284–90.
63. American Psychiatric Association. Diagnostic and statistical manual of mental disorders. 5th ed. Washington, DC: Author; 2013.
64. Nicholson RA, Houle TT, Rhudy JL, Norton PJ. Psychological risk factors in headache. Headache. 2007;47(3):413–26.
65. Beck AT, Steer RA, Garbin MG. Psychometric properties of the Beck Depression Inventory: twenty-five years of evaluation. Clin Psychol Rev. 1998;8:77–100.
66. Radloff LS. The CES-D scale: a self-report depression scale for research in the general population. Appl Psychol Meas. 1997;1:385–401.

67. Williams AC, Richardson PH. What does the BDI measure in chronic pain? Pain. 1993;55(2):259–66.
68. Geisser ME, Roth RS, Robinson ME. Assessing depression among persons with chronic pain using the Center for Epidemiological Studies-Depression Scale and the Beck Depression Inventory: a comparative analysis. Clin J Pain. 1997;13:163–70.
69. Kroenke K, Spitzer RL, Williams JB. The PHQ-9: validity of a brief depression severity measure. J Gen Intern Med. 2001;16:606–13.
70. Seo JG, Park SP. Validation of the patient health questionnaire-9 (PHQ-9) and PHQ-2 in patients with migraine. J Headache Pain. 2015;16:65–72.
71. Spitzer RL, Kroenke K, Williams JB, Lowe B. A brief measure for assessing generalized anxiety disorder: the GAD-7. Arch Intern Med. 2006;166:1092–7.
72. Seo JG, Park SP. Validation of the generalized anxiety disorder-7 (GAD-7) and GAD-2 in patients with migraine. J Headache Pain. 2015;16:97.
73. McCracken L, Dhingra L. A short version of the Pain Anxiety Symptoms Scale (PASS-20): preliminary development and validity. Pain Res Manag. 2002;7(1):45–50.
74. Suhr JA, Spickard B. Pain-related fear is associated with cognitive task avoidance: exploration of the cogniphobia construct in a recurrent headache sample. Clin Neuropsychol. 2012;26(7):1128–41.
75. Seng EK, Klepper JE. Development of the cogniphobia scale for headache disorders (CS-HD): a pilot study. Psychol Assess. 2017;29(10):1296–301. https://doi.org/10.1037/pas0000432.
76. Okifuji A, Turk DC, Curran SL. Anger in chronic pain: investigations of anger targets and intensity. J Psychosom Res. 1999;47:1–12.
77. Bruehl S, Burns JW, Chung OY, Chont M. Pain-related effects of trait anger expression: neural substrates and the role of endogenous opioid mechanisms. Neurosci Biobehav Rev. 2009;33:475–91.
78. Trost Z, Vangronsveld K, Linton SJ, Quartana PJ, Sullivan MJ. Cognitive dimensions of anger in chronic pain. Pain. 2012;153(3):515–7.
79. Spielberger CD. State-trait anger expression inventory, professional manual. Odessa: Psychological Assessment Resources; 1988.
80. Brown M, Dean S, Hay-Smith EJ, Taylor W, Baxter GD. Musculoskeletal pain and treatment choice: an exploration of illness perceptions and choices of conventional or complementary therapies. Disabil Rehabil. 2010;32(20):1645–57.
81. Gross DP, Deshpande S, Werner EL, Reneman MF, Miciak MA, Buchbinder R. Fostering change in back pain beliefs and behaviors: when public education is not enough. Spine J. 2012;12(11):979–88.
82. Thompson E, Broadbent J, Bertino MD, Staiger PK. Do pain-related beliefs influence adherence to multidisciplinary rehabilitation? A systematic review. Clin J Pain. 2016;32(2):164–78.
83. Seng EK, Buse DC, Klepper JE, Mayson SJ, Grinberg AS, Grosberg BM, et al. Psychological factors associated with chronic migraine and severe migraine-related disability: an observational study in a tertiary headache center. Headache. 2017;57(4):593–604. https://doi.org/10.1111/head.13021.
84. Jensen MP, Karoly P, Huger R. The development and preliminary validation of an instrument to assess patients' attitudes toward pain. J Psychosom Res. 1987;31(3):393–400.
85. Romano JM, Jensen MP, Turner JA. The chronic pain coping inventory-42: reliability and validity. Pain. 2003;104(1–2):65–73.
86. Rosenstiel AK, Keefe FJ. The use of coping strategies in chronic low back pain patients: relationship to patient characteristics and current adjustment. Pain. 1983;17:33–44.
87. Nicholas MK. The pain self-efficacy questionnaire: taking pain into account. Eur J Pain. 2007;11:153–63.
88. Nicholas MK, McGuire BE, Asghari A. A 2-item short form of the pain self-efficacy questionnaire: development and psychometric evaluation of PSEQ-2. J Pain. 2015;16(2):153–63.
89. McCracken LM, Vowles KE, Eccleston C. Acceptance of chronic pain: component analysis and a revised assessment method. Pain. 2004;107:159–66.

90. Skevington SM. A standardised scale to measure beliefs about controlling pain (BPCQ): a preliminary study. Psychol Health. 1990;4:221–32.
91. Martin NJ, Holroyd KA, Penzien DB. The headache-specific locus of control scale: adaptation to recurrent headaches. Headache. 1990;30(11):729–34.
92. Sullivan MJL, Bishop S, Pivik J. The pain catastrophizing scale: development and validation. Psychol Assess. 1995;7:524–32.
93. Severejins R, Vlaeyen JWS, van den Hout MA, Weber W. Pain catastrophizing predicts pain intensity, disability, and psychological distress independent of the level of physical impairment. Clin J Pain. 2001;17:165–72.
94. Burton AK, Tillotson KM, Main CJ, Hollis S. Psychosocial predictors of outcome in acute and subchronic low back trouble. Spine. 1995;20(6):722–8.
95. Butcher JN, Graham JR, Tellegen A, Kaemmer B. Manual for the restandardized Minnesota Multiphasic Personality Inventory: MMPI-2. Minneapolis: University of Minnesota Press; 1989.
96. Ben-Porath YS, Tellegen A. Minnesota Multiphasic Personality Inventory-2 Restructured Form: MMPI-2-RF. NCS Pearson, Incorporated; 2008.
97. Ziegler DK, Paolo AM. Headache symptoms and psychological profile of headache-prone individuals. A comparison of clinic patients and controls. Arch Neurol. 1995;52(6):602–6.
98. Manfredini D, Cerea S, Pavan C, Guarda-Nardini L. Personality traits are potentially associated with the presence of chronic temporomandibular joint pain in patients without effusion as determined by T-2 weighted magnetic resonance. Cranio. 2017;20:1–7.
99. Millon T, Antoni M, Millon C, Minor S, Grossman S. Millon behavioral medicine diagnostic. Minneapolis: National Computer Systems; 2006.
100. Bruns D, Disorbio JM. Assessment of biopsychosocial risk factors for medical treatment: a collaborative approach. J Clin Psychol Med Settings. 2009;16(2):127–47.
101. Block C, Cianfrini L. Neuropsychological and neuroanatomical sequelae of chronic non-malignant pain and opioid analgesia. NeuroRehabilitation. 2013;33(2):343–66.
102. Moriarty O, McGuire BE, Finn DP. The effect of pain on cognitive function: a review of clinical and preclinical research. Prog Neurobiol. 2011;93(3):385–404.
103. Randolph C, Tierney MC, Mohr E, Chase TN. The Repeatable Battery for the Assessment of Neuropsychological Status (RBANS): preliminary clinical validity. J Clin Exp Neuropsychol. 1993;20(3):310–9.
104. Folstein M, Folstein SE, McHugh PR. "Mini-mental state" a practical method for grading the cognitive state of patients for the clinician. J Psychiatr Res. 1975;12(3):189–98.
105. Seidenberg M, Haltiner A, Taylor MA, Hermann BB, Wyler A. Development and validation of a Multiple Ability Self-Report Questionnaire. J Clin Exp Neuropsychol. 1994;16(1):93–104.
106. Almoznino G, Benoliel R, Sharav Y, Haviv Y. Sleep disorders and chronic craniofacial pain: characteristics and management possibilities. Sleep Med Rev. 2017;33:39–50. https://doi.org/10.1016/j.smrv.2016.04.005.
107. Alsaadi SM, McAuley JH, Hush JM, Lo S, Bartlett DJ, Grunstein RR, et al. The bidirectional relationship between pain intensity and sleep disturbance/quality in patients with low back pain. Clin J Pain. 2014;30(9):755–65.
108. Sommer I, Lavigne G, Ettlin DA. Review of self-reported instruments that measure sleep dysfunction in patients suffering from temporomandibular disorders and/or orofacial joints. Sleep Med. 2015;16(1):27–38.
109. Johns MW. A new method for measuring daytime sleepiness: the Epworth Sleepiness Scale. Sleep. 1991;14:540–5.
110. Buysse DJ, Reynolds CF 3rd, Monk TH, Berman SR, Kupfer DJ. The Pittsburgh Sleep Quality Index: a new instrument for psychiatric practice and research. Psychiatry Res. 1989;28(2):193–213.
111. Sivertsen B, Lallukka T, Petrie KJ, Steingrimsdottir OA, Stubhaug A, Nielsen CS. Sleep and pain sensitivity in adults. Pain. 2015;156(8):1433–9.
112. Gass JJ, Glaros AG. Autonomic dysregulation in headache patients. Appl Psychophysiol Biofeedback. 2013;38(4):257–63.

113. Crider AB, Glaros AG. A meta-analysis of EMG biofeedback treatment of temporomandibular disorders. J Orofac Pain. 1999;13(1):29–37.
114. Chou R, Fanciullo GJ, Fine PG, Adler JA, Ballantyne JC, Davies P, et al. Clinical guidelines for the use of chronic opioid therapy in chronic noncancer pain. J Pain. 2009;10(2):113–30.
115. Moore TM, Jones T, Browder JH, Daffron S, Passik SD. A comparison of common screening methods for predicting aberrant drug-related behavior among patients receiving opioids for chronic pain management. Pain Med. 2009;10(8):1426–33.
116. Ewing JA. Detecting alcoholism: the CAGE questionnaire. JAMA. 1989;252:1905–7.
117. Skinner HA. The drug abuse screening test. Addict Behav. 1982;7(4):363–71.
118. Webster LR. Predicting aberrant behaviors in opioid-treated patients: preliminary validation of the opioid risk tool. Pain Med. 2005;6(6):432–42.
119. Butler SF, Fernandez K, Benoit C, Budman SH, Jamison RN. Validation of the revised screener and opioid assessment for patients in pain (SOAPPR). J Pain. 2008;9:360–72.
120. Butler SF, et al. Development and validation of the Current Opioid Misuse Measure. Pain. 2007;130(1–2):144–56.
121. Bass C, Halligan PW. Factitious disorders and malingering: challenges for clinical assessment and management. Lancet. 2014;383(9926):1422–32.
122. Bianchini KJ, Aguerrevere LE, Guise BJ, Ord JS, Etherton JL, Meyers JE, et al. Accuracy of the Modified Somatic Perception Questionnaire and Pain Disability Index in the detection of malingered pain-related disability in chronic pain. Clin Neuropsychol. 2014;28(8):1376–94.

Chapter 8
Diagnosis of Orofacial Pain of Dental Origin

John K. Jones

As is the case when evaluating other types of pain, the diagnosis of orofacial pain of dental origin requires a thorough and systematic approach. This includes establishing a chief complaint and history of the present illness, a review of past medical history, a history of any past interventions regarding the chief complaint, a physical examination, appropriate imaging and diagnostic testing (to include diagnostic local anesthesia blocks), and psychosocial evaluation. Oral hard tissues (teeth and bone) and oral soft tissue (gingiva and mucosa) can be sources of pain. Orofacial pain can be further categorized as odontogenic or non-odontogenic. Odontogenic pain is so prevalent that orofacial pain of dental origin should be presumed odontogenic in nature until ruled out. By far toothache or odontalgia represents the vast majority of orofacial pain complaints. Epidemiologic studies have revealed an incidence of 12–14% of the population reporting a toothache over the past 6 months [1]. A recent study of the burden of dental complaints on a level 1 hospital emergency department found an incidence of 4.3% [2]. Given the prevalence of odontalgia as a contributor to orofacial pain, it is important that the evaluation of orofacial pain includes early evaluation by a dental professional.

Odontogenic Dental Pain

Teeth are visceral components that function as part of the musculoskeletal system. Their attachment is called the periodontal ligament and is part of the musculoskeletal system. This is an important distinction when evaluating odontogenic pain.

J. K. Jones
Department of Otolaryngology/Head and Neck Surgery/Oral and Maxillofacial Surgery, University of Arkansas for Medical Sciences, Little Rock, AR, USA
e-mail: jjones353f@uams.edu

J. Y. Suen, E. Petersen (eds.), *Diagnosis and Management of Head and Face Pain*, https://doi.org/10.1007/978-3-319-90999-8_8

Being a visceral component, teeth exhibit a threshold painful response to noxious stimuli. Periodontal disorders manifest more as musculoskeletal pain and thus exhibit a graduated response. Of course odontogenic pain can be a combination of the two. It is this uniqueness that leads to the extreme variability in the nature of symptoms related to odontogenic sources of pain. There are fortunately "typical" presentations, and unlike many other orofacial pain entities, there are many times clinical and radiographic findings as well as diagnostic testing findings can confirm or rule out teeth and supporting structures as sources of pain.

Tooth Anatomy

Topographically teeth consist of a crown or coronal portion and a root or radicular portion. The crown and root are comprised of four distinct components (Fig. 8.1). Dentin and the dental pulp are present in the coronal and radicular elements. Enamel is the outermost layer of the crown and is insensate. Beneath the enamel lies the dentin which is comprised of tubules that radiate from the dental pulp and terminate at the dentin-enamel (crown) and dentin- cementum (root) junction. The dentin is sensate. The tubules are patent and thus fluid movement is possible as well as potential contamination of the dental pulp. The dental pulp is neurovascular tissue providing vitality to the tooth. The pulp is innervated by myelinated (A gamma) and unmyelinated (C) fibers from the trigeminal nerve. It is the pulp that is the source of

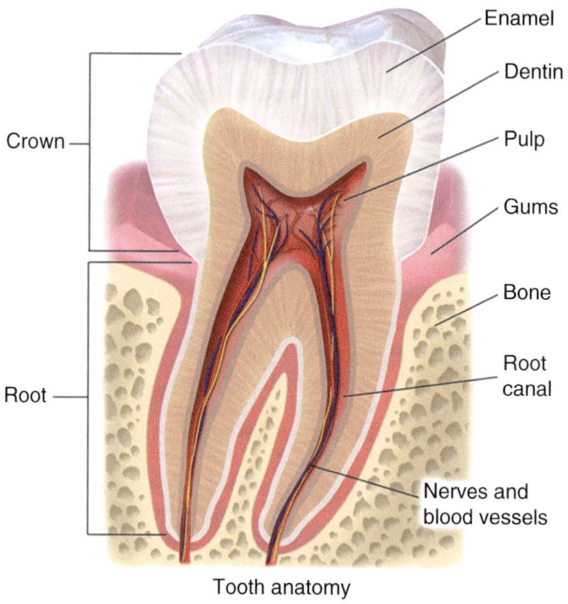

Fig. 8.1 Tooth anatomy. "Medical gallery of Blausen Medical 2014". *Wiki Journal of Medicine* **1** (2). DOI:10.15347/wjm/2014.010. ISSN 2002-4436

visceral pain when affected by contamination (caries), trauma, erosion, abrasion, or iatrogenic injury [3].

Pulpitis

Noxious stimulation of the pulp results in a visceral pain response. It is a threshold-mediated response and not necessarily easy to localize without physical, diagnostic, and radiographic findings. One of the hallmarks of pulpal pain is that it does not stay the same over time [4]. It is the end result of pulpal stimulation as a consequence of dentinal exposure. Pulpal pain or pulpitis is generally classified as reversible or irreversible. Reversible pulpitis resolves with removal of the noxious stimulus. Irreversible pulpitis results in pulpal necrosis. Because pulpitis symptoms are visceral in nature, percussion of the teeth is not useful for localization. Pain to percussion generally means that the periodontal structures are involved.

Reversible pulpitis is characterized by pain upon mechanical or thermal stimulation that is acute and sharp but that dissipates without lingering aching or discomfort. Irreversible pulpitis is characterized by the same symptoms at onset but followed by lingering and aching discomfort. Pulpitis does not result in radiographic changes to assist in diagnosis. Pulpitis can be detected and localized by thermal testing with hot and cold stimuli. Irreversible pulpitis results in pulpal necrosis. At this point the pulp becomes insensate and the pain becomes more musculoskeletal in nature due to involvement of the periodontal structures. Pain associated with pulpitis can be resolved by appropriate local anesthesia block or infiltration. Appropriate diagnostic use of local anesthesia can be very helpful regarding localization and inclusion/exclusion with regard to differential diagnosis.

Periodontitis

The musculoskeletal pain associated with involvement of the periodontal ligament can be localized by percussion of the involved tooth and with dental imaging. The typical findings on imaging are that of a widened periodontal ligament space and a later finding of a periapical radiolucency as a result of sterile abscess formation due to pulpal necrosis. It is the secondary bacterial contamination of this necrotic debris that leads to odontogenic abscess formation. Apical periodontitis can be classified as acute or chronic. Acute apical periodontitis is characterized by radiographic findings of periodontal ligament space widening at the apex or a periapical radiolucency associated with a tooth that exhibits throbbing, aching discomfort with pain elicited upon percussion, or movement of the tooth. Tooth mobility may also be present. Chronic apical periodontitis shares the same radiographic findings but is generally painless. Transition from acute apical periodontitis to chronic apical periodontitis and vice versa is possible. Periodontitis in the absence of pulpal necrosis can manifest with mild, episodic, or dull pain [3]. This is a graduated musculoskeletal type of pain response to inflammation within the periodontal tissues. Clinical signs of periodontitis are found in gingiva and include erythema, edema, recession, tooth mobility, and purulence emanating from the gingival sulcus.

Non-odontogenic Dental Pain

Non-odontogenic dental pain is much less common than odontogenic pain, thus the recommendation to first rule out odontogenic pain. It is varied in etiology and presentation and typically more difficult to accurately diagnose due to a relative lack of helpful diagnostic imaging and diagnostic testing. This pain can be due to inflammatory, infectious, systemic, neoplastic, autoimmune, and neuropathic conditions. It can be referred pain as well. As an example one widely known referral pattern is that of anginal pain manifesting as jaw pain. Some of the more common sources of non-odontogenic dental pain will be presented in this chapter.

Maxillary Sinusitis

Maxillary sinusitis frequently manifests as pain in the maxillary posterior dentition on the involved side(s). This is due to the proximity of the root apices to the sinus floor and the very thin osseous partition separating the apex and the floor of the sinus. The pain is musculoskeletal in nature. Typically multiple teeth are involved and are painful to percussion despite normal vitality testing and lack of periapical findings on dental radiographs. Fluid or sinus membrane edema may be seen on dental radiology. The pain in the teeth will resolve with resolution of the sinusitis. Just as importantly teeth can be the cause of maxillary sinusitis. This should be suspected especially when the sinusitis is unilateral and refractory to typical medical or surgical management. The contamination of the sinus is the end result of apical periodontitis that erodes the thin osseous partition at the root apex.

Temporomandibular Disorders

Temporomandibular pain complaints are quite common and can present a diagnostic challenge to the practitioner tasked with evaluating and treating orofacial pain. In one survey the prevalence was found to be 6% of the adult population. A complaint of preauricular pain accounted for another 6%. The prevalence is 1.5 times higher in women than in men, and greatest risk of onset of complaints is between the ages of 18 and 44 [5]. The anatomy and function of the temporomandibular is unique as an articulation. It is orthopedically classified as a ginglymoarthrodial joint exhibiting both hinge and gliding functions. It has two separate synovial spaces (inferior and superior) which are separated by the temporomandibular joint meniscus which is fibrous rather than cartilaginous. With its very significant gliding range of motion (translation), it is by orthopedic standards a very loose articulation. As such it has a very complex proprioceptive and positioning/movement system. Function is reliant on stability of the contralateral joint as well as the occlusion. While occlusion is thought to contribute to the relative risk for TMD symptomatology, many other contributing factors have been identified. Other identified factors are biologic, psychiatric, environmental, and cognitive [6].

Careful history taking is paramount in evaluating possible temporomandibular disorders. Associated symptomatology can make diagnosis challenging. Common associated symptoms are headache, ear fullness and tinnitus, and muscular, cervical, and orbital pain. A history of previous trauma as well as a history of parafunctional habits such as clenching or bruxism can raise suspicion. Clinical examination should include palpation of the muscles of mastication, auscultation of the TMJs, inspection of the dentition and occlusion, otologic examination, and recording of range of motion in protrusion, lateral excursions, and maximal opening.

Temporomandibular complaints are typically classified as articular and extra-articular (myofascial) or both. Both exhibit a graduated response typical of musculoskeletal pain. Typical findings of intraarticular derangement are preauricular pain to palpation on one or both sides, noise, and limited range of motion. Noise is typically classified as clicks that occur with joint translation indicating meniscal mobility problems or crepitus which is indicative of synovitis and/or degeneration. Intra-articular problems are best diagnosed on physical examination and can be imaged with TMJ arthrography or with magnetic resonance imaging. Degenerative changes can be detected by auscultation and confirmed with high resolution radiography or CT scanning.

Myofascial TMD Pain

Myofascial pain is classically described as a deep dull aching muscle pain that results in referral of the pain to the teeth. It is associated with trigger points in the muscle that when active can be identified within the muscle by careful evaluation via palpation. Three masticatory muscles have been found to refer pain to the teeth with patterns of referral having been identified [4]. The superior belly of the masseter refers pain to the maxillary posterior teeth. The inferior belly of the masseter refers pain to the mandibular posterior teeth. The anterior digastric muscle refers pain to the mandibular anterior teeth, and the temporalis muscle refers pain to the maxillary anterior or posterior teeth. The temporalis muscle and temporomandibular joint frequently refer pain to the teeth. Referred myofascial pain has characteristics, the presence of which should raise clinical suspicion. It is musculoskeletal in nature as a dull, aching, non-relenting pain when the trigger point is active. The involved teeth are found to be free of pulpal or periodontal disease. The pain is not altered by testing of the involved teeth. Painful trigger points are palpable in the muscles of mastication. The stimulation of the trigger point increases the tooth pain. The pain does not resolve with local anesthesia blockade of the teeth but does resolve with local anesthesia infiltration of the trigger point [5].

Neuropathic Pain

Neuropathic pain arises in neural tissue making the nerve itself the source of the pain. It is usually a diagnosis of exclusion. The most common neuropathic pain of dental origin is trigeminal neuralgia (also known as Tic Douloureux). It can present in many forms, but the classic form involves severe, lancinating, electric type pain localized to areas innervated by the trigeminal nerve. The mandibular branch is most commonly involved but maxillary branch involvement is possible also. It is characterized by having a trigger spot that when stimulated results in pain. The pain is out of proportion to the magnitude of stimulation. The trigger spot can be refractory temporarily. The teeth in the area of pain are found to be free of pulpal or periodontal disease. Local anesthesia block of the painful teeth does not eliminate the pain (except in rare cases when the tooth is the trigger). The trigger can be inactivated by local anesthesia block rendering the patient pain free for the duration of the action of the local anesthesia [7].

Mucosal Diseases

Mucosal diseases can be sources of non-odontogenic pain. They can be isolated to the oral cavity or be manifestations of systemic conditions that affect other mucous membranes. They can be infectious, inflammatory, or autoimmune in nature. Some examples are lichen planus, benign mucous membrane pemphigoid, pemphigus vulgaris, monoliasis, herpetic gingivostomatitis, benign migratory glossitis, and major aphthae. Typically there are physical examination findings of erythema, edema, leukoplakia, vesicle formation, ulceration, or necrosis that lead to the generation of a differential diagnosis. The pain results from the loss of epithelial protection (ulceration) and inflammation. Incisional and excisional biopsy can be necessary to establish a definitive diagnosis and direct therapeutic efforts.

Burning Mouth Syndrome

Burning mouth syndrome is idiopathic and thus a diagnosis of exclusion. The hallmark symptomatology is an intraoral burning sensation that is present despite the absence of clinical signs of injury or pathology. The pain may be restricted to the tongue and may be associated with dysesthesia, taste alteration, and a sensation of xerostomia [8]. Burning mouth syndrome disproportionately affects postmenopausal women [9]. Spontaneous improvement can be seen in 30–50% of cases [10]. The diagnostic criteria are oral pain recurring daily for more than 2 h per day for greater than 3 months. The pain is of a burning quality and is perceived superficially in the oral mucosa. Oral mucosa is of normal appearance and clinical examination including neurosensory testing is normal [8]. It is important to rule out mucosal diseases, xerostomia, nutritional deficiencies, and allergic stomatitis.

References

1. Lipton JA, Ship JA, Larach-Robinson D. Estimated prevalence and distribution of reported orofacial pain in the United States. J Am Dent Assoc. 1993;124:115–21.
2. McCormick AP, Abubaker AO, Laskin DM, et al. Reducing the burden of dental patients on the busy hospital emergency department. J Oral Maxillofac Surg. 2013;71:475–8.
3. Edens MH, Khaled Y, Napenas JJ. Intraoral pain disorders. Oral Maxillofac Surg Clin North Am. 2016;28:275–88.
4. Okeson JP. Bell's oral and facial pain. 7th ed. Chicago: Quintessence Publishing; 2014.
5. Macfarlane TV, Blinkhorn AS, Davies RM, et al. Oro-facial pain in the community: prevalence and associated impact. Community Dent Oral Epidemiol. 2002;30:52.
6. Solberg WK. Epidemiology, incidence and prevalence of temporomandibular disorders: a review. In: The President's Conference on the Examination, Diagnosis and Management of Temporomandibular Disorders. Chicago: American Dental Association; 1983. p. 30.
7. Simons DG, Travell JG, Simons LS. Travell and Simons' myofascial pain and dysfunction: a trigger point manual. 2nd ed. Baltimore: Williams and Wilkins; 1999.
8. Headache Classification Committee of the International Headache Society (IHS). The International Classification of Headache Disorders, 3rd edition (beta version). Cephalalgia. 2013;33:629.
9. Kohorst JJ, Bruce AJ, Torgerson RR, et al. A population-based study of the incidence of burning mouth syndrome. Mayo Clin Proc. 2014;89:1545.
10. Cranial neuralgias and central causes of facial pain. In: Lance JW, Goadsby PJ, editors. Mechanism and management of headache. Philadelphia: Elsevier Butterworth Heinemann; 2005. p. 333.

Chapter 9
Diagnostic Nerve Blocks

James Y. Suen and Chelsey Smith

Introduction

We feel most headaches and facial pain are related to the nerves that innervate the head and face. ***Diagnostic nerve blocks are one of the most important tools for the diagnosis and treatment of facial and head pain!*** When obtaining a history from the patient, it is critical to listen to the patient describe his or her pain. Especially important is where the pain starts and where, if any, the "trigger points" are [1]. As the examiner listens, he or she should think of the nerve innervation to those trigger points. It is common to find that if an isolated nerve off the trigeminal nerve triggers the pain, then other branches can begin to hurt. **Knowledge of the anatomy and nerve innervation is critical.**

Nerve blocks are an efficient, inexpensive, and low risk tool to diagnose peripheral trigeminal neuralgia. This is usually performed on the first clinic visit with a new patient and can provide important information. If done properly, it may also treat the pain for varying periods of time.

J. Y. Suen (✉)
Department of Otolaryngology—Head and Neck Surgery,
University of Arkansas for Medical Sciences, Little Rock, AR, USA
e-mail: suenjamesy@uams.edu

C. Smith
ENTcare, Dothan, AL, USA
e-mail: chelseyjsmith5@gmail.com

J. Y. Suen, E. Petersen (eds.), *Diagnosis and Management of Head and Face Pain*, https://doi.org/10.1007/978-3-319-90999-8_9

Applied Anatomy

The nerve supply to the face and head is from the trigeminal nerve, the greater occipital nerve, and the upper cervical plexus nerves. Knowing the anatomy and the nerve innervation to the face and head is the key to proper diagnosis and treatment of facial and head pain.

Trigeminal Nerve

The classic Type I, trigeminal neuritis is due to an artery adjacent to the takeoff of the trigeminal nerve from the brainstem and pulsating against the nerve. The underlying causes of atypical trigeminal neuritis have not been clearly defined, but we feel there are a number of etiologies for what we term "*peripheral trigeminal neuritis*." Some known common causes are herpes zoster and trauma with neuromas or entrapment of the nerve branch. More recently it is postulated that compression of the peripheral nerves at various points, such as, in a foramen, a tight notch, or through fascia can result in nerve pain and headaches [1–6]. In addition, ***we feel that there is a high likelihood that arteries which accompany these nerves can pulsate against peripheral nerves resulting in pain similar to the Type I trigeminal neuritis***.

The three divisions of the trigeminal nerve, commonly referred to as V1, V2, and V3, converge at the ganglion in Meckel's cave. It is important to know the branches of each of these three divisions and where they innervate the face and head (Fig. 9.1).

The first division, V1, is the ophthalmic nerve. It enters the orbit through the superior orbital fissure and has several nerves to eye structures and to the internal upper nose before branching into the *infratrochlear nerve* and the frontal nerve. The frontal nerve is the largest branch of V1, dividing into the supraorbital and supratrochlear branches as it exits the orbit (Fig. 9.2). *The supraorbital nerve* exits the orbit through the supraorbital notch or foramen, and it supplies the upper eyelid and the ipsilateral forehead to the vertex of the scalp. The notch or foramen can be a place where the supraorbital nerve can be compressed. A notch occurs about 83% of the time and is usually encircled by a ligamentous fascial band which encircles the nerve [7]. The *supratrochlear nerve* exits at the superior medial part of the orbit near the bridge of the nose and supplies the skin of the forehead near the midline. *Pain in V1 can be in the eyelid, the forehead, or the top of the head and can trigger headaches, commonly diagnosed as migraine headaches.*

The *infratrochlear nerve* supplies the skin over the bridge of the nose and the medial part of the lower eyelid.

The second division, V2, is called the maxillary branch, and it is primarily sensory in function. It is more complex and takes more study to understand the innervation and where pain from V2 can elicit. The main nerve of V2 is the *infraorbital nerve*, which goes in a groove in the floor of the orbit and exits through the

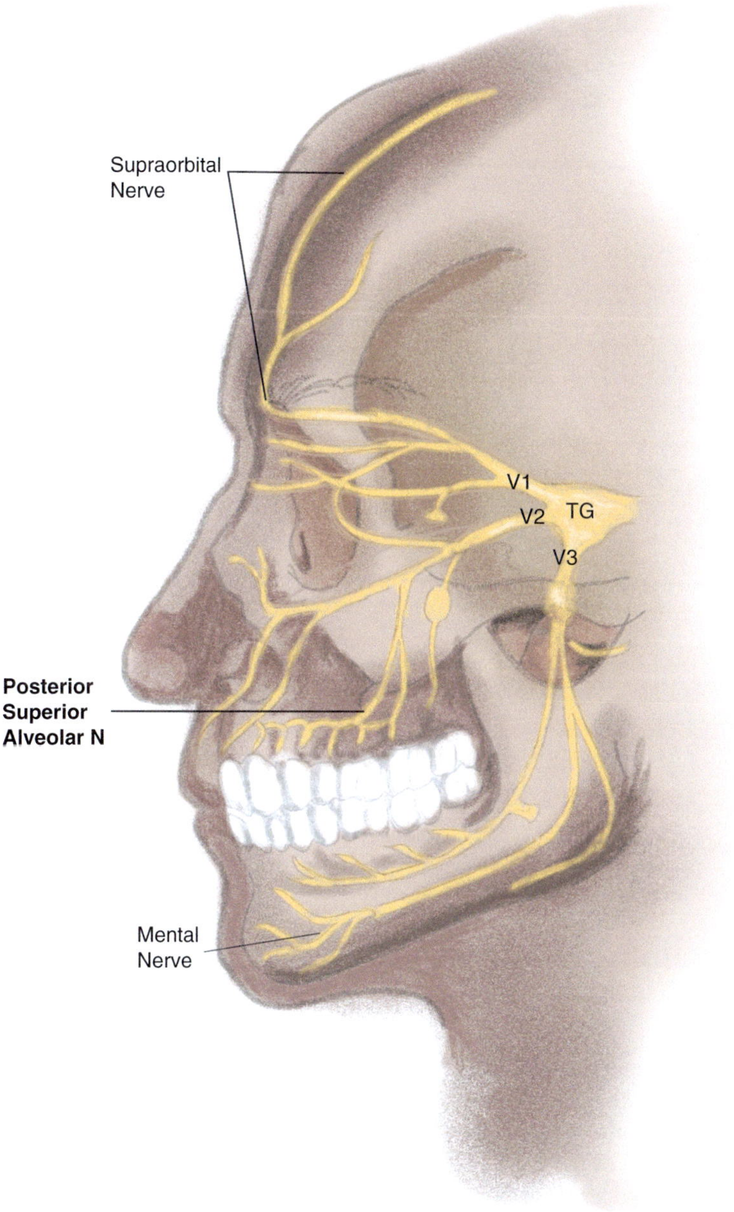

Fig. 9.1 Trigeminal nerve ganglion with the three divisions supplying the face

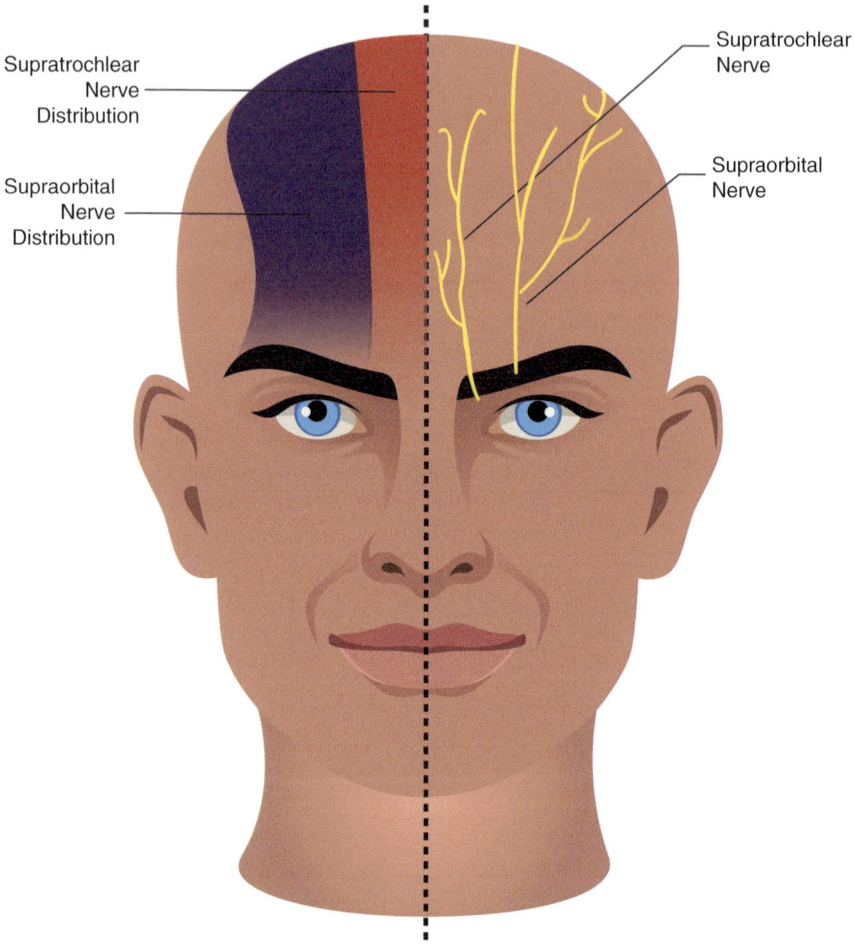

Fig. 9.2 Terminal branches of the frontal branch—supraorbital and supratrochlear nerves supplying the forehead

infraorbital foramen and supplies the midface. There are two other branches of this nerve that are important to know. One is the *posterior superior alveolar nerve* which comes off the V2 after it exits the foramen rotundum and wraps around the posterior-lateral wall of the maxilla where it enters the underlying bone and innervates the posterior upper teeth (Fig. 9.1). It is common for pain in this nerve to be diagnosed as dental pain and result in extractions with no pain relief.

The second important branch is the *zygomatico-temporal nerve* (ZTN) which leaves the infraorbital nerve in the floor of the orbit and goes into the zygoma bone and exits just lateral to or through the bone of the lateral orbital rim and goes to the anterior temporalis muscle area (Fig. 9.3). The foramen where the ZTN exits the

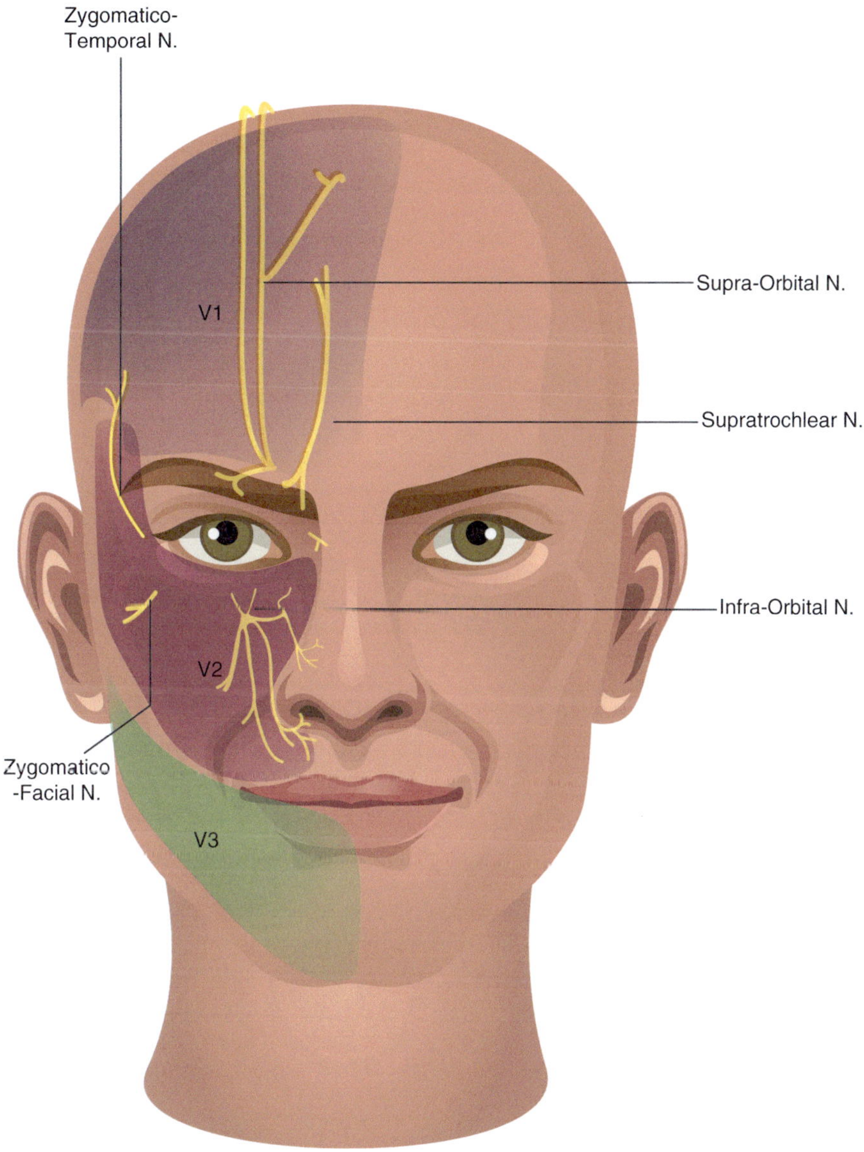

Fig. 9.3 Infraorbital nerve and the zygomaticotemporal nerve branch innervating anterior temporalis muscle area

zygoma is about 7 mm lateral to the lateral orbital rim and about 8 mm cranial to the lateral canthus [7]. It goes into the temporalis muscle or just superficial to it. Sometimes the ZTN comes out just lateral to the lateral orbital rim. *Pain in this nerve is quite common and can cause temporal headaches which are commonly called migraine headaches.*

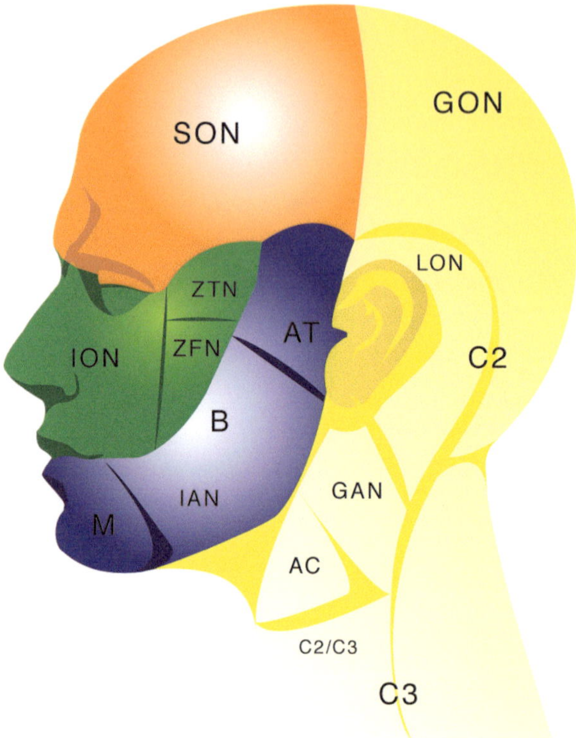

Fig. 9.4 The green shaded area is the innervation of the midface by the second division of the trigeminal nerve. ZTN is the area innervated by the zygomatico-temporal nerve branch. The purple shaded area is the innervation by the mandibular division and the AT area is supplied by the auriculotemporal nerve branch

The third division, V3, the mandibular branch (Fig. 9.1), has both sensory and motor function. The motor part supplies the muscles of mastication. The sensory branches go to three main areas: the lingual nerve, the inferior alveolar nerve, and the auriculotemporal nerve. The *lingual nerve* goes to the tongue. The *inferior alveolar nerve* goes into the mandible in the ascending ramus and supplies the lower jaw teeth, then exits the mental foramen to supply the chin and lower lip. The third branch is the *auriculotemporal nerve*, which exits just posterior to the mandibular condyle and goes superiorly to the area of the temple and above the ear (Fig. 9.4). Pain can occur in one or all of these branches. We feel the auriculotemporal nerve can also trigger migraine headaches [1].

Greater Occipital Nerve

This nerve arises from the dorsal roots of C2 off of the spinal cord and goes through the posterior neck muscles and fascia, emerging 3 cm below the occipital protuberance and about 2–3 cm lateral from the midline of the occiput and the going superiorly to the top of the scalp (Fig. 9.5) [8]. Occipital headaches are common, and most arise from the greater occipital nerve. ***There is a connection between the trigeminal nerves and the occipital nerves which is referred to as the trigeminocervical***

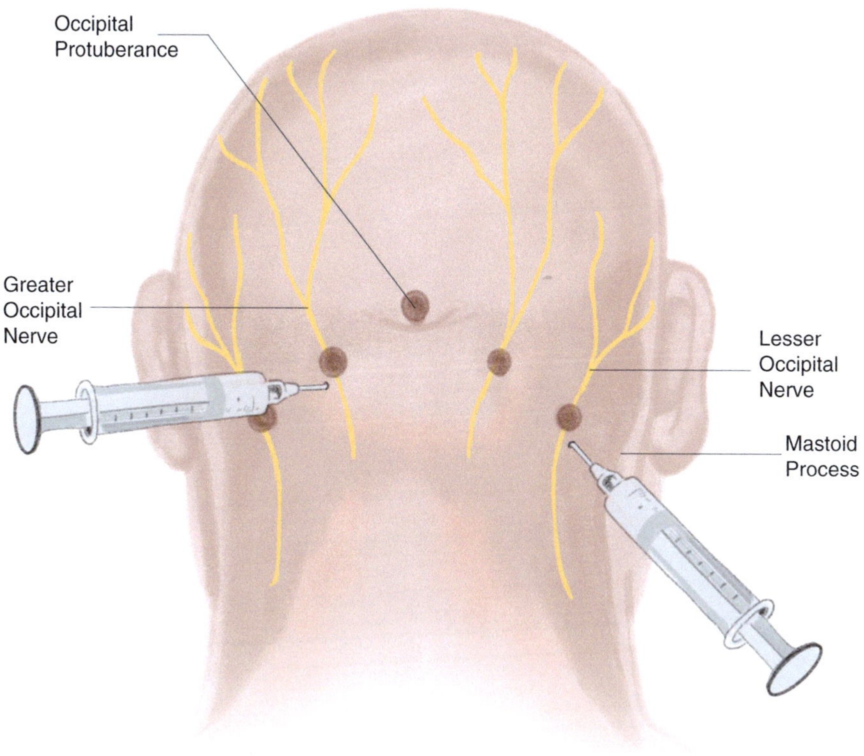

Fig. 9.5 Shows the terminal branches of the greater occipital and the lesser occipital nerves

complex, where there are interneuronal connections in the trigeminal spinal nucleus (Fig. 9.6). ***Pain in the greater occipital nerve distribution can trigger pain in the trigeminal nerve distribution and vice versa.***

Upper Cervical Plexus Nerves

These nerves include the *lesser occipital nerve*, which comes from C2 to C3 and goes from the posterior neck, under the posterior border of the upper sternocleidomastoid muscle and over the mastoid bone to the top of the ear. It also includes the *greater auricular nerve* which goes to and around the lower earlobe and an *anterior cervical branch* along the jawline (Fig. 9.7). *When patients describe pain in the jawline area, from the earlobe to chin, it is important to differentiate whether the pain is in the jaw and teeth (inferior alveolar nerve) or is the pain more superficial and from the cervical plexus nerves.*

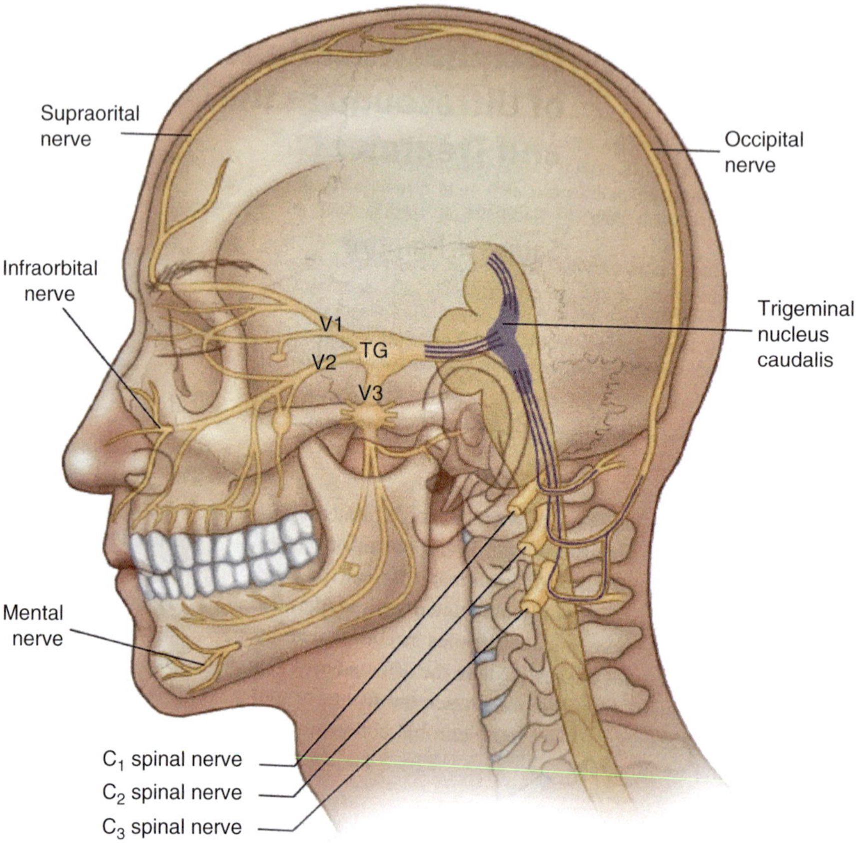

Fig. 9.6 Trigeminal cervical complex where there are interneuronal connections in the trigeminal spinal nucleus which connects the trigeminal and occipital nerves (with permission of Springer Nature)

Procedure Technique

Anesthetics: We use xylocaine 1% with epinephrine at 1:100,000 or 1:200,000 strength as the initial injection for diagnostic purposes. We prefer using a 1 or 1½ inch 25 Ga. needle. If the patient's pain is relieved with the xylocaine injection, then we follow with 0.5% bupivacaine for a longer effect.

Injection technique: Because of the sensitivity of the facial skin, we start by injecting, very quickly, about 1–1.5 mL of 1% xylocaine with epinephrine into the skin overlying the target nerve and let it absorb for about 5 min before injecting the nerve itself. This seems to be less painful for the patient. Ultrasound can be used by those not as familiar with the nerve anatomy; however we have not found it to be necessary if a clinician has good knowledge of the anatomy. *Our goal is to inject the*

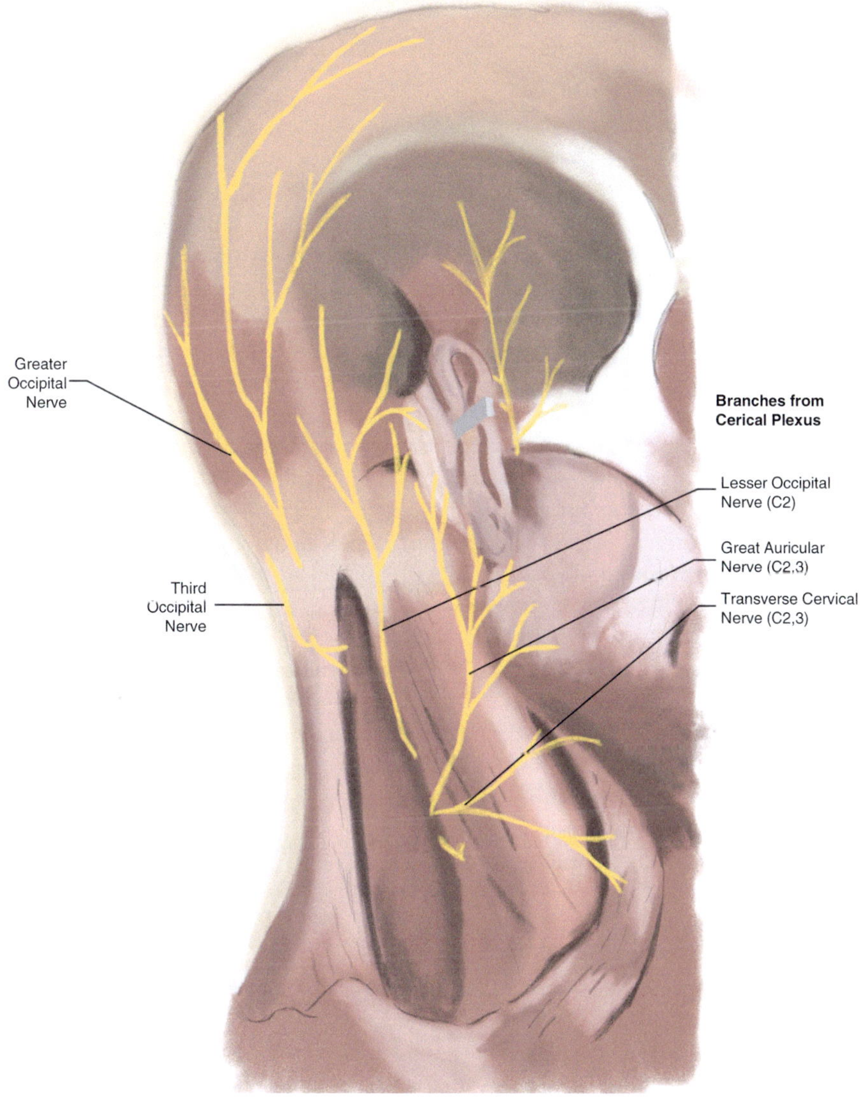

Fig. 9.7 The upper cervical plexus nerves include the lesser occipital, greater auricular, and transverse cervical nerves from C2 to C3

nerve itself or close enough that the anesthetic will include the nerve. We have never had an injury to the nerve with this technique in over a thousand nerve blocks.

The initial dose of the xylocaine is from 2 to 3 mL into the nerve area. Before injecting, we aspirate to be sure we are not in a blood vessel. For a larger area, such as the upper cervical plexus nerves, we use about 4 mL of the xylocaine.

If the patient obtains relief of pain, we follow the xylocaine with 3–4 mL of Marcaine 0.5% for longer effect.

Nerve Block Techniques

Supraorbital and Supratrochlear Nerve Blocks

These nerves can trigger migraine headaches and are easy to block for diagnostic purposes [5]. If a patient is having severe head pain in the frontal area and if, when the supraorbital and supratrochlear nerves are blocked with xylocaine, the pain or headaches subside or go away, it is diagnostic that those nerves are triggering the pain or headaches.

The nerves come out of the orbit separately: the supraorbital nerve comes out through a notch or foramen which is located just medial to the midline of the superior orbital rim [6] (Fig. 9.2). The notch or foramen can frequently be palpated. The supratrochlear nerve exits the orbit at the superior medial orbital rim near the nasal bridge. We aim for the nerves and feel that direct injection into the nerve is not harmful to the nerve, and the pain relief will last longer. If the nerve is hit with the needle, the patient will usually have a sharp pain sensation, and we tell the patient that the nerve block can be more effective. Even if the nerve is not directly hit, the xylocaine will anesthetize the nerves. We recommend injecting about 2–3 mL into each nerve and wait at least 5 min to see what happens to the pain or headache. If the patient obtains numbness and pain relief, we then inject the same amount of 0.5% bupivacaine into each nerve for longer term relief. The patients are told that there is a chance that the pain relief can be days, weeks, or months. If the nerve blocks using xylocaine and bupivacaine do not last more than a day or two, we add 0.5–1.0 mL of Kenalog (40 mg/mL) during subsequent nerve blocks and frequently have seen more prolonged pain relief.

Infraorbital Nerve Block

This nerve block is performed when patients have pain in the midface, side of the nose, and/or the upper lip. The infraorbital nerve comes out of the floor of the orbit about 1 cm below the middle of the inferior orbital rim (Fig. 9.3).

This nerve can be anesthetized in two different ways: one is directly through the skin over the nerve and the second is under the upper lip between the canine and first premolar teeth. We prefer to go transoral by placing some topical anesthetic (tetracaine, benzocaine, or 4% lidocaine) under the upper lip where the injection is to be done and let it sit for 5 min. Then we inject about 1–1.5 mL of 1% xylocaine with epinephrine submucosal and have the patient massage the skin over this area for 5 min.

Next we inject superiorly through this area where the infraorbital nerve is located using about 3 mL xylocaine.

We place a finger on the inferior orbital rim during the nerve injection to make sure the needle does not go to the eyeball.

After about 5 min, the patients should have pain relief; then, we inject 3 mL of 0.5% bupivacaine into the nerve area. We are not concerned about hitting the nerve with the needle because it is unlikely to cause permanent nerve injury and we feel there is better and longer pain relief if the nerve is injected directly. We frequently use 0.5–1 mL of Kenalog 40 mg/mL also.

Posterior Superior Alveolar Nerve Block

This nerve is part of the maxillary nerve and comes off the infraorbital nerve before it enters the floor of the orbit. It goes into the posterior-lateral maxillary sinus wall and goes anteriorly to give off branches to the molar and premolar teeth (Fig. 9.1). This nerve causes pain in the teeth and extracting the teeth does not relieve the pain. Patients will point to the area above the premolar and molar teeth where the pain is greatest.

To block this nerve, we use the same technique as for the infraorbital nerve except we also inject the submucosal area above the molar teeth. The same local anesthetics are used.

This nerve is more difficult to anesthetize because it is usually within the bone above the molar and premolar teeth.

Zygomaticotemporal Nerve Block

This nerve can be the trigger point for temporal headaches and is an important nerve to know how to block. It is located about 8 mm lateral to the lateral orbital rim and goes superiorly to the temporal area (Fig. 9.8). It lies just above the level of the lateral canthus. The zygomatic branch of the facial nerve innervates the orbicularis oculi muscle nearby and can be temporary paralyzed for several hours from the local anesthetics. The zygomaticotemporal nerve runs subcutaneous superiorly and into the temporalis muscle about 50% of the time. Usually we infiltrate the anterior part of the temporalis muscle with the nerve block to help headaches in this area. If there is relief of the pain or headache with the 3–4 mL xylocaine, we inject with the same of 0.5% bupivacaine.

Inferior Alveolar Nerve Block

This nerve is blocked trans-orally as the dentist does. The inferior alveolar nerve is a branch of the mandibular division (V3) after it exits the foramen ovale in the skull base. It enters the mandible through a foramen about the level of the lower teeth and

Fig. 9.8 Blocking the zygomaticotemporal nerve which exits the zygoma at the “x” and goes to the temporal muscle and temple

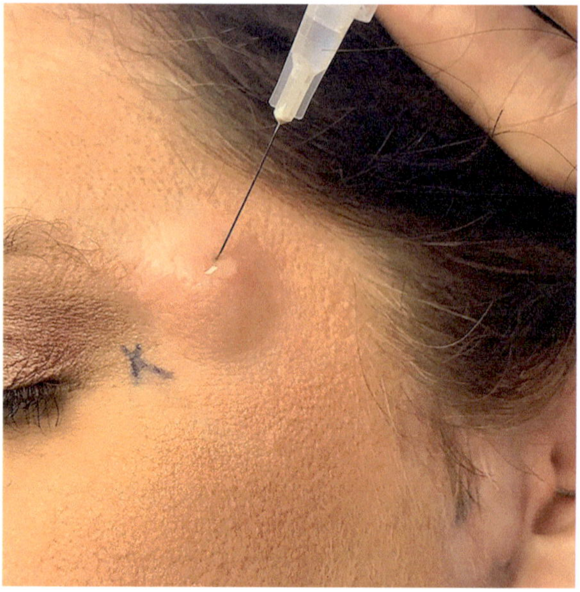

about 2 cm from the anterior edge of the ascending part of the mandible (Fig. 9.9). We use some topical anesthetic, 2% tetracaine, on the mucosa just posterior to the retromolar trigone area, and after about 5 min, we inject 4 mL of 1% xylocaine with 1:100,000 epinephrine submucosal and through the medial pterygoid muscle and hitting the mandible at the level of the teeth. We use a 25 Ga. 1 or 1½ inch needle and curve the needle so that it aims toward the bone, rather than going posterior where the internal carotid artery is located. If the nerve is hit, indicated by a sharp pain, we go ahead and inject since the anesthesia is greater and the duration of the numbing is longer. We have never had permanent injury to the nerve by injecting directly into the nerve. Most of the time, the anesthetic will diffuse around the nerve and anesthetize it. If the patient has relief of pain in his jaw, we follow with 4 mL 0.5% bupivacaine into the same area.

Mental Nerve Block

The mental nerve is the distal end of the inferior alveolar nerve and exits through the mental foramen of the horizontal ramus of the mandible just below the root of the second premolar tooth (Fig. 9.6). It is the sensory supply to the chin and lower lip. It is simple to block this nerve when it is the source of the facial pain. We use an intraoral approach by placing some topical tetracaine on the mucosa for several minutes then injecting 1% xylocaine between the mucosa and mandible just below the root of the second molar tooth. If the pain is relieved, we follow with 0.5% bupivacaine injection into the mental nerve.

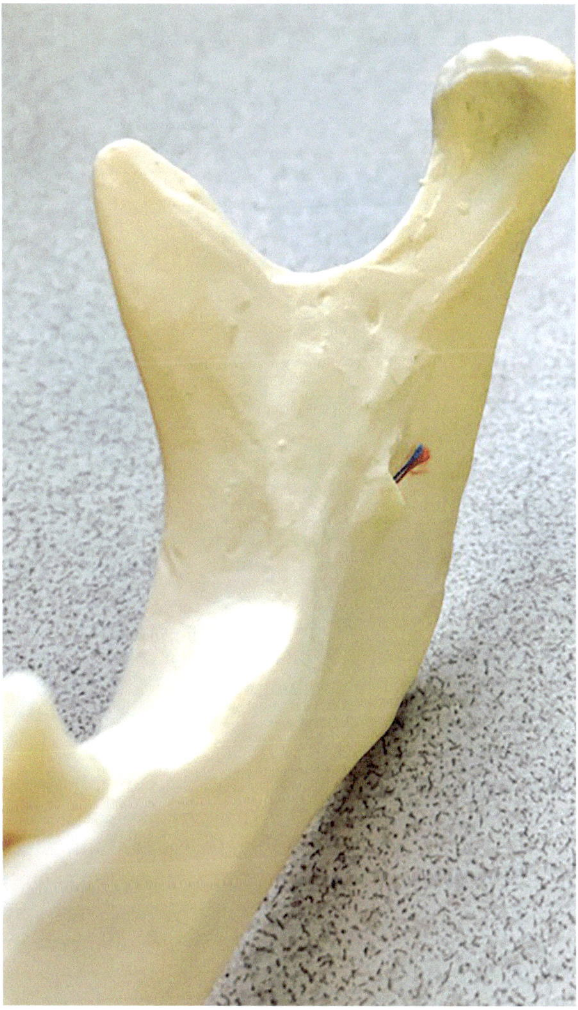

Fig. 9.9 Inferior alveolar nerve enters the mandible at the level of the lower teeth and about 2–2.5 cm from the anterior border of the ascending ramus

Auriculotemporal Nerve Block

This nerve is another nerve which commonly contributes to temporal headaches. It is easy to block the auriculotemporal nerve which is a branch of the mandibular division (V3) of the trigeminal nerve. When patients are having severe temporal headaches, this nerve can be blocked to see if it relieves the headache. The nerve comes off the third division of the trigeminal just after it leaves the foramen ovale and then goes between the mandibular condyle and the external auditory canal. From there, it goes superiorly to the temple area (Figs. 9.4 and 9.10).

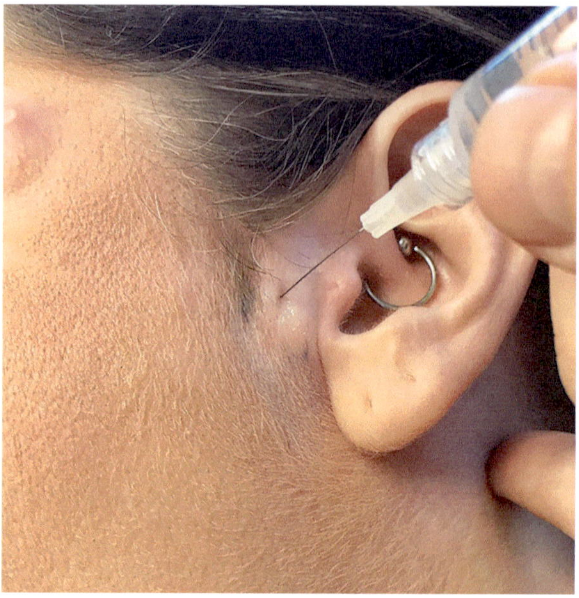

Fig. 9.10 Nerve block of auriculotemporal nerve between the TMJ and the tragus with jaw in open position

To locate the nerve, a finger is placed over the TMJ area, and the patient is asked to open their jaw. The depression from the condyle moving forward can be palpated and 1 mL xylocaine is injected quickly into the skin overlying the depression just anterior to the tragus of the external ear (Fig. 9.10). After about 5 min, the needle is passed perpendicular between the tragus of the ear and the TMJ for about 2 cm. Negative pressure is placed on the syringe plunger to be sure the needle tip is not in a blood vessel. If no blood is withdrawn, 2 mL of xylocaine is injected as the needle is withdrawn toward the skin. When the subcutaneous tissue is reached, the needle is then pointed subcutaneous superiorly, and about 2 mL of the xylocaine is injected alongside the nerve and superficial temporal artery toward the temporal muscle. If the patient is having a severe headache, we also inject 2–3 mL of xylocaine into the temporalis muscle. If the headache is improved after about 5 min, we follow up with the same amount of 0.5% bupivacaine in the same areas.

It is important to recognize that this nerve block can temporarily paralyze the forehead and the orbicularis oculi for about 5 h. The patient should be told that this can happen and that it will correct when the anesthetic wears off.

Greater Occipital Nerve Block

This nerve commonly contributes to occipital headaches which frequently progress to diffuse headaches. If the greater occipital nerve is blocked and the headache improves significantly, this indicates that the nerve is probably the trigger point and the nerve block can abort the headache.

The greater occipital nerve is from the dorsal root of C2 and supplies the posterior scalp from the occipital prominence to the top of the scalp. The nerve is located about 3 cm below and 2–3 cm lateral to the occipital protuberance and runs subcutaneous under the scalp to the vertex. We will inject about 2 cm lateral and below the occipital protuberance and go deep, about 2 cm, into the underlying muscles where the nerve is traversing. We will use about 2 mL of xylocaine into nerve area in the muscles, and then inject 3 mL toward the occipital scalp in a subcutaneous plane and fan it out in three different directions to be sure to inject the nerve (Fig. 9.5).

If the headache and pain improves after 5–10 min, then we follow with 0.5% bupivacaine in the same areas.

Lesser Occipital and Greater Auricular Nerve Block

These two nerves can be blocked together since they both originate from C2 to C3. The lesser occipital nerve innervates the posterior scalp behind the ear to the top of the ear. The greater auricular nerve supplies the skin of the lower earlobe and over the tail of the parotid and angle of the jaw (Fig. 9.7).

To block these nerves, we find the sternocleidomastoid (SCM) muscle and identify the posterior border and about 2 cm above the middle of the muscle between the mastoid and the clavicle (Fig. 9.7). We inject the overlying skin with about 1 mL of xylocaine and wait several minutes for the skin to numb. Then we inject about 3 mL of xylocaine into the subcutaneous tissues and about 2 cm deep to the posterior SCM muscle to catch the nerves as they curve around the muscle. Then we inject about 2 mL along the path of the lesser occipital nerve and about 2 mL subcutaneously toward the earlobe (greater auricular nerve) and slightly below (Fig. 9.7).

If the pain improves significantly, we follow by injecting with the same amount of bupivacaine into the same areas.

If we feel the pain is coming from the proximal upper cervical plexus nerves, we inject about 1½ inches deep under the SCM muscle in several directions to catch the nerves deeper in the neck. It is important to aspirate the syringe to be sure the needle is not in the jugular vein.

Discussion

It is critical to find the trigger point for the patient's pain because the nerve that innervates that area is commonly the cause of the pain or headache [1]. There may be more than one trigger point that needs to be injected to control the pain. **If blocking the nerve with xylocaine stops the pain, then it is diagnostic and will give future options for control of the pain.** (See Chap. 13.)

Possible side effects of the nerve blocks should be discussed with the patient and listed on the consent form. For example, with the nerve block of the zygomatico-temporal or auriculotemporal nerves, part of the facial nerve may be weak for the duration of the anesthetics. With the cervical plexus nerve blocks, it is common to affect the spinal accessory nerve with shoulder weakness and also the vagus nerve with hoarseness for the duration of the anesthetics.

References

1. Janis JE, Dhanik A, Howard JH. Validation of the peripheral trigger point theory of migraine headaches: single-surgeon experience using botulinum toxin and surgical decompression. Plast Reconstr Surg. 2011;128:123–31.
2. Guyuron B, Kriegler JS, Davis J, et al. Five-year outcome of surgical treatment of migraine headaches. Plast Reconstr Surg. 2011;127:603–8.
3. Guyuron B, Reed D, Kriegler JS, et al. A placebo-controlled surgical trial of the treatment of migraine headaches. Plast Reconstr Surg. 2009;124:461–8.
4. Lee M, Lineberry K, Reed D, et al. The role of the third occipital nerve in surgical treatment of occipital migraine headaches. J Plast Reconstr Aesthet Surg. 2013;66:1335–9.
5. Ducic I, Felder JM III, Khan N, et al. Greater occipital nerve excision for occipital neuralgia refractory to nerve decompression. Ann Plast Surg. 2014;72:184–7.
6. Chepla KJ, Oh E, Guyruon B. Clinical outcomes following supraorbital foraminotomy for treatment of frontal migraine headache. Plast Reconstr Surg. 2012;129:656e–62e.
7. Fallucco M, Janis JE, Hagan RR. The anatomical morphology of the supraorbital notch: clinical relevance to the surgical treatment of migraine headaches. Plast Reconstr Surg. 2012;130:1227–33.
8. Janis JE, Hatef DA, Thakar H, et al. The zygomaticotemporal branch of the trigeminal nerve: part II. Anatomical variations. Plast Reconstr Surg. 2010;126:435–42.

Chapter 10
Interventional Approach to the Diagnosis of Head and Face Pain

Vikas Agarwal and Ryan T. Fitzgerald

Cervicogenic Headache

Cervicogenic headache is head pain referred from either the bony or soft tissue structures of the neck innervated by the upper three cervical spinal nerves [1]. Common sources of cervicogenic headaches therefore include the atlanto-occipital joint, the atlantoaxial joint, and the C2–C3 facet (zygapophyseal) joint. In most cases, careful history and physical examination can lead to the diagnosis using established diagnostic criteria from the Cervicogenic Headache International Study Group [2]. Given that clinical features of cervicogenic headaches may overlap and even mimic those associated with primary headache disorders, diagnosis can be challenging. Response to image-guided blockade is therefore an important consideration in the diagnosis of cervicogenic headache.

The atlanto-occipital joint is a synovial joint formed by the articulation of the superior articular process of the C1 vertebral body (atlas) and the occiput. It can therefore be thought of as a modified facet (zygapophyseal) joint since it is positioned anterolateral to the spinal canal as opposed to true facet (zygapophyseal) joints which are positioned posterolateral [3]. Injection into the atlanto-occipital joint is performed using fluoroscopic guidance in the prone position with the patient's neck slightly flexed. A major consideration when targeting the atlanto-occipital joint for injection is that the vertebral artery overlies the medial one third of the joint before turning medially and diagonally to enter the foramen magnum.

V. Agarwal (✉)
Department of Radiology, University of Pittsburgh Medical Center,
Pittsburgh, PA, USA
e-mail: agarwalv@upmc.edu

R. T. Fitzgerald
Department of Radiology, University of Arkansas for Medical Sciences,
Little Rock, AR, USA

J. Y. Suen, E. Petersen (eds.), *Diagnosis and Management of Head and Face Pain*, https://doi.org/10.1007/978-3-319-90999-8_10

Therefore the target site for injection is along the lateral third of the joint superiorly.

The atlantoaxial joint is a synovial joint formed by the articulation of the superior articulating processes of the C2 vertebral body (axis) and the inferior articulating processes of the C1 vertebral body (atlas). Injection into the atlantoaxial joint is performed using fluoroscopic guidance in the prone position with the patient's neck slightly flexed. As with the atlanto-occipital joint injections, the major consideration when targeting the atlantoaxial joint is the vertebral artery which is located lateral to the joint as it courses through the C2 and C1 foramen. Therefore the target site for injection is medial to the junction of the lateral one third and medial two thirds of the joint space.

The C2–C3 facet (zygapophyseal) joint is innervated by the third occipital nerve which arises from the medial branch of the dorsal ramus of C3. Injection into the C2–C3 facet joint is performed using fluoroscopic guidance and can be performed using either a posterior or lateral approach.

Headache Related to Intracranial Hypotension

Spontaneous intracranial hypotension (SIH) is an underdiagnosed cause of persistent and debilitating headaches. Patients typically present with orthostatic headaches in the setting of decreased CSF volume and low CSF pressure without a history of spinal instrumentation or penetrating trauma [4]. The underlying pathophysiology of SIH is not well understood complicating both diagnosis and treatment. The majority of patients with SIH are successfully treated with conservative management including bed rest, high fluid intake, and caffeine [5]. When medical management fails to resolve symptoms, image-guided epidural blood patches have been shown to be effective for treating the CSF leak. In cases where a single or even multiple sites of CSF leakage are identified on spinal imaging, a targeted epidural blood patch is performed to induce a dural tamponade and seal the site of CSF leak [6]. In many patients the location of a CSF leakage is not identified on imaging, and a nontargeted epidural blood patch is performed. For this technique, a lumbar approach is utilized with the patient in the Trendelenburg position facilitating spread of the blood to the cervicothoracic region restricting CSF flow, reducing CSF absorption, and subsequently causing re-equilibration of CSF pressure [7–10].

Facial Pain

Facial pain can be caused by a variety of etiologies. Careful history and physical examination can lead to the diagnosis using established diagnostic criteria from the International Association for the Study of Pain (IASP) or the International Headache Classification [11, 12]. Peripheral nerve blocks can provide valuable diagnostic information to help determine the site of origin of facial pain. Potential targets for temporary nerve blockade include the supra- and infraorbital nerves, supratrochlear nerve, inferior alveolar nerve, mental nerve, auriculotemporal nerve, greater auricular nerve, maxillary nerve, mandibular nerve, and glossopharyngeal nerve. While the majority of these can be performed without image guidance using established landmarks, ultrasound and fluoroscopy are now increasingly used for guidance. For indications and techniques of peripheral nerve blockade, please refer to Chaps. 8 and 9.

References

1. Sjaastad O, Saunte C, Hovdahl H, Breivik H, Gronback E. "Cervicogenic" headache. A hypothesis. Cephalalgia. 1983;3:249–56.
2. Sjaastad O, Fredriksen TA, Pfaffenrath V. Cervicogenic headache: diagnostic criteria. Headache. 1998;38:442–5.
3. Ogoke BA. The management of the atlanto-occipital and atlanto-axial joint pain. Pain Physician. 2000;3:289–93.
4. Schievink WI. Spontaneous spinal cerebrospinal fluid leaks and intracranial hypotension. JAMA. 2006;295:2286–96.
5. Schievink WI, Meyer FB, Atkinson JL, et al. Spontaneous spinal cerebrospinal fluid leaks and intracranial hypotension. J Neurosurg. 1996;84:598–605.
6. Beards SC, Jackson A, Griffiths AG, et al. Magnetic resonance imaging of extradural blood patches: appearances from 30 min to 18 h. Br J Anaesth. 1993;71:182–8.
7. Su CS, Lan MY, Chang YY, et al. Clinical features, neuroimaging and treatment of spontaneous intracranial hypotension and magnetic resonance imaging evidence of blind epidural blood patch. Eur Neurol. 2009;61:301–7.
8. Franzini A, Messina G, Nazzi V, et al. Spontaneous intracranial hypotension syndrome: a novel speculative physiopathological hypothesis and a novel patch method in a series of 28 consecutive patients. J Neurosurg. 2010;112:300–6.
9. Ferrante E, Arpino I, Citterio A. Is it a rational choice to treat with lumbar epidural blood patch headache caused by spontaneous cervical CSF leak? Cephalgia. 2006;26:1245–6.
10. Ferrante E, Arpino I, Citterio A, et al. Epidural blood patch in Trendelenburg position premedicated with acetazolamide to treat spontaneous intracranial hypotension. Eur J Neurol. 2010;17:715–9.
11. Merskey H, Bogduk N. Classification of chronic pain. Descriptors of chronic pain syndromes and definitions of pain terms. 2nd ed. Seattle: IASP Press; 1994.
12. Headache Classification Committee of the International Headache Society. The International Classification of Headache Disorders, 3rd edition (beta version). Cephalalgia. 2013;33:629–808.

Part III
Management and Treatment

Chapter 11
Medical Management of Head and Face Pain

Johnathan H. Goree, Christopher S. Fiedorek, Ruben G. Alexander, and Boris Spektor

Non-opiate Analgesics

(a) Introduction
No longer regarded as a potent, universal remedy for all pain, opiates have fallen out of favor in the most recent pain literature. Increases in addiction, rising overdose deaths, systemic side effects, and the discovery of opiate induced-hyperalgesia have illuminated the need for non-opiate alternatives for all chronic pain disorders. During this chapter we will explore the literature behind many of these alternative, non-opiate medications, and their use for nonmalignant pain of the head and neck.

Antiepileptics

Carbamazepine

(a) Mechanism of Action
Carbamazepine is a first-generation anticonvulsant. It binds voltage-dependent sodium channels during the inactivated phase and slows the recovery rate.

J. H. Goree (✉) · C. S. Fiedorek
Department of Anesthesiology, University of Arkansas for Medical Sciences, Little Rock, AR, USA
e-mail: Jhgoree@uams.edu; cfiedorek@uams.edu

R. G. Alexander · B. Spektor
Department of Anesthesiology, Emory University School of Medicine, Atlanta, GA, USA
e-mail: ruben.gerard.alexander@emory.edu; bspekto@emory.edu; boris.spektor@emoryhealthcare.org

J. Y. Suen, E. Petersen (eds.), *Diagnosis and Management of Head and Face Pain*, https://doi.org/10.1007/978-3-319-90999-8_11

This prevents the generation of rapid action potentials in neuronal cells by prolonging the cells' inactivated state [1].

(b) Evidence for Trigeminal Neuralgia
Carbamazepine was first shown to have some benefit for the relief of pain from trigeminal neuralgia 3years after its introduction as an anticonvulsant [2]. Its efficacy was subsequently confirmed in four placebo-controlled studies containing 147 total patients [3–6]. The effective dose of carbamazepine ranges from 100 to 600 mg twice daily and should be titrated gradually to attainment of pain relief. Robust treatment responses were demonstrated in these trials with 1.7–1.8 being the number needed to treat to achieve clinically significant pain relief. Carbamazepine decreases both the intensity and frequency of paroxysmal pain and is equally efficacious on spontaneous and trigger-evoked attacks [3]. The American Academy of Neurology and the European Federation of Neurological Societies (AAN-EFNS) guidelines on trigeminal neuralgia management conclude that carbamazepine is a standard of care for controlling pain in patients with this disease [7].

(c) Adverse Effects
Common side effects include hypotension, pruritus (8%), rash (7%), constipation (10%), nausea (29%), vomiting (18%), xerostomia (8%), anemia (IV, 7%), asthenia (8%), ataxia (15%), dizziness (bipolar disorder, 44%; seizures, 9%), somnolence (bipolar disorder, 32%; seizures, 5%), blurred vision (5–6%), and nystagmus [8]. Serious reactions include cardiac dysrhythmias, hyponatremia (oral, 4–22%; IV, less than 2%), liver failure, renal failure, pulmonary hypersensitivity, aplastic anemia, agranulocytosis, pancytopenia, and toxic epidermal necrolysis and Stevens-Johnson syndrome, particularly in patients with the inherited allelic variant HLA-B15:02 who are almost exclusively of Asian ancestry [8]. The frequency of adverse reactions, particularly in elderly patients with trigeminal neuralgia, limits the use of carbamazepine. The number needed to harm is 3.4 for minor and 24 for severe adverse events [9–11].

Gabapentin

(a) Mechanism of Action
Gabapentin is an antiepileptic originally designed as a structural analog of gamma aminobutyric acid (GABA). The original intention was that it would cross the blood-brain barrier and enhance GABA-mediated inhibition of neuronal firing [12]. While current evidence suggests that gabapentin does have limited action on the GABAergic neurotransmitter system as well as voltage-gated potassium channels [13–16], the primary molecular target is

the $\alpha 2\delta$-1 subunit of voltage-gated calcium channels on nociceptor nerve terminals [17]. Binding to $\alpha 2\delta$-1 subunits inhibits membrane trafficking of the $\alpha 1$ subunit of calcium channels from the endoplasmic reticulum to the plasma membrane [18] and anterograde (axonal) transport of $\alpha 2\delta$-1 subunits from the dorsal root ganglion to the primary afferent nerve terminals in the dorsal horn [19]. Gabapentin thus decreases the density of calcium channels in the presynaptic terminals, leading to decreased release of neurotransmitters such as glutamate, substance P, and calcitonin gene-related peptide and decreased postsynaptic excitability [20, 21]. Other targets currently being investigated include β subunits, NMDA receptors, protein kinase C, transient receptor potential ion channels, and descending inhibitory spinal tracts [22].

(b) Evidence for Postherpetic Neuralgia
Gabapentin is among the first-line agents for postherpetic neuralgia. Eight placebo-controlled trials of gabapentin for postherpetic neuralgia have been conducted demonstrating at least 50% pain intensity reduction in 34% of patients and achievement of a reduction in Patient Global Impression of Change (PGIC) of "much" or "very much improved" in 39% of patients [23]. Admittedly, the total daily dosing in these trials varied between 1800 and 3600 mg. Unfortunately, there is insufficient dosing regimen data to establish a dose-response relationship.

(c) Evidence for Trigeminal Neuralgia
There is limited evidence for the use of gabapentin for classical trigeminal neuralgia with only small open-label studies showing some therapeutic benefit. For symptomatic trigeminal neuralgia, there are likewise no placebo-controlled studies. Three open-label studies including 19 total patients with trigeminal neuralgia associated with multiple sclerosis report a beneficial effect [24–26]. The AAN-EFNS guidelines conclude that there is insufficient evidence to support or refute the effectiveness of gabapentin for classical or symptomatic trigeminal neuralgia.

(d) Evidence for Post-traumatic Trigeminal Neuropathy (Anesthesia Dolorosa)
No trials of gabapentin for post-traumatic trigeminal neuropathy have been conducted. One case report described relief with dosing of 1200 mg daily [27].

(e) Evidence for Trigeminal Trophic Syndrome
Gabapentin has been used as first-line therapy for symptoms of trigeminal trophic syndrome but with limited efficacy based on case reports in the literature [28].

(f) Evidence for Burning Mouth Syndrome
Evidence for the use of gabapentin for burning mouth syndrome is limited and conflicting. A case report described benefit from 900 mg daily as monotherapy [29], while an open-label pilot study showed little or no effect [30]. The combination of alpha lipoic acid and gabapentin was more effective than either drug alone in a randomized controlled trial [31].

(g) Adverse Effects
Common side effects include peripheral edema (5–12%), increased appetite (5%), weight gain (3.3–12%), constipation (4–8%), xerostomia (2–11%), asthenia (5–10%), ataxia (3–15%), dizziness (9–43%), headache (5–9%), incoordination (2–10%), somnolence (10–36%), tremor (1–11%), blurred vision (3–10%), diplopia (2–9%), disturbance in thinking (2–8%), euphoria (2–6%), nasopharyngitis (8%), and fatigue (7–11%) [8]. Serious adverse effects include jaundice, hypersensitivity reaction, increased creatine kinase level (1.5–2.7%), suicidal thoughts, and angioedema [8].

Pregabalin

(a) Mechanism of Action
Pregabalin, like gabapentin, is thought to act as a specific ligand of the α2-δ subunits of voltage-gated calcium channels on presynaptic endings of neurons in the brain and spinal cord. The pharmacologic effect is believed to be primarily via the α2δ-1 subunit [32, 33]. By binding to the α2δ-1 subunit, pregabalin alters its molecular interaction with the α1 pore-forming subunit that normally leads to stabilization of the channel [34]. This results in reduced calcium influx at the presynaptic neuronal membrane, which subsequently reduces glutamate and other neurotransmitter release [21]. Pregabalin thus reduces nociceptive responses, particularly in conditions involving central sensitization [35] and nerve injury, in which α2-δ-1 expression is upregulated [36]. Another antinociceptive mechanism of pregabalin involves an effect on the descending noradrenergic and serotonergic pathways that modulates pain transmission in the spinal cord [37].

(b) Evidence for Postherpetic Neuralgia
Two randomized controlled trials involving over 400 patients have been conducted showing pregabalin improves sleep and decreases mean pain scores in patients with postherpetic neuralgia at doses ranging from 150 mg daily to the maximum dose of 600 mg daily [38, 39]. The total daily dose should be divided into two or three doses and titrated based on effect and tolerability.

(c) Evidence for Use in Other Types of Facial Pain
In a systematic review of randomized, double-blind trials on the analgesic effect of pregabalin, doses of 300, 450, and 600 mg daily were effective in patients with postherpetic neuralgia, painful diabetic neuropathy, central neuropathic pain, and fibromyalgia (19 studies, 7003 participants) [40]. Due to this beneficial effect on neuropathic pain conditions, pregabalin is frequently prescribed for various types of facial pain, but evidence is scant. No literature was found regarding the efficacy of pregabalin for painful post-traumatic trigeminal neuropathy (anesthesia dolorosa), burning mouth syndrome, and persistent idiopathic facial pain.

(d) Adverse Effects
The most commonly reported adverse events (AEs) are dizziness (9.1–42.7%), somnolence (10.2–28.1%), weight gain (4–12%), xerostomia (2.3–10.1 %), and peripheral edema (5–12%) [8]. Serious adverse effects include angioedema [8].

Phenytoin

(a) Mechanism of Action
Phenytoin is a barbiturate derivative with anticonvulsant properties whose mechanism is not completely understood. Recent studies have described its action at an ever-increasing number of receptor sites, but most important are its inhibitory effects on a variety of sodium and calcium channels [41, 42]. Evidence suggests its effect on persistent sodium current inactivation is primarily responsible for its anticonvulsant effect [43]. Phenytoin suppresses high-frequency repetitive firing of depolarized neurons while allowing normal activity due to poor blockade of slow firing rates [44].
(b) Evidence for Use in Facial Pain
The evidence supporting the use of phenytoin in facial pain is limited. One early report exists of its use for facial neuralgia [45]. Subsequent small trials have been performed with mixed results regarding its use in other types of neuropathic pain [46–48]. In a 2012 systematic review of literature, occasional use for refractory trigeminal neuralgia was found, but the review concluded that no evidence of sufficient quality to support the use of phenytoin in chronic neuropathic pain currently exists [49].
(c) Adverse Effects
Common adverse effects include rash, constipation, gingival hyperplasia, nausea, vomiting, ataxia, coordination problem, nystagmus, slurred speech, confusion, and anxiety [8]. Serious adverse effects include bullous dermatosis, purpuric rash, Stevens-Johnson syndrome, toxic epidermal necrolysis, agranulocytosis, granulocytopenic disorder, leukopenia, pancytopenia, thrombocytopenia, toxic hepatitis, lupus erythematosus, and nephrotoxicity [8]. Phenytoin is contraindicated in pregnancy because of teratogenicity and should not be taken by women of childbearing age.

Topiramate

(a) Mechanism of Action
Topiramate has multiple molecular targets within the shared pathogenic mechanism of migraine and epilepsy [50]. Topiramate diminishes frequency of neuronal action potentials by enhancing neuronal inhibition and decreasing

neuronal excitation. It modulates potassium channels [51] and blocks voltage-dependent sodium and calcium channels [52, 53]. Topiramate inhibits glutamate-induced excitation at the kainate and AMPA glutamate receptor subtypes [54, 55]. It also enhances $GABA_A$-mediated reduction of excitability [56] and alters neurotransmitter release, including the reduction of extracellular glutamate and aspartate in conditions of excess concentrations [57]. Despite these many known molecular mechanisms with theoretical effects, the precise mode or modes of action involved in the prophylaxis of migraines is not currently known [58].

(b) Evidence for Migraine Prophylaxis

Multiple open-label and controlled trials suggest the efficacy of topiramate for migraine prophylaxis. Two large randomized, controlled trials involving 970 patients demonstrate a significant decrease in mean monthly migraine frequency in patients receiving topiramate dosed at either 100 or 200 mg/day compared with placebo. In these two studies, 50% of patients achieved a greater than 50% reduction in mean migraine frequency [59, 60]. A systematic review of the literature identified 17 unique randomized, controlled trials showing benefit, with a reduction of headache frequency by about 1.2 attacks per 28 days as compared to placebo and approximately double the number of responders compared to placebo [61, 62]. Meta-analysis of studies including more than one dose of topiramate suggests that 200 mg is no more effective than 100 mg [61, 62]. The AAN and AHS guidelines on migraine prophylaxis recommend the use of topiramate as a first-line agent [63].

(c) Evidence for Trigeminal Neuralgia

One small study including six patients with multiple sclerosis reported efficacy of topiramate for trigeminal neuralgia [64]. A study of eight patients with classical trigeminal neuralgia reported at least moderate benefit in six patients [65]. A meta-analysis of six randomized, controlled trials including 354 patients showed no significantly different overall effectiveness or tolerability between topiramate and carbamazepine in the treatment of classic TN [66]; however, the results were limited due to the poor methodological quality of these trials [67]. Thus, while there is some recent suggestion of some benefit, the conclusion remains as in the 2008 AAN-EFNS that insufficient evidence exists to support or refute the effectiveness of topiramate for trigeminal neuralgia [7].

(d) Evidence for Persistent Idiopathic Facial Pain

There are no trials supporting the use of topiramate for persistent idiopathic facial pain. However, one case report found benefit with topiramate titrated to 125 mg two times a day [68].

(e) Adverse Effects

Common adverse events include anorexia (4–24%), fatigue (14–30%), memory problems (5–14%), nausea (6–14%), paresthesia (2–51%), taste disturbance (3–15%), weight loss (6–21%), and disorder of language (6–10%) [8, 69]. The cognitive symptoms involving word-finding, slowed thinking, decreased concentration, and memory deficits may be amenable to altering pharmacokinetic profile such as reduced dose or rate of drug introduction [70]. Serious adverse events include erythema multiforme, Stevens-Johnson syndrome, toxic epidermal necrolysis, fever, hyperhidrosis, hyperammonemia, metabolic acidosis, liver failure, glaucoma, myopia, depression, suicidal ideation, mood disorder, and nephrolithiasis [8].

Valproate

(a) Mechanism of Action
Valproate, by several distinct mechanisms, modulates nociceptive neurotransmission including the pain systems involved in the complex pathophysiology of migraine [71, 72].
Valproic acid, sodium valproate (the solid salt that results from valproic acid reacting with sodium hydroxide), or a mixture of the two (divalproex sodium) will here be referred to collectively as "valproate."
Valproate has several effects involved in modulation of nociception and migraine prophylaxis including inhibition of GABA transaminase (thereby enhancing the neurotransmission of GABA), blockade of voltage-gated sodium channels, and blockade of T-type calcium channels. Increased GABA and stabilization of neuronal cell membranes likely result in reduction pain processing and signal transduction [73]. Investigations indicate a potential beneficial effect at nine different stages of the migraine headache [74], but the precise mechanism is not known [61, 62].
(b) Evidence for Migraine Prophylaxis
Multiple randomized controlled trials have shown the benefit of valproate for migraine prophylaxis, and it has been approved for this use since 1996. It is recommended as a first-line agent by both the Quality Standards Subcommittee of the American Academy of Neurology (AAN) and the American Headache Society (AHS) [63] and the EFNS guidelines [75]. In a 2013 systematic review, ten randomized controlled trials were identified as similar in basic design. Meta-analysis revealed a robust conclusion of efficacy over placebo. Patients were more than twice as likely to have a greater than 50% reduction in headache frequency with valproate than placebo, and mean headache frequency was reduced by approximately four headaches per month [61, 62]. The doses of valproate investigated ranged from 400 to 1500 mg/day, but no direct dose-response relationship was observed.
(c) Evidence for Use in Facial Pain
Two randomized, controlled trials of valproate for neuropathic pain (diabetic neuropathy and postherpetic neuralgia) showed statistically greater improvements in pain scores with active treatment compared with placebo [76, 77]. However, both studies were limited due to small sample size. A 2014 systematic

review concluded that there is insufficient evidence to recommend first-line use of valproate for neuropathic pain. It is currently reserved for cases where other proven treatment options have failed [78].

(d) Adverse Effects
Clinically significant adverse effects include asthenia/fatigue, dizziness/vertigo, nausea, tremor, and weight gain with number needed to harm ranging from 7 to 14 [61, 62]. Serious adverse effects include palpitations (1% to less than 5%); tachycardia (1% to less than 5%); hyperammonemia; hematemesis (1% to less than 5%); thrombocytopenia, dose-related (1–27%); immune hypersensitivity reaction (rare); ototoxicity (deafness) (1% to less than 5%); pleural effusion (rare); and pulmonary hemorrhage (rare) [8].

Anti-inflammatory Medications

Nonsteroidal Anti-inflammatory Drugs (NSAIDs)

(a) Mechanism of Action
NSAIDs are one of the most commonly used drug classes in the United States accounting for 70 million prescriptions annually [79]. They were first discussed during the fifth century BC when Hippocrates wrote about willow bark's multiple medical applications [80]. While one might consider this a significant advance in modern medicine, the active ingredient, salicin, was not isolated until 1829 [81]. Felix Hoffman later converted this compound into acetylsalicylic acid by 1897. This new synthetic compound continues to be successfully marketed as aspirin by the Bayer Corporation to this day [81]. In the past 50 years, many different NSAIDs have been created due to their wide market acceptance and multiple functions. While these medications are often employed for their antipyretic effects, in this chapter, we will explore their anti-inflammatory and analgesic effects.
The primary mechanism of action of NSAIDs is inhibition of the cyclooxygenase enzymes (COX). These enzymes are essential to the pro-inflammatory pathway and are catalysts in the conversion of arachidonic acid to prostaglandins and thromboxanes. These inflammatory mediators regulate a number of processes including smooth muscle constriction and platelet activity.

(b) Evidence for Temporomandibular Joint Disease (TMJ) in Adults
The majority of positive studies published for the effectiveness of NSAIDs in nonmalignant diseases of the head and neck are found in the TMJ literature. In a double-blind, randomized trial, patients with primary TMJ were treated with either celecoxib 100 mg twice per day, naproxen 500 mg twice per day, or placebo. Naproxen was found to have the most efficacy with a 75% decrease in pain scores. This was noticed after 3 weeks of treatment, and results were maintained at 6 weeks. Celecoxib, on the other hand, showed no significant difference when compared directly to placebo [82]. In a more recent study, the

efficacy of sodium diclofenac 50 mg twice per day was compared to placebo in 18 adult volunteers wearing a rigid occlusive splint. A statistically significant difference in pain control was found for patients using sodium diclofenac over placebo [83]. While multiple studies have shown benefit with use of systemic NSAID treatment for TMJ, studies have shown little benefit with the use of topical NSAIDs for the same condition [84].

(c) Adverse Effects
The most common adverse reactions to NSAIDs occur in the GI tract. NSAIDs reduce prostaglandins in the GI tract which stimulate protective mucus production and decrease acid production. This can cause a number of adverse effects including ulcers, gastritis, diarrhea, and others. NSAIDs have been proven to increase the risks of myocardial infarction and stroke and are also associated with a dramatic increase in symptoms in patients previously diagnosed with congestive heart failure [85]. It is often recommended to avoid the use of these medications in patients with diagnosed heart conditions. The same is true for patients with renal conditions. Since prostaglandins are essential to the regulation of renal blood flow, prolonged use of these medications can cause elevated creatinine and altered renal function. Other common side effects of oral NSAIDS include abdominal pain (3–9%), ecchymosis (3–9%), pruritus (3–9%), anemia (1–3%), and tinnitus (3–9%) [8].

Corticosteroids

(a) Mechanism of Action
These medications were first used in the 1930s when Kendall and Reichstein isolated and synthesized cortisol [86]. Shortly after, Philip Hench described the efficacy of this treatment for patients with rheumatoid arthritis [86]. These three men were subsequently awarded the Nobel Prize for Medicine and Physiology in 1950 [86]. Over the subsequent 50 years, various corticosteroid medications were adapted from the cortisol molecule and marketed for treatment of many inflammatory conditions.

The primary mechanism of action of corticosteroids is the activation of the glucocorticoid receptor on the cell membrane. This causes increased trans-activation of anti-inflammatory mediators and trans-repression of inflammatory markers [86].

(b) Evidence for Giant Cell Arteritis (GCA)
Corticosteroids are the first-line treatment for this GCA. Since the progression of this disease can cause devastating sudden visual loss and the effectiveness of treatment has been well established, randomized placebo-controlled trials were never conducted. During the 1980s and 1990s, observational studies by Delecoeuilerie and Lundberg showed a decrease in pain and lack of progression to blindness after treatment with corticosteroids [87, 88]. After this revelation, corticosteroids became standard of care for this condition. The current recommended dosage for ophthalmic GCA is IV methylprednisolone 15 mg/kg/day

for 3–5 days or until erythrocyte sedimentation rate and C reactive protein are normal. The dose then decreases to 1–1.5 mg/kg/day of oral prednisone followed by a prolonged taper [89]. For non-ophthalmic cases of GCA, the current recommended treatment is 1 mg/kg/day of oral prednisone followed by a prolonged taper [89].

(c) Evidence for Treatment of Optic Neuritis

In a landmark trial by The Optic Neuritis Study Group published in 1992, the use of corticosteroids for the treatment of optic neuritis was studied in a randomized, multicenter trial including 15 centers and 457 patients. Patients were randomized to either oral prednisone (1 mg/kg) for 14 days, intravenous methylprednisolone (1 g/day) for 3 days followed by oral prednisone (1 mg/kg) for 11 days, or placebo. In the original study, visual function was assessed over a 6 month follow up period. Reversal of visual field defects was found to recover faster in the methylprednisolone group ($p = 0.0001$) [90]. At 6 months, the improvement of visual fields, contrast sensitivity, and color vision were also all better in the intravenous group [90]. There was no difference between the oral group and placebo except for a higher rate of new episodes of this disease in the oral prednisone group [90]. Visual function on a visual analog scale was examined in a smaller, single center study in which 60 patients were randomized to treatment with placebo vs. 500 mg oral methylprednisolone for 5 days followed by a 10 days taper. Oral methylprednisolone showed a significant VAS score at 3 weeks ($p = 0.008$), but VAS scores at 8 weeks were comparable to placebo [91].

(d) Evidence for Tolosa-Hunt Syndrome

Due to the low incidence of this disease and the early identification of dramatic improvement with corticosteroids through case reports in the 1960s [92], there have been no high-quality randomized controlled trials providing evidence for steroids as the treatment of this condition. In the largest observational study of 20 patients, 15 patients were treated with steroids of varying doses, and all had improvement of pain and variable improvement of ophthalmoplegia [93]. The current recommended dose based on observational data is 80 mg daily for 3 days followed by a taper if pain has resolved [94, 95].

(e) Evidence for Ophthalmoplegic Migraine

There have been a number of case reports which demonstrate the benefit of steroid treatment for ophthalmoplegia with migraine in the adult population. In a case study of 62 patients which was published in 2009, it was found that there is a statistically significant hastened recovery in patients with this disease who were treated with steroids [96]. There is no consensus dose because throughout the literature, the doses have varied significantly.

(f) Adverse Effects

Common side effects of corticosteroids are hypertension, impaired glucose tolerance, weight gain, loss of bone density, and mood disturbances [8]. Long-term use of corticosteroid can cause a decrease in endogenous production, aseptic necrosis of the femoral head, or iatrogenic Cushing's syndrome. While the adverse effects of long-term steroids are well known in the medical community, there are also increased risks for patients who take high dose steroids for inflammatory diseases like GCA. In a cohort study of 125 patients with

GCA treated with high dose IV steroids, 86% of patients were found to have an adverse event including cataracts (41%), infection (31%), hypertension (22%), development of diabetes (9%), or fracture (38%) [97].

Muscle Relaxants

Baclofen

(a) Mechanism of Action
Baclofen is a centrally acting muscle relaxant analog of the inhibitory neurotransmitter gamma aminobutyric acid (GABA). It has antispasmodic action which is derived from activation of $GABA_B$ receptors [98]. This has multiple downstream effects including inhibition of calcium channels, direct inhibition of neurons in the dorsal horn and spinal trigeminal nucleus, and inhibition of pain transmission in the thalamus [98, 99].

(b) Evidence for Trigeminal Neuralgia (TN)
In a small randomized, double-blind controlled crossover trial of ten patients with classic trigeminal neuralgia, 70% of patients experienced a statistically significant reduction in frequency and severity of attacks relative to placebo. Importantly, 88% of patients who were unable to tolerate carbamazepine benefitted from baclofen treatment, and 83% of those who had become refractory to carbamazepine achieved analgesia with this drug [98]. Six of the ten patients controlled their symptoms with baclofen monotherapy [98]. A further open-label study of 50 patients with trigeminal neuralgia showed that 37 of 50 patients (74%) experienced reduced attack frequency and severity [98]. Starting baclofen dose in both of these studies was 10 mg three times daily, with dosage increased by 10 mg/day every other day to goal of 60–80 mg a day in three to four divided doses. Based on the above evidence from a single small RCT, the American Academy of Neurology and the European Federation of Neurological Societies have deemed baclofen possibly effective for controlling facial pain in TN [7].

(c) Adverse Effects
Common side effects of oral baclofen include constipation (2–6%), nausea (4–12%), and sedation (10–63%) [8]. Of importance, chronic (>2 month) baclofen users should not suddenly discontinue the drug due to possibility of developing hallucinations, seizures, or both; rather, baclofen dosage should be progressively reduced by 5–10 mg per day at weekly intervals [98].

Tizanidine

(a) Mechanism of Action
Tizanidine is an alpha-2 adrenergic agonist that inhibits release of norepinephrine at both the brainstem and spinal cord. This results in both central muscle

relaxation as well as an independent antinociceptive effect that is unrelated to serotonin, dopamine, endogenous opioids, or GABA [100].

(b) Evidence for Chronic Tension-Type Headache
In a randomized, double-blind, placebo-controlled crossover trial of 37 women with chronic tension-type headaches, tizanidine was initiated at a dose of 2 mg three times daily and gradually up-titrated to 6 mg three times daily. The tizanidine group experienced statistically significant reductions versus placebo in pain intensity visual analog scale, verbal rating scale, use of analgesics, and Beck Depression Inventory scores [101, 102]. Mechanistically, this favorable result did not correlate with trapezius electromyographic activity measured during the trial [101].

(c) Evidence for Chronic Daily Headache (CDH) Prophylaxis
Saper and colleagues randomized 134 patients who reported at least 15 days of headache per month for at least 3 months (CDH comprising migraine, migrainous, and tension-type headaches) to 12 weeks of scheduled treatment with tizanidine versus placebo. Tizanidine dosing was initially 2 mg before sleep titrated up in 3-day intervals to maximum 8 mg three times daily. The tizanidine group experienced statistically significant reductions in mean headache days per week, average headache intensity, and mean headache duration [100]. There was no difference in benefit for patients with migraine versus tension-type headaches [100].

(d) Adverse Effects
Common side effects of tizanidine include hypotension (16–33%), xerostomia (49–88%), somnolence (48–92%), and dizziness (16–45%) [8]. A serious but rare side effect is hepatotoxicity with elevation of liver enzymes to more than three times normal in about 5% of treated patients [100].

Serotonin-Norepinephrine Reuptake Inhibitors (SNRI)

Venlafaxine

(a) Mechanism of Action
Venlafaxine blocks the presynaptic reuptake of both serotonin and norepinephrine. While both neurotransmitters are affected, there is a 30-fold higher affinity for serotonin-reuptake inhibition relative to norepinephrine [103]. The norepinephrine reuptake is thought to contribute most to analgesia, occurring dose-dependently above 100 mg/day [103].

(b) Evidence for Migraine Prophylaxis as Monotherapy
The 2012 American Academy of Neurology guideline on pharmacologic migraine prophylaxis classifies the evidence supporting venlafaxine as level B: probably effective and should be considered for migraine prevention [63]. In a single randomized placebo-controlled blinded study, venlafaxine XR (extended release formulation) dose-dependently reduced the number of headache days:

150 mg (−4 days), 75 mg (−2 days), and placebo (−1 day), $p < 0.006$ [63]. When efficacy was compared against amitriptyline for migraine prophylaxis in a randomized study, both were effective in reducing migraine attack frequency without clear superiority [63].

(c) Adverse Effects

Common side effects include the following: hypertension (3–13%), sweating (7–25%), weight loss (3–47%), nausea (21–58%), dry mouth (12–22%), constipation (8–15%), headache (25–38%), insomnia (14–24%), somnolence (14–26%), and erectile dysfunction (2–6%) [8]. Hyponatremia and hepatitis are rare complications [8]. Of note, drug-drug interactions are possible as venlafaxine is liver metabolized by CYP-2D6 and CYP-3A3/4 [103].

Duloxetine

(a) Mechanism of Action

Duloxetine also prevents presynaptic reuptake of serotonin and norepinephrine, but duloxetine has a tenfold selectivity favoring serotonin over norepinephrine [104].

(b) Evidence for Chronic Burning Mouth Syndrome (BMS) and Atypical Odontalgia (AO)

There are unfortunately no current randomized controlled studies of SNRI's in atypical odontalgia or burning mouth syndrome. However, in an open-label, prospective study evaluating 20–40 mg daily duloxetine in 29 patients over 12 weeks, VAS levels were significantly decreased from 55.4 to 26.4, with significance first achieved at 2 weeks of medication use. At 12 weeks, 51.7% of patients achieved 50% analgesia, and analgesia was found to be unrelated to depression levels [105].

(c) Adverse Effects

Common side effects include the following: hypertension (2%), diaphoresis (up to 6%), constipation (9–10%), nausea (18–23%), dry mouth (11–14%), headache (13–18%), and hypersomnia/insomnia (7–10%). Liver failure is a very rare but serious adverse effect. Increased depression has also rarely occurred but should be monitored by the prescribing physician.

Milnacipran

(a) Mechanism of Action

Unlike venlafaxine and duloxetine, milnacipran blocks the reuptake of serotonin and norepinephrine with almost equal affinity [104].

(b) Evidence for Chronic Burning Mouth Syndrome (BMS) and Atypical Odontalgia (AO)

There are unfortunately no current randomized controlled studies of SNRI's in atypical odontalgia or burning mouth syndrome. However, in an open-label, prospective study evaluating 15–100 mg daily milnacipran in 32 patients over 12 weeks, VAS levels were significantly decreased from 46.7 to 27.7, and analgesia was found to be unrelated to depression levels [106].

(c) Adverse Effects
Common side effects include the following: hypertension (5–18%), tachycardia (6–8%), diaphoresis (9%), constipation (16%), nausea (37%), dry mouth (5%), headache (18%), and insomnia (12%). Liver failure is a very rare but serious adverse effect. Increased depression has also rarely occurred and should be monitored by the prescribing physician

Tricyclic Antidepressants (TCAs)

Amitriptyline

(a) Mechanisms of Action
Tricyclic antidepressants (TCAs) achieve pain control through a complex array of mechanisms. The descending bulbospinal inhibitory pathway is harnessed through blocking reuptake of both norepinephrine and serotonin [104, 107]. The noradrenergic effect is thought to be the primary analgesic mechanism. The increased levels of norepinephrine and serotonin at the synaptic cleft augment inhibitory action on secondary pain neurons at the spinal cord. This decreases nociception [108]. Additionally TCAs block adenosine reuptake and antagonize sodium channels. Amitriptyline possesses the greatest potency among this class of medications for sodium channel blockade [104]. Tricyclic antidepressants also variably block histaminic and cholinergic (both muscarinic and nicotinic) receptors. This greatly contributes to their side effect profile [104]. Tertiary amine TCAs such as amitriptyline have greater antihistamine and anticholinergic effects relative to secondary amines such as nortriptyline or desipramine [104]. Importantly, analgesic properties of TCA's are independent of their antidepressant effect, with their pain-relieving benefit occurring more rapidly and at lower doses relative to mood improvement [104].

(b) Evidence for Migraine Prophylaxis as Monotherapy
The 2012 American Academy of Neurology guideline on pharmacologic migraine prophylaxis classifies the evidence supporting amitriptyline as level B: probably effective and should be considered for migraine prevention. It was downgraded from prior level A rating (established as effective) due to supportive studies having >20% dropout rates [63].

(c) Evidence for Postherpetic Neuralgia (PHN)
While PHN may affect facial trigeminal regions, no randomized study has focused exclusively on facial pain patients. Instead most studies included a mixed population with varied dermatomal involvement. Moore and colleagues reviewed five randomized studies in a 2015 Cochrane analysis comprising 227 total patients;

the longest study duration was 8 weeks [109]. In the active controlled studies, amitriptyline was found to be equally efficacious to nortriptyline or desipramine. Placebo-controlled trials revealed improved analgesia with amitriptyline [109].

(d) Adverse Effects
TCA side effects are secondary to their effects on various neurotransmitter systems. Tertiary amines like amitriptyline cause more sedation attributable to the antihistamine impact. This can be beneficial for patients suffering from insomnia [108]. Orthostasis and dizziness are secondary to effects on adrenergic receptors. Dry mouth, constipation, and urinary retention are due to anticholinergic side effects. Tachyarrhythmia and prolonged QTc are also rare but noteworthy possibilities. Amitriptyline should be used with caution in fragile elderly patients due to risk of over sedation and mental status changes [108].

Nortriptyline

(a) Mechanism of Action
Nortriptyline is a tricyclic antidepressant active metabolite of amitriptyline [107]. Unlikely amitriptyline, nortriptyline has a secondary amine chemical structure with less activity at acetylcholine, histamine, and alpha-adrenergic receptors [104]. Its mechanism of action is similar to that of amitriptyline, except nortriptyline is less effective at sodium channel blockade [104].

(b) Evidence for Migraine Prophylaxis with Combination Therapy
Krymchantowski and colleagues evaluated 80 chronic migraineurs with less than 50% headache frequency improvement at 8 weeks using prophylactic monotherapy with either topiramate 50 mg bid or nortriptyline 30 mg nightly. For the baseline topiramate group, addition of nortriptyline resulted in at least 50% reduction in headache frequency in 70% of patients. This is compared to an improvement of 47% in patients treated with placebo ($p = 0.04$) [110].

(c) Adverse Effects
The most common side effects include constipation, dry mouth, dizziness, orthostatic hypotension, and fatigue. TCA's also increase the corrected QT (QTc) interval. At clinical doses, nortriptyline is thought to have a minor effect on QTc, though drug overdose can result in lethal arrhythmia from QTc prolongation [111].

Topicals

Lidocaine

(a) Mechanism of Action
Lidocaine is an amide local anesthetic that provides analgesic benefits from reduction of signal transmission via blockade of sodium channels on the neuronal surface. Decreased permeability of neuronal membranes to sodium

influx halts the propagation of pain signaling [112]. Lidocaine also functions in a use-dependent fashion. This may underlie its clinical utility for different pathologic conditions. Topical lidocaine has been shown in certain disease processes to have analgesic effects without anesthetizing the skin [112].

(b) Evidence for Migraines
Intranasal lidocaine is believed to work for headaches by blocking signaling from the Vidian nerve, sphenopalatine ganglion (SPG), or maxillary branch of trigeminal nerve [113]. One randomized control trial showed a two-point reduction on the visual analog scale in patients with migraines and tension-type headaches after the use of intranasal lidocaine compared to placebo [113]. This effect was noted at 1 min post-inhalation and persisted for a 30 min follow-up period.

(c) Evidence for Autonomic Cephalgias: (Cluster Headache, Paroxysmal Hemicrania, and Short-Lasting Unilateral Neuralgiform Headache with Conjunctival Injection and Tearing)
Given the acute nature of these attacks, lidocaine has been used as an abortive treatment with moderate success. Intranasal lidocaine has been found to be effective for almost one-third of patients with cluster headaches, while additionally 27% obtained mild relief [114]. A recent review highlights that intranasal lidocaine (4 and 10%) has been effective as an abortive therapy for these headache syndromes [115].

(d) Evidence for Trigeminal Neuralgia
Recent case reports have shown that 5% topical lidocaine is effective for about half of patients with trigeminal neuropathic pain. Patients with allodynia, hyperalgesia, and neuropathic pain secondary to facial postherpetic neuralgia all have improved outcomes when topical lidocaine is a component of their analgesic regimen [116]. Continuous pain was more responsive to topical lidocaine compared to episodic pain. In a small series, 85% of patients reported benefit with topical use of 5% lidocaine for their orofacial pain [117]. Eleven out of 14 patients had a pain reduction of greater than two points on the visual analog scale, and 9 of 14 patients were able to decrease the use of adjuvant medications.

(e) Side Effects
Topical application of lidocaine is associated with generally low risk of adverse events. When used as directed, the most common side effects are application site erythema and pruritus [112, 118]. Systemic absorption is possible, although usually minimal. IN such a case, systemic toxicity leading to cardiovascular effects (bradycardia, hypotension, arrest) and central nervous system effects (seizures, confusion, visual changes, tinnitus, and unconsciousness) have been reported [118].

Capsaicin

(a) Mechanism of Action
Capsaicin is a component of plants from the nightshade variety. It is thought to exert its effects via the agonist activity at the TRPV1 receptor on Aδ and C fibers. This leads to the release of substance P and calcitonin gene-related peptide.

Topical application results in nerve fiber degeneration beneath the application site [112].

(b) Evidence for Migraines

A small randomized control trial showed that patients using intranasal capsaicin had fewer headaches and less severe headaches when compared to placebo [119]. In this study, 3% capsaicin was used intranasally for 7 days, and patients in the treatment group had an average decrease in pain score of over 2.5 points on a 10-point scale

(c) Evidence for Cluster Headaches

There is little evidence that capsaicin may be effective for cluster headaches. Application of capsaicin to the ipsilateral nostril appears to be more effective than application to the contralateral side for patients with acute cluster attacks, but due to local irritation, this treatment was poorly tolerated [120].

(d) Side Effects

The most common side effect is local skin irritation [112]. The burning sensation may lessen with repeated use. Erythema (63%) at the application site, pain (42%), nausea/vomiting (5%), and hypertension (2%) are the most common adverse effects [118]. Additionally, treated skin may be more sensitive to heat following capsaicin use.

Migraine Prophylactics

Botulinum Toxin

(a) Mechanism of Action

Botulinum toxin is derived from the naturally occurring toxin produced by various strains of *Clostridium botulinum*. The toxin is a metalloproteinase that cleaves certain peptide bonds that are necessary for vesicle fusion at the neuron terminal [121]. The primary mechanism of action is inhibition of acetylcholine release at neuromuscular junctions. The result is impairment of neuromuscular transmission and flaccid paralysis of the targeted muscle. Botulinum toxin is believed to work for migraine prophylaxis through prevention of the release of calcitonin gene-related peptide and substance P, by cleaving membrane peptides necessary for vesicle fusion and release [121].

(b) Evidence

Stereotyped injection of botulinum into the facial and neck muscles has been shown in multiple studies to provide substantial prevention of chronic migraine headaches. Total headache days per month and severity of headache episodes were decreased for patients treated with botulinum toxin injection versus placebo [122]. Studies also show that in nonresponders to initial treatment, there has been benefit derived with a second series of injections [122].

(c) Side Effects

Neck pain (8.7%) and muscular weakness (5.5%) along with injection site irritation are among the most common adverse effects from botulinum toxin injection for migraine prevention [122]. Less severe side effects include eyelid ptosis and myalgia of injected muscles.

Beta-Blockers

(a) Mechanism of Action
Beta-blockers are the name given to a class of medications that antagonize beta-adrenergic receptors. While there are three forms of beta receptors which have various distinct functions, nonselective medications and medications that are selective for beta-1 receptors are effective in migraine treatment. Beta-blockers aid in migraine prevention through modulation of the central nervous system catecholamines as well as interaction with serotoninergic receptors. It is also believed that propranolol may have membrane-stabilizing effects which may contribute to its analgesic properties [123].

(b) Evidence
Propranolol, timolol, and metoprolol have been approved for migraine prevention according to evidence-based guidelines from the American Association of Neurology [63]. All of these medications have shown to decrease migraine days or frequency of attack by 50%. Several randomized controlled trials show that each agent is effective for reduction of headache days, duration of headaches, and headache severity. [63, 124]. In the review, Silberstein gives a level A (highest) recommendation for the use of propranolol, timolol, and metoprolol for migraine prophylactic treatment.

(c) Side Effects
Adverse effects from this class of medications include fatigue (1–10%), sleep disorders, depression (5%), decreased exercise tolerance, orthostatic hypotension, significant bradycardia, and impotence [118]. Contraindications include acute congestive heart failure, asthma, and insulin-dependent diabetes, although metoprolol may be suitable in asthma and DM due to its preserved beta-1 selectivity [124].

Calcium Channel Blockers

(a) Mechanism of Action
Calcium channel blockers antagonize the binding of calcium to receptors located in the heart, vascular smooth muscle, neuronal cells, and adrenal gland. The benefit in migraine treatment is believed to be related to elicited vasodilation and the prevention of cerebral vasospasm as well as neurotransmitter modulation [125].

(b) Evidence
While calcium channel blockers have been studied for migraine prophylaxis, evidence shows that they do not have benefit versus placebo for migraine prevention and are likely not effective [63].

(c) Side Effects
Known adverse effects of calcium antagonists include dizziness (4–23%), hypotension (4%), headache (>10%), constipation (2–9%), peripheral edema (>10%), flushing (>10%), and mood changes (7%) [118].

ACE Inhibitors/ARB Blockers

(a) Mechanism of Action
Angiotensin-converting enzyme inhibitors (ACE-I) and angiotensin II receptor blockers (ARB) both function by disrupting the renin-angiotensin-aldosterone system. The resultant action is vasodilation, modulation of sympathetic activity, and alteration of neurotransmitter processing (substance P, dopamine, encephalin, and serotonin). These actions are believed to underlie the effective migraine reduction attributable to ACE-I and ARB [126].
(b) Evidence
Recent studies have looked at lisinopril, candesartan, and telmisartan for migraine prophylaxis. Positive evidence for lisinopril and candesartan shows reduction in headache severity and headache days compared to placebo [63]. Telmisartan, on the other hand, did not show benefit for migraine prevention [63].
(c) Side Effects
Common side effects from this class of drug include cough (4–9%), muscle cramps, fatigue, dizziness, and headache (4–6%) [118]. More severe reactions include angioedema of the face, lips, throat, or GI tract as well as pancreatitis, mood changes, and bone marrow suppression [118].

Migraine Abortives

Triptans

(a) Mechanism of Action
Triptans are agonists of the serotonin type 1B and type 1D receptors (5HT 1B/D). Triptans are potent vasoconstrictors that work via extracerebral vasoconstriction and inhibition of transmitter release via the trigeminovascular network [124].
(b) Evidence
Sumatriptan is the oldest of the triptans and has strong evidence to its efficacy in abortive treatment for migraines. Available in a variety of delivery mechanisms (oral, subcutaneous, transdermal), sumatriptan has been shown to be effective in degree of pain reduction, time to maximal pain reduction, as well as prevention of migraine recurrence [124, 127]. Sumatriptan has proven to be superior to ergot derivatives and with a safer side effect profile.

Second-generation triptans include zolmitriptan, naratriptan, rizatriptan, almotriptan, eletriptan, and frovatriptan. In multiple trials, these agents have proven effective in acute migraine treatment. These drugs have been shown to be more efficacious than placebo and work in patients that have not responded to NSAIDs [124].

(c) Side Effects
Triptans side effects include a variety of unsettling feelings characterized as "triptan sensations" [127]—paresthesias (5–14%), flushing, tingling, neck pain, and mild transient chest pressure (2–5%). Other known side effects include dizziness (12%), abdominal distress (1%), as well as cardiovascular complications (vasospasm, hypertension, palpitations, and arrhythmias) [118].

Ergot Derivatives

(a) Mechanism of Action
Ergotamine and dihydroergotamine are synthetic agonists of the 5HT receptor. This class of drugs is a potent intracranial and extracerebral vasoconstrictor as well as an inhibitor of trigeminal neurotransmission. This action is very similar to that of triptans [124].

(b) Evidence
Ergot derivatives were the first approved drugs for acute migraine treatment. Ergotamine and dihydroergotaminc are effective in the terminating headaches but carry a weak recommendation for their use due to the severity of side effects [124, 127]. When compared to aspirin and other NSAIDs, these drugs showed greater initial response and more sustained response but had a higher side effect profile.

(c) Side Effects
Ergot derivatives are known to have various side effects related to activity at not only serotonergic receptors but also dopaminergic and adrenergic receptors. Severe adverse reactions include cardiovascular effects (angina, hypertension, vascular spasm, and tachycardia) as well as peripheral ischemia [118]. These medications are also associated with rebound headaches, fatigue, and potential for spontaneous fetal abortion. Due to the significant side effects, ergot derivatives are currently not considered the drug of choice for acute migraine treatment.

Cannabinoids

(a) Mechanism of Action
The endocannabinoid system is postulated to play a role in the pathophysiology of migraines and is important in acute and chronic pain states such as

central and peripheral neuropathic conditions [128]. Currently, there are two known receptor targets in this system, CB1 and CB2. The CB1 receptor is localized primarily in the central nervous system. The CB2 receptor is primarily found in the periphery. The CB1 receptor is known to be important in the modulation of pain transmission through inhibition of neurotransmitters including dopamine, glutamine, and serotonin [129]. Current data demonstrates that the CB2 receptor is the more important mediator of anti-nociception as well as anti-inflammation. Tetrahydrocannabinol (THC) and cannabidiol (CBD) have been shown to have analgesic effects related to a reduction in hyperalgesic pathways and anti-inflammatory mechanisms that are independent of cyclooxygenase [130]. These same substances have been shown to have neuroprotective effects that relate to inhibition of glutamate toxicity and antioxidant properties [130].

(b) Evidence for Pain States
Cannabinoids that work at the CB2 receptor show efficacy for models of migraine and trigeminal neuropathic states [129]. Cannabinoids are believed to be more effective in pain states that involve hyperalgesia and inflammation, such as HIV and peripheral neuropathy, multiple sclerosis, and rheumatoid arthritis [131]. Sativex is a specific combination of THC and CBD which is delivered as an oral spray. It is not currently approved in the United States; however, it has been shown to be useful in central pain and peripheral neuropathic pain states with allodynia [130].

(c) Side Effects
The side effect profile of currently available cannabinoids may limit more widespread adoption. In addition, the legality of their wide commercial use is currently being debated. Dronabinol, a drug currently approved for chemotherapy-induced nauseas/vomiting, has been shown in the literature to have modest analgesic effects [130], but it has a high side effect profile. These include somnolence, paranoia, depression/emotional lability, dizziness, and cognitive dysfunction. Nabilone has a high incidence of vertigo (52%), sedation (52%), euphoria/dysphoria (11%), sleep disturbance (11%), and visual changes (13%) as listed adverse effects [118]. The adverse effects of Sativex may be milder. These include dry mouth/poor taste (<10%), nausea (<10%), fatigue (>10%), and euphoria (<10%) [118, 132]. While cannabinoids are not currently approved for nonmalignant chronic pain syndromes, future indications may include pain states such as trigeminal neuralgia, cluster headaches, and migraines.

References

1. Ambrosio AF, Soares-da-Silva P, Carvalho CM, Carvalho AP. Mechanisms of action of carbamazepine and its derivatives, oxcarbazepine, BIA 2-093, and BIA 2-024*. Neurochem Res. 2002;27(1):121–30.
2. Blom S. Tic douloureux treated with new anticonvulsant. Experiences with G32883. Arch Neurol. 1963;9:285–90.

3. Campbell FG, Graham JG, Zilkha KJ. Clinical trial of carbamazepine (tegretol) in trigeminal neuralgia. J Neurol Neurosurg Psychiatry. 1966;29(3):265–7.
4. Rockliff BW, Davis EH. Controlled sequential trials of carbamazepine in trigeminal neuralgia. Arch Neurol. 1966;15(2):129–36.
5. Killian JM, Fromm GH. Carbamazepine in the treatment of neuralgia. Use of side effects. Arch Neurol. 1968;19(2):129–36.
6. Nicol CF. A four year double-blind study of tegretol in facial pain. Headache. 1969;9(1):54–7.
7. Cruccu G, et al. AAN-EFNS guidelines on trigeminal neuralgia management. Eur J Neurol. 2008;15:1013–28.
8. Micromedex Drug Reference Essentials App; 2017; micromedex.com/mobile.
9. McQuay H, Carroll D, Jadad AR, et al. Anticonvulsant drugs for management of pain: a systematic review. BMJ. 1995;311:1047–52.
10. Wiffen P, Collins S, Carroll D, et al. Anticonvulsant drugs for acute and chronic pain. Cochrane Database Syst Rev. 2005;(3):CD001133.
11. Wiffen P, McQuay H, Moore R. Carbamazepine for acute and chronic pain. Cochrane Database Syst Rev. 2005;(3):CD005451.
12. Dougherty JA, Rhoney DH. Gabapentin: a unique anti-epileptic agent. Neurol Res. 2001;23:821–9.
13. Errante LD, Williamson A, Spencer DD, Petroff OAC. Gabapentin and vigabatrin increase GABA in the human neocortical slice. Epilepsy Res. 2002;49:203–10.
14. Petroff OAC, Rothman DL, Behar KL, Lamoureux D, Mattson RH. The effect of gabapentin on brain gamma-aminobutyric acid in patients with epilepsy. Ann Neurol. 1996;39:95–9.
15. Whitworth TL, Quick MW. Upregulation of γ-aminobutyric acid transporter expression: role of alkylated γ-aminobutyric acid derivatives. Biochem Soc Trans. 2001;29:736–41.
16. Freiman TM, Kukolja J, Heinemeyer J, Eckhardt K, Aranda H, Rominger A, Dooley DJ, Zentner J, Feuerstein TJ. Modulation of K+-evoked [3H]-noradrenaline release from rat and human brain slices by gabapentin: involvement of KATP channels. Naunyn Schmiedebergs Arch Pharmacol. 2001;363:537–42.
17. Jaggi AS, Singh N. Role of different brain areas in peripheral nerve injury-induced neuropathic pain. Brain Res. 2011;1381:187–201.
18. Jarvis SE, Zamponi GW. Trafficking and regulation of neuronal voltage gated calcium channels. Curr Opin Cell Biol. 2007;19:474–82.
19. Morimoto S, Ito M, Oda S, Sugiyama A, Kuroda M, Adachi-Akahane S. Spinal mechanism underlying the antiallodynic effect of gabapentin studied in the mouse spinal nerve ligation model. J Pharmacol Sci. 2012;118:455–66.
20. Yaksh TL. Calcium channels as therapeutic targets in neuropathic pain. J Pain. 2006;7(1 Suppl 1):S13–30.
21. Taylor CP. The biology and pharmacology of α2-δ proteins. CNS Drug Rev. 2004;10:183–8.
22. Kukkar A, Bali A, Singh N, et al. Arch Pharm Res. 2013;36:237.
23. Moore RA, Wiffen PJ, Derry S, Toelle T, Rice ASC. Gabapentin for chronic neuropathic pain and fibromyalgia in adults. Cochrane Database Syst Rev. 2014;(4):CD007938.
24. Khan OA. Gabapentin relieves trigeminal neuralgia in multiple sclerosis patients. Neurology. 1998;51:611.
25. Solaro C, Lunardi GL, Capello E. An open-label trial of gabapentin treatment of paroxysmal symptoms in multiple sclerosis patients. Neurology. 1998;51:609–11.
26. Solaro C, Messmer Uccelli M, et al. Low-dose gabapentin combined with either lamotrigine or carbamazepine can be useful therapies for trigeminal neuralgia in multiple sclerosis. Eur Neurol. 2000;44:45–8.
27. Rozen TD. Relief of anesthesia dolorosa with gabapentin. Headache. 1999;39:761.
28. Sawada T, Asai J, Nomiyama T, Masuda K, Takenaka H, Katoh N. Trigeminal trophic syndrome: report of a case and review of the published work. J Dermatol. 2014;41:525–8.
29. White TL, Kent PF, Kurtz DB, Emko P. Effectiveness of gabapentin for treatment of burning mouth syndrome. Arch Otolaryngol Head Neck Sug. 2004;130:786–8.

30. Heckmann SM, Heckman JG, Ungethum A, Hujoel P, Hummel T. Gabapentin has little or no effect in the treatment of burning mouth syndrome—results of an open-label pilot study. Eur J Neurol. 2006;13:e6–7.
31. López-D'Alessandro E, Escovich L. Combination of alpha lipoic acid and gabapentin, its efficacy in the treatment of burning mouth syndrome: a randomized, double-blind, placebo controlled trial. Med Oral Patol Oral Cir Bucal. 2011;16(5):e635–40.
32. Li Z, et al. Pregabalin is a potent and selective ligand for α(2)δ-1 and α(2)δ-2 calcium channel subunits. Eur J Pharmacol. 2001;667:80–90.
33. Lotarski SM, et al. Anxiolytic-like activity of pregabalin in the Vogel conflict test in α2δ-1 (R217A) and α2δ-2 (R279A) mouse mutants. J Pharmacol Exp Ther. 2011;338:615–21.
34. Dolphin AC. Calcium channel auxiliary alpha2delta and beta subunits: trafficking and one step beyond. Nat Rev Neurosci. 2012;13:542–55.
35. Tuchman M, et al. Central sensitization and Ca(V)α2δ ligands in chronic pain syndromes: pathologic processes and pharmacologic effect. J Pain. 2010;11:1241–9.
36. Bauer CS, et al. The anti-allodynic alpha(2)delta ligand pregabalin inhibits the trafficking of the calcium channel alpha(2)delta-1 subunit to presynaptic terminals in vivo. Biochem Soc Trans. 2010;38:525–8.
37. Takeuchi Y, et al. Pregabalin, S-(+)-3-isobutylgaba, activates the descending noradrenergic system to alleviate neuropathic pain in the mouse partial sciatic nerve ligation model. Neuropharmacology. 2007;53:842–53.
38. Dworkin RH, Corbin AE, Young JP Jr, Sharma U, LaMoreaux L, Bockbrader H, Garofalo EA, Poole RM. Pregabalin for the treatment of postherpetic neuralgia: a randomized, placebo-controlled trial. Neurology. 2003;60(8):1274.
39. Sabatowski R, Gálvez R, Cherry DA, Jacquot F, Vincent E, Maisonobe P, Versavel M. Pregabalin reduces pain and improves sleep and mood disturbances in patients with post-herpetic neuralgia: results of a randomised, placebo-controlled clinical trial. Pain. 2004;109(1–2):26.
40. Moore RA, Straube S, Wiffen PJ, Derry S, McQuay HJ. Pregabalin for acute and chronic pain in adults. Cochrane Database Syst Rev. 2009;(3):CD007076.
41. Tunnicliff G. Basis of the antiseizure action of phenytoin. Gen Pharmacol. 1996;27(7):1091–7.
42. Patejdl R, Leroux AC, Noack T. Phenytoin inhibits contractions of rat gastrointestinal and portal vein smooth muscle by inhibiting calcium entry. Neurogastroenterol Motil. 2015;27(10):1453–65.
43. Colombo E, Franceschetti S, Avanzini G, Mantegazza M. Phenytoin inhibits the persistent sodium current in neocortical neurons by modifying its inactivation properties. PLoS One. 2013;8(1):e55329.
44. Thorn CF, Whirl-Carrillo M, Leeder JS, Klein TE, Altman RB. Phar-mGKB summary: phenytoin pathway. Pharmacogenet Genomics. 2012;22(6):466–70.
45. Bergouignan M. Cures heureuses de nevralgies faciales essentielles par le diphenylhydantoinate de soude. Rev Laryngol Otol Rhinol. 1942;63:34–41.
46. Chadda VS, Mathur MS. Double blind study of the effects of diphenylhydantoin sodium on diabetic neuropathy. J Assoc Physicians India. 1978;26(5):403–6.
47. Saudek CD, Werns S, Reidenberg MM. Phenytoin in the treatment of diabetic symmetrical polyneuropathy. Clin Pharmacol Ther. 1977;22(2):196–9.
48. McCleane GJ. Intravenous infusion of phenytoin relieves neuropathic pain: a randomized, double-blinded, placebo-controlled, crossover study. Anesth Analg. 1999;89(4):985–8.
49. Birse F, Derry S, Moore RA. Phenytoin for neuropathic pain and fibromyalgia in adults. Cochrane Database Syst Rev. 2012;(5):CD009485.
50. Galletti F, Cupini LM, Corbelli I, Calabresi P, Sarchielli P. Pathophysiological basis of migraine prophylaxis. Prog Neurobiol. 2009;89:176–92.
51. Herrero AI, Del Olmo N, Gonzalez-Escalada JR, Solis JM. Two new actions of topiramate: inhibition of depolarizing GABA(a)-mediated responses and activation of a potassium conductance. Neuropharmacology. 2002;42:210–20.

52. Sun GC, Werkman TR, Battefeld A, Clare JJ, Wadman WJ. Carbamazepine and topiramate modulation of transient and persistent sodium currents studied in HEK293 cells expressing the Na(v)1.3 alpha-subunit. Epilepsia. 2007;48:774–82.
53. Kuzmiski JB, Barr W, Zamponi GW, MacVicar BA. Topiramate inhibits the initiation of plateau potentials in CA1 neurons by depressing R-type calcium channels. Epilepsia. 2005;46:481–9.
54. Gibbs JW 3rd, Sombati S, DeLorenzo RJ, Coulter DA. Cellular actions of topiramate: blockade of kainate-evoked inward currents in cultured hippocampal neurons. Epilepsia. 2000;41:S10–6.
55. Poulsen CF, Simeone TA, Maar TE, Smith-Swintosky V, White HS, Schousboe A. Modulation by topiramate of AMPA and kainate mediated calcium influx in cultured cerebral cortical, hippocampal and cerebellar neurons. Neurochem Res. 2004;29:275–82.
56. Braga MFM, Aroniadou-Anderjaska V, Li H, Rogawski MA. Topiramate reduces excitability in the basolateral amygdala by selectively inhibiting GluK1 (GluR5) kainate receptors on interneurons and positively modulating GABAa receptors on principal neurons. J Pharmacol Exp Ther. 2009;330:558–66.
57. Kanda T, Kurokawa M, Tamura S, et al. Topiramate reduces abnormally high extracellular levels of glutamate and aspartate in the hippocampus of spontaneously epileptic rats (SER). Life Sci. 1996;59:1607–16.
58. Edvinsson L, Linde M. New drugs in migraine treatment and prophylaxis: telcagepant and topiramate. Lancet. 2010;376(9741):645–55.
59. Brandes JL, Saper JR, Diamond M, Couch JR, Lewis DW, Schmitt J, Neto W, Schwabe S, Jacobs D. Topiramate for migraine prevention: a randomized controlled trial. JAMA. 2004;291(8):965.
60. Silberstein SD, Neto W, Schmitt J, Jacobs D. Topiramate in migraine prevention: results of a large controlled trial. Arch Neurol. 2004;61(4):490.
61. Linde M, Mulleners WM, Chronicle EP, McCrory DC. Topiramate for the prophylaxis of episodic migraine in adults. Cochrane Database Syst Rev. 2013;(6):CD010610.
62. Linde M, Mulleners WM, Chronicle EP, McCrory DC. Valproate (valproic acid or sodium valproate or a combination of the two) for the prophylaxis of episodic migraine in adults. Cochrane Database Syst Rev. 2013;(6):CD010611.
63. Silberstein SD, et al. Evidence-based guideline update: pharmacologic treatment for episodic migraine prevention in adults (Report of the quality standards subcommittee of the American Academy of Neurology and the American Headache Society). Neurology. 2012;78:1337–45.
64. Zvartau-Hind M, Din MU, Gilani A, et al. Topiramate relieves refractory trigeminal neuralgia in MS patients. Neurology. 2000;55:1587–8.
65. Domingues RB, Kuster GW, Aquino CC. Treatment of trigeminal neuralgia with low dose topiramate. Arq Neuropsiquiatr. 2007;65(3B):792–4.
66. Wang QP, Bai M. Topiramate versus carbamazepine for the treatment of classical trigeminal neuralgia: a meta-analysis. CNS Drugs. 2011;25:847–57.
67. Al-Quliti KW. Update on neuropathic pain treatment for trigeminal neuralgia: the pharmacological and surgical options. Neurosciences. 2015;20(2):107–14.
68. Volcy M, Rapoport AM, Tepper SJ, et al. Persistent idiopathic facial pain responsive to topiramate. Cephalalgia. 2006;26:489.
69. Adelman J, Freitag FG, Lainez M, et al. Analysis of safety and tolerability data obtained from over 1,500 patients receiving topiramate for migraine prevention in controlled trials. Pain Med. 2008;9:175–85.
70. Silberstein SD. Topiramate in migraine prevention: a 2016 perspective. Headache. 2017;57:165–78.
71. Silberstein SD, Saper J, Berenson F, Somogyi M, McCague K, D'Souza J. Oxcarbazepine in migraine headache: a double-blind, randomized, placebo-controlled study. Neurology. 2008;70(7):548–55.

72. Wiffen PJ, Collins S, McQuay HJ, Carroll D, Jadad A, Moore RA. Anticonvulsant drugs for acute and chronic pain. Cochrane Database Syst Rev. 2010;(1):CD001133.
73. Toth M. The epsilon theory: a novel synthesis of the underlying molecular and electrophysiological mechanisms of primary generalized epilepsy and the possible mechanism of action of valproate. Med Hypotheses. 2005;64(2):267–72.
74. Cutrer FM, Limmroth V, Moskowitz MA. Possible mechanisms of valproate in migraine prophylaxis. Cephalalgia. 1997;17(2):93–100.
75. Evers S, Afra J, Frese A, Goadsby PJ, Linde M, May A, et al. European Federation of Neurological Societies. EFNS guideline on the drug treatment of migraine—revised report of an EFNS task force. Eur J Neurol. 2009;16(9):968–81.
76. Kochar DK, Garg P, Bumb RA, Kochar SK, Mehta RD, Beniwal R, et al. Divalproex sodium in the management of post-herpetic neuralgia: a randomized double-blind placebo-controlled study. QJM. 2005;98(1):29–34.
77. Kochar DK, Rawat N, Agrawal RP, Vyas A, Beniwal R, Kochar SK, et al. Sodium valproate for painful diabetic neuropathy: a randomized double-blind placebo-controlled study. QJM. 2004;97(1):33–8.
78. Gill D, Derry S, Wiffen PJ, Moore RA. Valproic acid and sodium valproate for neuropathic pain and fibromyalgia in adults. Cochrane Database Syst Rev. 2011;(10):CD009183.
79. Green GA. Understanding NSAIDs: from aspirin to Cox-2. Clin Cornerstone. 2001;3(5):50–60.
80. Brogan S, et al. Non-opiate analgesics. In: Hemmings H, Egan T, editors. Pharmacology and physiology for anesthesia: foundations and clinical application (Chapter 16). 1st ed. 2013. Saunders: Elsevier.
81. Minor J, Hofhines A. The discovery of aspirin's antithrombotic effects. Tex Heart Inst J. 2007;34(2):179–86.
82. Ta LE, Dionne RA. Treatment of painful temporomandibular joints with a cyclooxygenase-2 inhibitor: a randomized placebo-controlled comparison of celecoxib to naproxen. Pain. 2004;111(1–2):13–21.
83. Varoli F, et al. Analgesia evaluation of 2 NSAID drugs as adjuvant in management of chronic temporomandibular disorders. Sci World J. 2015;2015:359152.
84. Senye M, et al. Topical nonsteroidal anti-inflammatory medications for treatment of temporomandibular joint degenerative pain: a systematic review. J Orofac Pain. 2012;26(1):26–32.
85. Page J, Henry D. Consumption of NSAIDs and the development of congestive heart failure in elderly patients: an underrecognized health problem. Arch Intern Med. 2000;160(6):777–84.
86. Barnes P. How corticosteroids control inflammation: Quintiles Prize Lecture 2005. Br J Pharmacol. 2006;148(3):245–54.
87. Delecoeuillerie G, et al. Polymyalgia rheumatica and temporal arteritis: a retrospective analysis of prognostic features and different corticosteroid regimens. Ann Rheum Dis. 1988;47(9):733–9.
88. Lundberg I, Hedfors E. Restricted dose and duration of corticosteroid treatment in patients with polymyalgia rheumatica and temporal arteritis. J Rheumatol. 1990;17(10):1340–5.
89. Jivraj I, Tamhankar M. The treatment of giant cell arteritis. Curr Treat Options Neurol. 2017;19(1):2.
90. Beck RW, et al. A randomized, controlled trial of corticosteroids in the treatment of acute optic neuritis. The OpticNeuritis Study Group. N Engl J Med. 1992;326(9):581–8.
91. Sellebjerg F, et al. A randomized, controlled trial of oral high-dose methylprednisolone in acute optic neuritis. Neurology. 1999;52(7):1479–984.
92. Smith JL, Taxdal DS. Painful ophthalmoplegia. The Tolosa-Hunt syndrome. Am J Ophthalmol. 1966;61(6):1466–72.
93. Hannerz J. Recurrent Tolosa-Hunt syndrome. Cephalalgia. 1992;12(1):45–51.
94. Cakirer S. MRI findings in Tolosa-Hunt syndrome before and after systemic corticosteroid therapy. Eur J Radiol. 2003;45(2):83–90.
95. Zurawski J, Akhondi H. Tolosa-Hunt syndrome—a rare cause of headache and ophthalmoplegia. Lancet. 2013;382(9895):912.

96. Lal V, et al. Ophthalmoplegia with migraine in adults: is it ophthalmoplegic migraine? Headache. 2009;49(6):838–50.
97. Proven A, et al. Glucocorticoid therapy in giant cell arteritis: duration and adverse outcomes. Arthritis Care Res. 2003;49(5):703–8.
98. Fromm GH, et al. Baclofen in the treatment of trigeminal neuralgia: double-blind study and long-term follow-up. Ann Neurol. 1984;15:240–4.
99. Yomiya K, et al. Baclofen as an adjuvant analgesic for cancer pain. Am J Hosp Palliat Med. 2009;26(2):112–8.
100. Saper JR, et al. Chronic daily headache prophylaxis with tizanidine: a double-blind, placebo-controlled, multicenter outcome study. Headache. 2002;42:470–82.
101. Fogelholm R, Murros K. Tizanidine in chronic tension type headache: a placebo controlled double blind crossover study. Headache. 1992;32:509–13.
102. Freitag FG. Preventative treatment for migraine and tension-type headaches: do drugs having effects on muscle spasm and tone have a role? CNS Drugs. 2003;17(6):373–81.
103. Aiyer R, et al. Treatment of neuropathic pain with venlafaxine: a systematic review. Pain Med. 2016;18(10):1999–2012.
104. Smith HS, et al. Antidepressants as analgesics. In: Benzon H, Rathmell JP, editors. Practical management of pain (Chapter 38). 5th ed; 2014.
105. Nagashima W, et al. Effectiveness of duloxetine for the treatment of chronic nonorganic facial pain. Clin Neuropharmacol. 2012;35:273–7.
106. Ito M, et al. Effectiveness of milnacipran for the treatment of chronic pain in the orofacial region. Clin Neuropharmacol. 2010;33:79–83.
107. Derry S, et al. Nortriptyline for neuropathic pain in adults (review). Cochrane Database Syst Rev. 2015;(1):CD011209.
108. Pettengill CA, Reisner-Keller L. The use of tricyclic antidepressants for the control of chronic orofacial pain. J Craniomandibular Pract. 1997;15(1):53–6.
109. Moore RA, et al. Amitriptyline for neuropathic pain in adults (review). Cochrane Database Syst Rev. 2015;(7):CD008242.
110. Krymchantowski AV, et al. Topiramate plus nortriptyline in the preventive treatment of migraine: a controlled study for nonresponders. J Headache Pain. 2012;13:53–9.
111. Jeon SH, et al. Effects of nortriptyline on QT prolongation: a safety pharmacology study. Hum Exp Toxicol. 2011;30(10):1649–56.
112. Peppin JF, Albrecht PJ, Argoff C, et al. Skin matters: a review of topical treatments for chronic pain. Part Two: treatments and applications. Pain Therapy. 2015;4(1):33–50.
113. Mohammadkarimi N, Jafari M, Mellat A, Kazemi E, Shirali A. Evaluation of efficacy of intra-nasal lidocaine for headache relief in patients refer to emergency department. J Res Med Sci. 2014;19(4):331–5.
114. Robbins L. Intranasal lidocaine for cluster headache. Headache. 1995;35:83–4.
115. Costa A, Antonaci F, Ramusino MC, Nappi G. The neuropharmacology of cluster headache and other trigeminal autonomic cephalalgias. Curr Neuropharmacol. 2015;13(3):304–23.
116. Kern K-U, Nalamachu S, Brasseur L, Zakrzewska JM. Can treatment success with 5% lidocaine medicated plaster be predicted in cancer pain with neuropathic components or trigeminal neuropathic pain? J Pain Res. 2013;6:261–80.
117. Khawaja N, Yilmaz Z, Renton T. Case studies illustrating the management of trigeminal neuropathic pain using topical 5% lidocaine plasters. Br J Pain. 2013;7(2):107–13.
118. Medscape Mobile Application. Copyright WebMD, LLC, 1994-2016.
119. Marks DR, Rapoport A, Padla D, Weeks R, Rosum R, Sheftell F, Arrowsmith F. A double-blind placebo-controlled trial of intranasal capsaicin for cluster headache. Cephalalgia. 1993;13(2):114–6.
120. Matharu M. Cluster headache. BMJ Clin Evidence. 2010;2010:1212.
121. Szok D, Csáti A, Vécsei L, Tajti J. Treatment of chronic migraine with OnabotulinumtoxinA: mode of action, efficacy and safety. Toxins. 2015;7(7):2659–73. https://doi.org/10.3390/toxins7072659.

122. Finkel AG. Botulinum toxin and the treatment of headache: a clinical review. Toxicon. 2015;107(Pt A):114–9. https://doi.org/10.1016/j.toxicon.2015.09.008.
123. Wang DW, Mistry AM, Kahlig KM, Kearney JA, Xiang J, George AL. Propranolol blocks cardiac and neuronal voltage-gated sodium channels. Front Pharmacol. 2010;1:144.
124. Antonaci F, Ghiotto N, Wu S, Pucci E, Costa A. Recent advances in migraine therapy. Springerplus. 2016;5:637.
125. Negoro K. Calcium antagonists in the prophylactic treatment of migraine. Brain Nerve. 2009;61(10):1135–41.
126. Schrader H, Stovner LJ, Helde G, Sand T, Bovim G. Prophylactic treatment of migraine with angiotensin converting enzyme inhibitor (lisinopril): randomised, placebo controlled, crossover study. Br Med J. 2001;322(7277):19.
127. Orr SL, Aubé M, Becker WJ, Davenport WJ, Dilli E, Dodick D, Giammarco R, Gladstone J, Leroux E, Pim H, Dickinson G, Christie SN. Canadian Headache Society systematic review and recommendations on the treatment of migraine pain in emergency settings. Cephalalgia. 2015;35(3):271–84.
128. Lynch ME, Campbell F. Cannabinoids for treatment of chronic non-cancer pain; a systematic review of randomized trials. Br J Clin Pharmacol. 2011;72(5):735–44.
129. Greco R, Mangione AS, Sandrini G, Nappi G, Tassorelli C. Activation of CB2 receptors as a potential therapeutic target for migraine: evaluation in an animal model. J Headache Pain. 2014;15(1):14.
130. Russo EB. Cannabinoids in the management of difficult to treat pain. Ther Clin Risk Manag. 2008;4(1):245–59.
131. Fine PG, Rosenfeld MJ. The Endocannabinoid System, cannabinoids, and pain. Eisenberg E, Vulfsons S, editors. Rambam Maimonides Med J. 2013;4(4):e0022. Cannabinoids in the management of difficult to treat pain.
132. Sativex Product Insert. http://www.medicines.org.uk/emc/medicine/23262#companyDetails

Chapter 12
Management of Pain of Oral-Dental Origin: An Evidence-Based Approach

John K. Jones

Management of pain of oro-dental origin begins with accurate diagnosis. The cornerstones are chief complaint, history of present illness, review of past history, history of past interventions, examination, and appropriate testing and imaging. Once a provisional or final diagnosis is made, efforts can be transitioned to management. There is currently a significant emphasis on evidence-based management decisions based on available publications and the level of evidence they represent (Table 12.1).

Evidence-Based Management of Oral-Dental Pain

Pain is by definition subjective in nature. It also often lacks associated physical findings to help in diagnosis and management. Because of the subjective nature of pain, frequent lack of objective physical and imaging findings, highly variable presentation, and low prevalence of many of the chronic pain entities, high levels of evidence for many management strategies are lacking. Despite the relative dearth of information, there are some noteworthy and applicable systematic reviews to present that may be helpful especially in the most difficult and refractory cases [1].

Acupuncture: An Alternative Therapy and in Dentistry and Its Potential Applications. Naik PN, Kiran RA, Yalamanchal, Kumer, VA, Goli, S Vashist N. Oral Surg, Oral Med Oral Pathol Oral Radiol Endid. 2011 Feb;111(2): e7–11

J. K. Jones
Department of Otolaryngology/Head and Neck Surgery/Oral and Maxillofacial Surgery, University of Arkansas for Medical Sciences, Little Rock, AR, USA
e-mail: jjones353f@uams.edu

J. Y. Suen, E. Petersen (eds.), *Diagnosis and Management of Head and Face Pain*, https://doi.org/10.1007/978-3-319-90999-8_12

Table 12.1 Evidence-based management decisions based on available publications and the level of evidence they represent

Level of evidence (LOE)	Description
Level I	Evidence from a systematic review or meta-analysis of all relevant RCTs (randomized controlled trial) or evidence-based clinical practice guidelines based on systematic reviews of RCTs or three or more RCTs of good quality that have similar results
Level II	Evidence obtained from at least one well-designed RCT (e.g., large multisite RCT)
Level III	Evidence obtained from well-designed controlled trials without randomization (i.e., quasi-experimental)
Level IV	Evidence from well-designed case-control or cohort studies
Level V	Evidence from systematic reviews of descriptive and qualitative studies (meta-synthesis)
Level VI	Evidence from a single descriptive or qualitative study
Level VII	Evidence from the opinion of authorities and/or reports of expert committees

This level of effectiveness rating scheme is based on the following: Ackley, B. J., Swan, B. A., Ladwig, G., & Tucker, S. (2008). *Evidence-based nursing care guidelines: Medical-surgical interventions.* (p. 7). St. Louis, MO: Mosby Elsevier

Level of Evidence: V

Traditional Chinese acupuncture has a history dating back more than 2500 years. It is a very well know alternative or complementary therapy. Skillfully applied acupuncture has the ability to alter the processing and perception of pain by stimulating the sensory cortex resulting in the release of natural endorphins. It has a proven efficacy in oro-dental facial pain. This article should be considered a systematic review of 40 articles that met the authors' criteria for inclusion. After careful review, they were able to conclude that acupuncture certainly has valid applications in the management of oral-dental facial pain. As such it should be considered as an alternative and/or complementary therapy for oral-dental facial pain.

Botulinum Toxin in the Treatment of Muscle Specific Oro-Facial Pain: A Literature Review. Dutt, CS. Ramnani P. Thakur, D. Pandit M. J Maxillofac Surg 2015 Jun: 14 (2): 171–175

Level of Evidence: V

Because of the prevalence of temporomandibular complaints and the varied presentations, management of temporomandibular joint-related pain is not dogmatic. Sources of pain can be intra-articular, extra-articular, or both. Extra-articular pain is generally muscular in nature. Muscle pain can be detected by palpation. When tender musculature or trigger points are identified on examination, injection of the muscle with botulinum toxin type A (Botox) can be considered and has been found to have significant efficacy. It works by blocking the acetylcholine receptors on skeletal muscle cell membranes, thus preventing depolarization and contraction. The authors reviewed 36 articles which consisted mostly of case series and case reports. They found treatment with botulinum toxin type A to be efficacious in the treatment of temporomandibular disorder pain as well as pain related to parafunctional clenching and bruxism, masseteric hypertrophy, chronic temporomandibular joint dislocation, orofacial dystonias, and painful chronic myogenous orofacial trigger points.

Medication Treatment Efficacy and Chronic Orofacial Pain. Clark GT. Padilla M. Dionne. R. Oral Maxillofacial Surg Clin N Am 28 (2016) 409–421

Level of Evidence: V

This chapter in the Oral and Maxillofacial Clinics of North America is a systematic review of 52 publications on the pharmacologic management of chronic orofacial pain. They specifically discuss the management of four separate chronic orofacial pain entities. The entities discussed are neuropathic pain, chronic headaches, myofascial pain, and osteoarthritis.

For neuropathic pain the pharmacologic choices found to have efficacy are gabapentinoids, tricyclic antidepressants, selective serotonin-norepinephrine reuptake inhibitors, and topical anesthetics. Three medications were found to have reasonable therapeutic efficacy for prophylaxis of chronic daily headaches. Those medications are beta-blockers, tricyclic antidepressants, and various anti-seizure medications.

There are three FDA-approved medications for myofascial pain/fibromyalgia, but none of them are considered to be significantly efficacious. The approved medications are pregabalin, duloxetine, and milnacipran. Regarding chronic pain associated with osteoarthritis, NSAIDs have proven efficacy. Corticosteroid injections are efficacious and can be used when NSAIDs are causing gastritis symptoms.

Interventional Procedures for Facial Pain. Vorenkamp K. Current Pain and Headache Roports. January 2013, 17:308

Level of Evidence: V

This article is a compilation of 45 articles regarding the treatment of trigeminal neuralgia and persistent idiopathic facial pain. Trigeminal neuralgia is the most common diagnosis regarding neuropathic pain in the face. Its prevalence is ten times greater than persistent idiopathic facial pain. Percutaneous interventions involving injection or ablation of the gasserian ganglion and its branches have proven efficacy in providing relief especially when pharmacologic management has been unsuccessful. The sphenopalatine ganglion block is efficacious in refractory cases of persistent idiopathic facial pain.

Burning Mouth Syndrome: A Review on Diagnosis and Treatment. Coculescu EC. Radu A. Coculescu BI. J Med Life v.7(4) Oct-Dec 201

Level of Evidence: V

This article reviews 22 publications regarding the diagnosis and treatment of burning mouth (tongue) syndrome. This entity remains enigmatic and is a diagnosis of exclusion when all organic causes have been ruled out. Its hallmark is the presence of burning pain of the oral mucosa or tongue in the absence of any clinical signs of disease. Being poorly understood as a pain entity treatment is also poorly understood. Nevertheless some therapeutic guidelines are proposed based on review of available literature. Treatment is frequently unsuccessful and is important that realistic expectations are conveyed at the outset. Therapeutic strategies have included benzodiazepines, tricyclic antidepressants, anticonvulsants, serotonin receptor inhibitors, capsaicin, alpha-lipoic acid, benzydamine hydrochloride, hormone replacement therapy, vitamins, and supplements such as iron and zinc. Acupuncture has been used as an adjunctive therapy.

Dental Management of Tooth-Related Pain

Dental management of tooth-related facial pain is well established. As mentioned in another chapter, odontogenic pain is so prevalent that pain of oral-dental origin should be presumed odontogenic (tooth-related) until ruled out [1]. Management of tooth-related pain is amenable to randomized clinical trials due to its prevalence, standard presentation, and objective physical and imaging findings. It is the ability to do randomized clinical trials that creates the highest levels of evidence for evidence-based management.

Non-odontogenic pain of oral-dental origin lacks the level of evidence made possible by the prevalence and objective findings associated with most odontogenic pain entities. Because of the low prevalence, subjective nature of pain, and the frequent lack of objective physical and imaging findings associated with the pain, high levels of evidence for many management strategies are limited to level V. Helpful information may still be gleaned from reviews of large series.

Tooth-Related (Odontogenic) Pain

Tooth-related (odontogenic) pain can be either due to pulpal diseases or to diseases of the supporting structures (periodontal). Pulpal disease tends to be visceral in nature and thus not graduated or variable [2]. Pulpitis can frequently be remedied by timely and appropriate dental intervention in the form of tooth restoration to insulate the pulp from the noxious stimulus and reestablish integrity to the crown. Irreversible pulpitis requires removal of the pulpal tissue (root canal) rendering the tooth insensate or by removal of the tooth. This is typically followed by an appropriate restoration to restore crown integrity and protect the crown from fracture.

Periodontal Pain

Diseases of the periodontal tissues result in a musculoskeletal type of pain response and thus are graduated and variable in presentation. They can be either primary (disease of the supporting structures of gingiva and/or bone) or secondary to pulpal necrosis. Management involves nonsurgical and surgical therapy to decrease infection and inflammation in the periodontal tissues to limit or halt progression of disease. Ideally this results in preservation of the bone and gingiva and attachment within the bone and gingiva. Of course tooth removal can also be therapeutic.

It is very important to recognize that tooth-related (odontogenic pain) and periodontal pain can mimic other pain entities in their presentation and refer pain to other areas of the face and head. For this reason referral to a dental professional for a thorough dental history and examination should be considered early in the management algorithm.

Non-odontogenic Oral-Dental Pain

Maxillary Sinusitis

Musculoskeletal pain in the maxillary posterior dentition, unilateral or bilateral, is frequently the result of maxillary sinusitis. On examination one finds pain to tapping or percussion of the teeth, membrane thickening or an air-fluid level radiographically, foul postnasal drip, and foul odor. Upon dental examination the involved teeth usually test positive for pulpal vitality and are radiographically free of apical disease. Treatment is initially medical in nature with prescription of appropriate antibiotic therapy. If medical therapy does not result in resolution, surgery can be necessary. Typically surgery involves accessing and lavaging the sinus with expansion of the maxillary ostium to encourage drainage. If the maxillary sinusitis is suspected to be caused by a non-vital tooth, then appropriate treatment of the tooth is also necessary for complete resolution.

Temporomandibular Disorders

Temporomandibular disorders are quite prevalent and in one study were found to afflict as much as 6% of the adult population [3]. They are extremely variable in presentation and have significant overlap with other common pain entities. Because of the extremely variable presentation, history taking is paramount. Fortunately there are many objective findings to aid diagnosis and thus direct management strategies. For this reason appropriate examination techniques are very helpful. Examination of the suspected TMD patient should include palpation in the preauricular area for pain when palpating over the temporomandibular joint. Auscultation will frequently reveal clicks and or crepitus. Palpation of the muscles of mastication will elicit pain. Examination of the occlusion may reveal instability. Mandibular range of motion may be decreased and elicit pain.

Management is typically referral to an appropriate dental provider or specialist for evaluation and treatment. The disorder is typically classified as intra-articular (internal derangement), extra-articular (muscular and ligamentous), or both. Classification directs management. Extra-articular disorders are generally managed orthotically to decrease muscle-related pain and improve stability by simulating orthopedic stability in the occlusion. Intra-articular disorders can be acute or chronic. Acute intra-articular disorders should be treated as dislocations and reduced or referred expeditiously. Chronic intra-articular disorders are very frequently associated with extra-articular findings. Typically the extra-articular disorder is managed initially with reevaluation of the internal derangement being planned at follow-up. Surgical intervention can be required to resolve pain related to internal derangement. The widely accepted interventions are arthrocentesis, arthroscopy, and arthrotomy which enjoy similar success rates as an initial surgical intervention. Arthrocentesis has no cumulative morbidity if a second procedure is necessary. Arthroscopy has little cumulative morbidity and can be repeated if necessary. Arthrotomy has significant cumulative morbidity thus the trend toward less invasive initial management of internal derangements. Because of the lack of standardized techniques regarding surgical management, high levels of evidence do not exist for careful comparison [2, 4].

Myofascial TMD Pain

Myofascial pain is characterized by deep dull aching pain that results in referral of pain to the teeth. It is elicited by and exacerbated by the palpation of painful trigger points in the muscle that when stimulated refer pain to the teeth. Of course dental evaluation of the involved teeth is necessary to rule out primary tooth-related disease. The teeth are typically found to have normal vitality. There are well-known pain referral patterns from masticatory muscles to particular areas of the dentition [5]. Local anesthesia injection of the teeth fails to resolve the pain when the trigger points are stimulated. Injection of the trigger points in the muscle results in at least temporary resolution of the pain. Short-acting local anesthetics can be used diagnostically and therapeutically. Longer-acting local anesthetics can be used to provide sustained relief of discomfort that can outlast the duration of action of the agent [6]. Injectable steroids and botulinum toxin have also been used to treat trigger points refractory to traditional management with local anesthetics.

Neuropathic Pain

Neuropathic pain has in common with myofascial pain the presence of a "trigger." In the case of neuropathic pain, the trigger is typically a sensate area of the face or oral cavity that when stimulated classically results in severe, stabbing, electric type pain that is most commonly localized to areas innervated by the trigeminal nerve. The most common neuropathic pain of dental origin is trigeminal neuralgia or tic douloureux. It is commonly a diagnosis of exclusion, but the response can many times be blocked by local anesthetic injection of the trigger providing assistance in diagnosis and at least temporary relief. Initial therapy is typically medical. Referral to a neurologist to help with diagnosis and medical management can be considered. Anticonvulsant medications such as carbamazepine, gabapentin, and pregabalin have some proven efficacy. When medical management fails to provide adequate relief, surgical intervention can be considered. Surgical interventions can be central or peripheral, resective or ablative. When neuropathic pain is in the area of a foramen or bony canal nerve decompression can be considered. Because prior surgical intervention has been suspected of contributing to the development of anesthesia dolorosa, surgical intervention is generally reserved for those patients that fail medical management.

Mucosal Diseases

Mucosal diseases can be infectious, oncologic, inflammatory, or autoimmune in nature. They fortunately have physical findings to aid in diagnosis. Involvement of extraoral mucous membranes should be investigated to aid in diagnosis as well. Clinical appearance and incisional biopsy are often diagnostic and thus can direct management. Oncologic disease can mimic almost any other mucosal disease and should always be on the differential diagnosis. Malignancies involving the tongue are very typically painful. Examples of common infectious mucosal diseases are candidiasis and herpetic gingivostomatitis. These will respond favorably to antifungal and antiviral therapy, respectively. Inflammatory and autoimmune mucosal diseases are typically managed palliatively, and the mainstay of therapy has been the use of topical or systemic steroid therapy to modulate immune system function. Newer immune system modulators may prove efficacious in refractory cases but at this time can only be used off-label regarding indications.

References

1. Lipton JA, Ship JA, Larach-Robinson D. Estimated prevalence and distribution of reported orofacial pain in the United States. J Am Dent Assoc. 1993;124:115–21.
2. Okeson JP. Bell's oral and facial pain. 7th ed. Chicago: Dental Pains. Quintessence Publishing; 2014. Chapter 12
3. Macfarlane TV, Blinkhorn AS, Davies RM, et al. Oro-facial pain in the community: prevalence and associated impact. Commuity Dent Oral Epidemiol. 2002;30:52.
4. Israel H. Internal derangement of the temporomandibular joint: new perspectives on an old problem. Oral Maxillofaxial Surg Clin N Am. 2016;28:313–33.
5. Graff-Redford SB, Abbott JJ. Temporomandibular disorders and headache. Oral Maxillofacial Surg Clin N Am. 2016;28:335–49.
6. Simons DG, Travell JG, Simons LS. Travel and Simons' myofascial pain and dysfunction: a trigger point manual. 2nd ed. Baltimore: Williams and Wilkins; 1999.

Chapter 13
Therapeutic Nerve Blocks

James Y. Suen and Chelsey Smith

Introduction

This is really a continuation of Chap. 9, Diagnostic Nerve Blocks.

With the history and physical exam, we look for a "trigger point" or where the pain or headache seems to start. This can identify which nerves innervate that area. The sensory nerves which innervate the face and head are actually easy to learn and we feel can help diagnose the nerves involved and allow treatment for the pain.

We have found that nerve blocks can be diagnostic and therapeutic.

Nerve blocks have been used for many years by some physicians to help pain, but it is interesting that many other physicians do not think of nerve blocks and start with medications which often have significant side effects. If a single or several nerves can be identified as the source of the pain, we do diagnostic nerve blocks first, and if effective, we use them for treatment. With the problems of addiction and abuse of the narcotics, we feel the nerve blocks should play a major role in the control of facial and head pain. If nerve blocks are effective in relieving the pain for a while, but the pain continues to recur, there are other options that may provide prolonged or permanent pain relief.

Several plastic surgeons noted that following surgery for forehead rejuvenation procedures, a large number of patients with history of migraine headaches noted improvement in their headaches [1–4]. These findings have led to a number of

J. Y. Suen (✉)
Department of Otolaryngology—Head and Neck Surgery, University of Arkansas for Medical Sciences, Little Rock, AR, USA
e-mail: suenjamesy@uams.edu

C. Smith
ENTcare, Dothan, AL, USA
e-mail: chelseyjsmith5@gmail.com

J. Y. Suen, E. Petersen (eds.), *Diagnosis and Management of Head and Face Pain*, https://doi.org/10.1007/978-3-319-90999-8_13

surgical procedures to stop facial pain and headaches and will be discussed in the chapter on surgical management of migraine headaches and facial pain.

Applied Anatomy

The nerve supply to the face and head is from the trigeminal nerves, the greater occipital nerve, and the upper cervical plexus nerves. Knowing the anatomy and the nerve innervation to the face and head is the key to proper diagnosis and treatment of facial and head pain (Fig. 13.1).

Trigeminal Nerve

The classic type I trigeminal neuritis is due to an artery adjacent to the takeoff of the trigeminal nerve from the brain stem and pulsating against the nerve. Management of the classic trigeminal neuritis is addressed in Chap. 19. We feel there are a number of etiologies for "peripheral trigeminal neuritis." Some known common causes

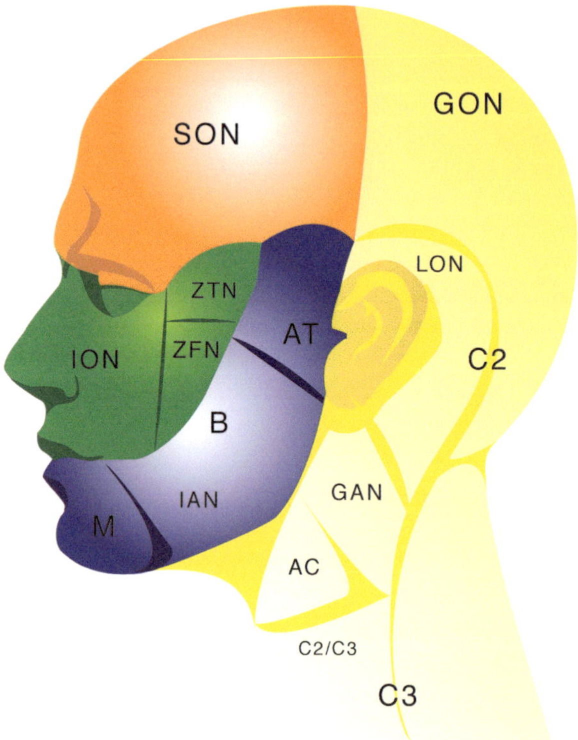

Fig. 13.1 Innervation of the face and head. Note that the zygomaticotemporal (ZTN) and auriculotemporal (ATN) nerves innervate most of the temporalis muscle and temple area

are herpes zoster, trauma with neuromas or entrapment of the nerve branch, and perineural involvement from cancer. More recently it has been postulated that compression of the peripheral nerves at various points, such as in a foramen, a tight notch, or through fascia, can result in nerve pain and headaches [1–4]. In addition we feel that there is a high likelihood that arteries which accompany these nerves can pulsate against peripheral nerves resulting in pain similar to the type I trigeminal neuritis.

There are three divisions of the trigeminal nerve that arise from the ganglion in the wall of the cavernous sinus, commonly referred to as V1, V2, and V3. It is important to know the branches of each of these three divisions and where they innervate the face and head (Fig. 13.2).

The first division, V1, is fairly simple in that it exits the skull through the orbit and divides into the supraorbital, supratrochlear, and infratrochlear nerve branches (Fig. 13.2). The supraorbital nerve exits the orbit through the supraorbital notch or foramen, and it supplies the upper eyelid and the ipsilateral forehead to the vertex of the scalp. The supratrochlear nerve exits at the superior-medial part of the orbit near the bridge of the nose and supplies the skin of the forehead near the midline to the top of the scalp. Pain in V1 can be in the eyelid, the forehead, or the top of the head and can trigger headaches, commonly diagnosed as migraine headaches.

There are also some branches which leave the main branch inside the orbit and go intranasal to the ethmoid sinus areas. These are the posterior and anterior ethmoid nerves. These also can cause headaches from intranasal origin.

The second division, V2, is more complex and takes more thought to understand where pain from V2 can elicit. The main nerve of V2 is the infraorbital nerve, which goes in a groove and foramen in the floor of the orbit and supplies the midface. There are two other branches of this nerve which are important to know. One is the *posterior superior alveolar nerve* which comes off the V2 after it exits the foramen rotundum and wraps around the posterior-lateral wall of the maxilla and enters the bony wall and innervates the posterior upper teeth (Fig. 13.3). It is common for pain in this nerve to be diagnosed as dental pain and result in extractions with no pain relief.

The second important branch is the *zygomaticotemporal nerve* which leaves the infraorbital nerve in the floor of the orbit and goes into the zygoma bone and exits just lateral to the lateral orbital rim and goes to the anterior temple area (Fig. 13.2). It frequently goes into the temporalis muscle or just superficial to it [5]. Pain in this nerve is quite common and can cause temporal headaches.

The third division, V3, has both sensory and motor function. The motor part supplies the muscles of mastication. The sensory branches go to three main areas: the *lingual nerve* to the tongue; the *inferior alveolar nerve* going into the mandible and supplies the lower jaw teeth and exits the mental foramen and supplies the chin and lower lip (Fig. 13.1); and the third branch is the *auriculotemporal nerve* which exits just posterior to the mandibular condyle and goes superiorly to the area of the temple and above the ear (Fig. 13.1). Pain can occur in one or all of these branches. We feel the auriculotemporal nerve is common to trigger migraine headaches. V3 nerves are the most common nerves to be involved with the classic trigeminal neuritis related to vascular compression of the main trunk at the brain stem.

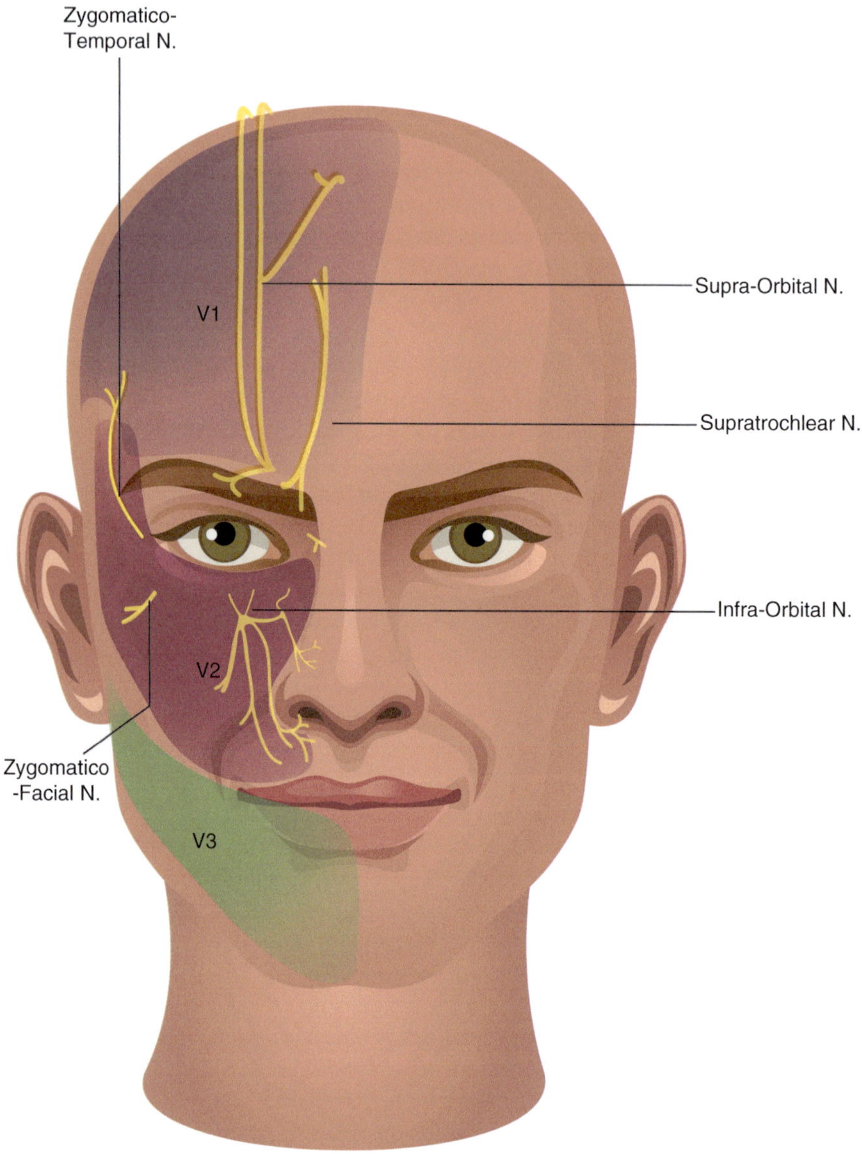

Fig. 13.2 The three divisions of the trigeminal nerve to the face

Greater Occipital Nerve

This nerve arises from C2 off of the spinal cord and goes through the posterior neck muscles and fascia about 2 cm lateral to the midline of the occiput and goes superiorly to the top of the scalp [4] (Fig. 13.4). Occipital headaches are common and

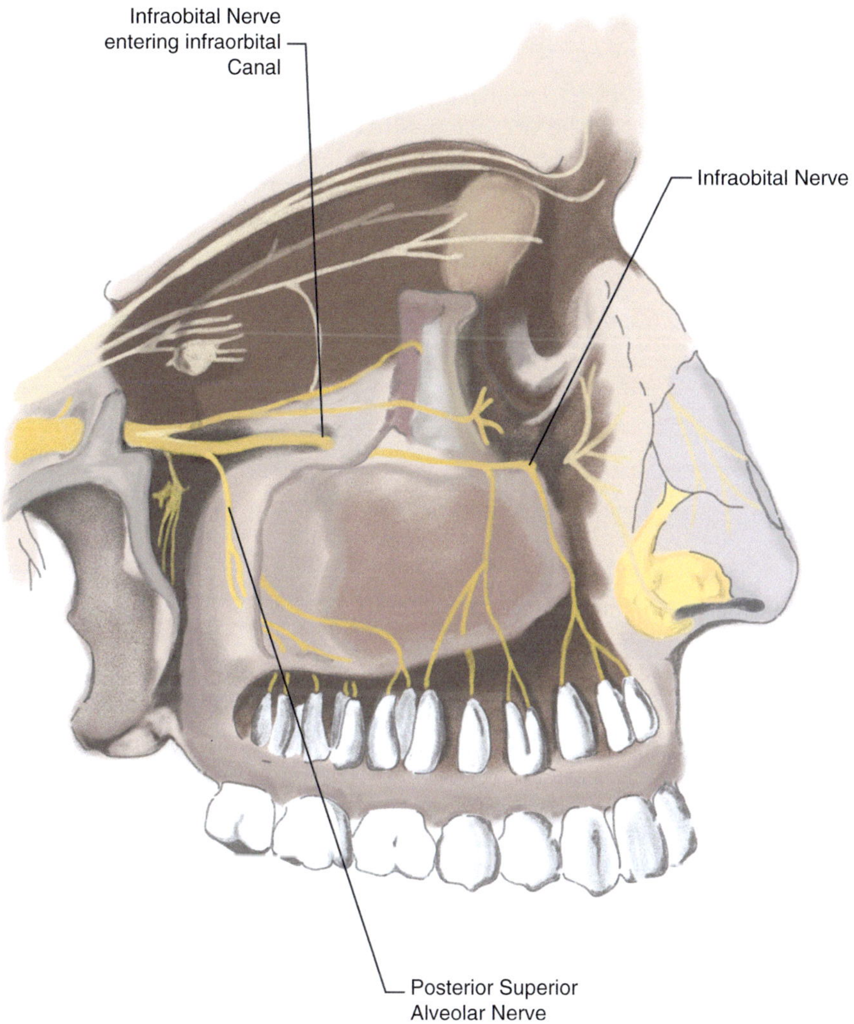

Fig. 13.3 The posterior superior alveolar nerve is a branch of the maxillary division of the trigeminal nerve and supplies the posterior teeth

most arise from the greater occipital nerve. There is a connection between the trigeminal nerve branches and the greater occipital nerve which is referred to as the trigeminocervical complex [6, 7]. Pain in the greater occipital nerve distribution can trigger pain in the supraorbital nerve distribution and vice versa.

Upper Cervical Plexus Nerves

These nerves include the l*esser occipital nerve* which comes from C2 to 3 and goes from the posterior neck and over the mastoid bone to the top of the ear. It also includes the *greater auricular nerve* and an anterior branch, *the transverse cervical branch* which goes to the lower earlobe and along the jawline (Fig. 13.4). When

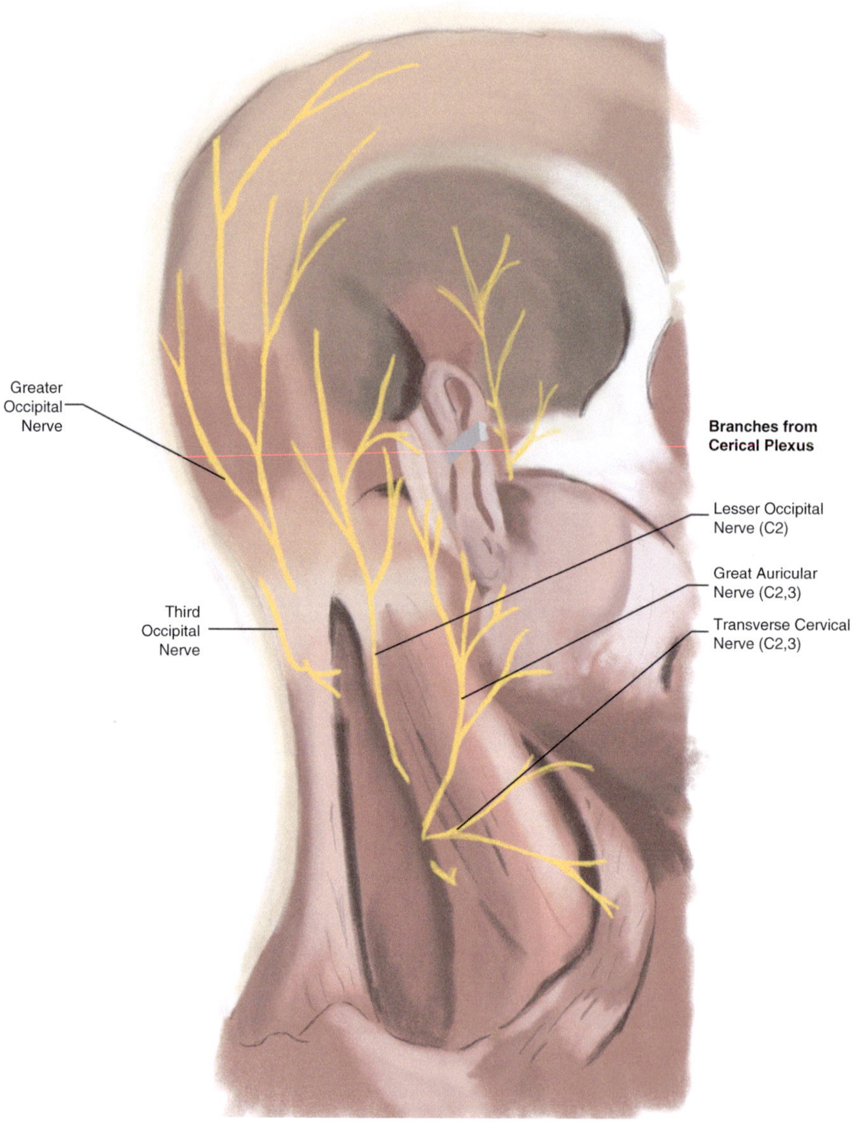

Fig. 13.4 Nerve distribution of the greater occipital and upper cervical plexus nerves

patients describe pain in the jawline area—from the earlobe to chin—it is important to differentiate whether the pain is in the jaw and teeth (inferior alveolar nerve) or is the pain more superficial and from the cervical plexus nerves.

Procedure Technique

Anesthetics: We use 3–4 mL of 1% Xylocaine with epinephrine at 1:100,000 or 1:200,000 strength as the initial injection for diagnostic purposes. We prefer using a 1 or 1 ½ in. 25 Ga. Needle. If the patient's pain is relieved after the block, then we follow with 2–4 mL of 0.5% bupivacaine for a longer effect.

Injection technique: Because of the sensitivity of the facial skin, we start by injecting, very quickly, about 1–1.5 mL of the 1% Xylocaine with epinephrine into the skin overlying the target nerve and let it absorb for about 5 min before injecting the nerve itself. This seems to be less painful for the patient. Because of our knowledge of the anatomy, we do not use ultrasound to localize the nerve being blocked. The use of ultrasound can be used by those not as familiar with the nerve anatomy. We do not feel that injecting directly into the nerve is harmful and actually can improve the therapeutic effect of the anesthetic.

The initial dose of the Xylocaine is from 2 to 3 mL into the nerve area. For a larger area, such as the upper cervical plexus nerves, we use about 4 mL of the Xylocaine.

If the patient obtains relief of pain, we follow the Xylocaine with the Marcaine for longer effect.

We have tried off-label use of bupivacaine in a liposomal preparation, which results in a slower release of up to 72 h. It is approved for infiltration after surgery to decrease pain and has been used many times with joint replacement surgery to allow patients to ambulate earlier. It is approved for use in patients who are 18 years old and older. We have treated over 25 patients with facial and head pain with the liposomal bupivacaine for the nerve blocks. With the use of this preparation, we have seen about 50% of the patients get prolonged pain relief from their chronic pain—some as long as 3–6 months. This is compared to only 1–2 weeks using the Xylocaine and Marcaine. We used 3–4 mL of liposomal bupivacaine to block the nerves.

The dose-response curve in facial and head pain is not known, but the dosage of the liposomal bupivacaine used has made a difference in the amount of pain control in patients after joint replacement surgery. It is possible that our results would have improved with higher doses.

It is important to know that the use of Xylocaine first can neutralize the liposomal bupivacaine. Therefore plain bupivacaine can be used to anesthetize the skin overlying the nerves prior to using the liposomal form.

We also use Kenalog (40 mg/mL) to inject the nerves if the Xylocaine and bupivacaine do not last but a few hours or days, and it seems to prolong the pain relief. The dose is 0.5–1.0 mL per nerve.

After a therapeutic nerve block with Xylocaine and bupivacaine, most patients complained of significant soreness after the numbness wore off and the soreness would last 1 or 2 days and then their pain would improve if the blocks were effective. We found that with using the liposomal bupivacaine, the "soreness" from the nerve block was insignificant because the postinjection numbness helped them through that time period.

We need to stress that liposomal bupivacaine is not approved by the FDA for nerve blocks but only for infiltration after a surgical procedure. However, if a patient has severe face and head pain which does not respond to medical therapy or nerve blocks with Xylocaine and bupivacaine, a physician can choose to use the liposomal preparation, off-label, if they feel the benefits outweigh the minimal risks.

Discussion

We cannot stress the importance of localizing the "trigger point(s)" from the history and physical exam, because that may be the key to deciding therapy. Once the trigger points are identified, we do *diagnostic nerve blocks* using Xylocaine 1% with epinephrine (strength depends on patient's cardiovascular condition and anxiety level). If the patient's pain is significantly reduced or disappears, there is a high likelihood that those nerves are the cause of the pain or headache. We then follow the Xylocaine with 0.5% bupivacaine, 2–4 mL into the same nerve area for a more prolonged effect. We have found that this regimen can provide pain relief for days, weeks, or even months. We tell the patients that every patient is different and we cannot predict the duration of pain relief until one or more nerve blocks. Because the pain is chronic, severe and disabling, we have the patients return 1 week later to reevaluate the results of the nerve blocks. If they had a few days of relief and the pain has recurred, we repeat the nerve block and add 0.5–1.0 mL of Kenalog (40 mg/mL) to the block. This can prolong the pain relief for days or weeks. We also stress to the patients that it commonly requires several different nerve blocks in hopes of getting prolonged relief. Having treated over 100 patients for facial and head pain, we feel that nerve blocks have a major role in the control of facial and head pain. We have seen pain relief for months and even years with only a few nerve blocks.

Not every patient responds to nerve blocks, but the majority do. It is common for our patients to return at regular intervals (weeks or months) to get nerve blocks because they feel the blocks are so helpful. Many patients are able to significantly decrease their pain medications or even stop them after several nerve blocks.

As described in the chapter on diagnostic nerve blocks, it is important to let the patients know that they may have temporary side effects of the nerve blocks, such as facial paralysis, shoulder weakness, or hoarseness.

If patients get relief of pain for only days or weeks from the nerve blocks and they would like more prolonged or permanent relief, we recommend decompressing or resecting the nerves which we feel are causing the pain. There are several studies on nerve decompression procedures which have significantly decreased or eliminated migraine headaches [1–5]. Most patients with chronic pain that undergo resection of the nerves will accept the permanent numbness if the pain is gone.

There are various methods of decompressing the nerves and even destroying the nerves.

We recommend decompressing the nerves in question by surgery, where we expose the nerves and look for compression points. We also will destroy the accompanying arteries because of the possibility of vascular compression of the nerves. It is common to find an artery directly against the nerve or even wrapped around the nerve. Our success rate with this method has been excellent to control the pain or headaches. Again, we stress the importance of a thorough history and physical exam to pinpoint the trigger points and the nerves innervating those areas.

References

1. Guyuron B, Varghai A, Michelow BJ, Thomas T, Davis J. Corrugator supercilii muscle resection and migraine headaches. Plast Reconstr Surg. 2000;106:429–34.
2. Janis JE, Hatef DA, Ducic I, et al. Anatomy of the auriculotemporal nerve: variations in its relationship to the superficial temporal artery and implications for the treatment of migraine headaches. Plast Reconstr Surg. 2010;126:1563–72.
3. Janis JE, Hatef DA, Hagan R, et al. Anatomy of the supratrochlear nerve: implications for the surgical treatment of migraine headaches. Plast Reconstr Surg. 2013;131:743–50.
4. Janis JE, Hatef DA, Reece EM, McCluskey PD, Schaub TA, Guyuron B. Neurovascular compression of the greater occipital nerve: implications for migraine headaches. Plast Reconstr Surg. 2010;126:1996–2001.
5. Janis JE, Hatef DA, Thakar H, et al. The zygomaticotemporal branch of the trigeminal nerve: part II. Anatomical variations. Plast Reconstr Surg. 2010;126:435–43.
6. Bartsch T, Goadsby PJ. Stimulation of the greater occipital nerve induces increased central excitability of dural afferent input. Brain. 2002;125(1):496–509.
7. Bartsch T, Goadsby PJ. Increased responses in trigeminocervical nociceptive neurons to cervical input after stimulation of the dura mater. Brain. 2003;126(1):801–13.

Chapter 14
Botox for Migraine Headaches and Facial Pain

Rachel Kaye, William J. Binder, and Andrew Blitzer

Abbreviations

BoNT	Botulinum neurotoxin
BoNT-A	Botulinum neurotoxin type A
BoNT-B	Botulinum neurotoxin type B
CGRP	Calcitonin gene-related peptide
FDA	US Food and Drug Administration
HA	Headache
NSF	*N*-ethylmaleimide-sensitive factor
SNAP	Soluble NSF attachment protein
SNARE	Soluble NSF attachment protein receptor
TMD	Temporomandibular disorder

R. Kaye
Rutgers New Jersey Medical School, Newark, NJ, USA

New York Center for Voice and Swallowing Disorders, New York, NY, USA

W. J. Binder
David Geffen School of Medicine, Los Angeles, CA, USA

Department of Head and Neck Surgery, University of California-Los Angeles, Los Angeles, CA, USA

A. Blitzer (✉)
Rutgers New Jersey Medical School, Newark, NJ, USA

New York Center for Voice and Swallowing Disorders, New York, NY, USA

Head and Neck Surgical Group, New York, NY, USA

Department of Otolaryngology-Head and Neck Surgery, Columbia University College of Physicians and Surgeons, New York, NY, USA

Department of Otolaryngology, Icahn School of Medicine at Mt. Sinai, New York, NY, USA

J. Y. Suen, E. Petersen (eds.), *Diagnosis and Management of Head and Face Pain*, https://doi.org/10.1007/978-3-319-90999-8_14

TN	Trigeminal neuralgia
TRPV1	Transient receptor potential vanilloid subfamily member 1
VAMP	Vesicular-associated membrane protein

Part I: Botulinum Toxin

Part Ia: History of Botulinum Toxin

Food-borne botulism has likely affected mankind for thousands of years but has only recently been identified. In the late eighteenth century, outbreaks of "sausage poisoning" in Southern Germany prompted early investigation into a possible causative agent. This search sparked the interest of Justinus Kerner (1786–1862) who was a German poet and district medical officer (Fig. 14.1). He subsequently reported accurate and complete accounts of botulism toxicity in monographs between 1817 and 1822 [1–4]. He also correctly deduced that the offending toxin acts by

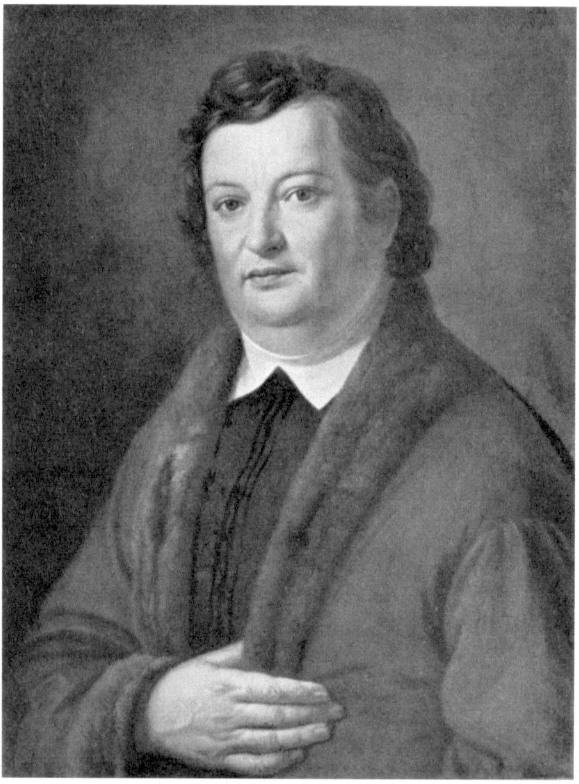

Fig. 14.1 Dr. Justinus Kerner. Oil painting by Alexander Bruckmann 1844. Retrieved from https://commons.wikimedia.org/wiki/File:Justinus_Kerner_1844.jpg

interrupting signal transmission in peripheral and autonomic nerves and sparing sensory transmissions. Kerner was intrigued with the possibility of therapeutic uses of such a toxin and performed extensive experimentation on animals and heroic self-experimentation but was unable to isolate the toxin [5]. After renewed interest in the matter due to a botulism outbreak stemming from a funeral dinner of smoked ham, microbiologist Emile Pierre van Ermengem discovered *Bacillus botulinus* (later named *Clostridium botulinum*) as the causative pathogen in 1895 [6]. It was named as such due to its association with consumption of spoilt sausages (botulus meaning sausage in Latin). Although originally thought to occur only in meat and fish products, an outbreak due to canned beans in 1904 leads to the isolation of a different strain that produced a serologically distinct toxin [7]. Again, a surge of public health interest led Tchitchikine to deduce in 1905 that *C. botulinum* produces a neurotoxin [8], and Georgina Burke designated the toxins into their present alphabetical serological subtypes by naming them A and B in 1919 [9]. During World War II, Edward J. Schantz (Fig. 14.2) purified and crystallized the toxin as a

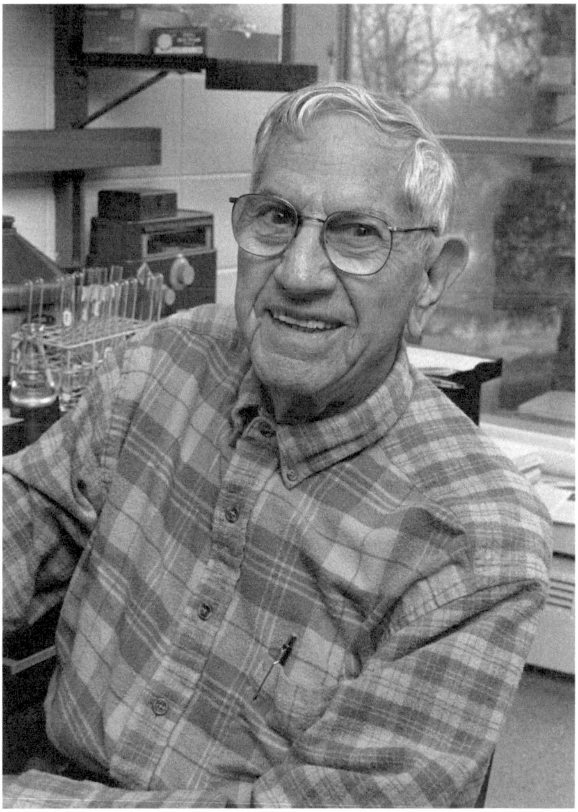

Fig. 14.2 Dr. Edward Schantz. Photo by Wolfgang Hoffmann/University of Wisconsin-Madison College of Agricultural and Life Sciences in 1994

potential biological weapon for the US Army and later worked to pioneer therapeutic chemodenervation with Alan B. Scott through experiments on monkeys [10] and humans [11] for use in strabismus and blepharospasm in the 1970s. Other clinical trials began to evaluate the utility of botulinum toxin (BoNT) for other focal dystonias, including torticollis, oromandibular, spasmodic dysphonia, and Meige syndrome. The successful use of botulinum toxin in treating blepharospasm and strabismus led the US Food and Drug Administration (FDA) to approve the first batch of botulinum toxin type A (BoNT-A) in 1989 as the orphan drug "Oculinum" which Allergan renamed Botox® in 2004 [12]. Similar and competing efforts by the Porton International company in the United Kingdom led to the commercialization of their BoNT-A product which was named Dysport® in 1984. Botulinum toxin type B (BoNT-B) formulation was produced under the name Myobloc™ in the United States and NeuroBloc® in Europe [13]. In 2005, Merz produced a BoNT-A preparation that is free of complex nontoxic proteins named Xeomin® [14]. Due to sustained continued interest, other serotypes are also currently under investigation for potential therapeutic benefit.

Part Ib: Mechanism of Action of Botulinum Toxin

Clostridium botulinum is a rod-shaped, gram-positive bacterium that is found ubiquitously in soil and water. Seven distinct neurotoxin serotypes were originally identified (A, B, C_1, D, E, F, G) with multiple subtypes (A_1–A_6, B_1–B_7, etc.) [15–17]. Although the serotypes have similar molecular structures, they differ significantly in their function and immunogenicity.

The botulinum toxin is produced by the bacterium as inactive polypeptide chains (150 kDa) which is cleaved by bacterial proteases into heavy (100 kDa) and light (50 kDa) chains that are joined by a disulfide bond. There are three domains of the polypeptide chain: the light chain (L), the N-terminus of the heavy chain (H_N), and the C-terminus of the heavy chain (H_C) [18]. The neurotoxins exist as complexes in nature and are thus accompanied by hemagglutinin and nontoxic proteins. These compounds are thought to preserve the potency of the neurotoxin when exposed to the gastrointestinal system.

The sequence of BoNT's neurotoxicity involves binding, internalization, neuromuscular blockade, and finally reinnervation. The first step begins when BoNT irreversibly binds to the presynaptic neuron via its H_C region. Through receptor-mediated endocytosis, the neurotoxin is internalized within endocytic vesicles that also contain an ATPase proton pump. This in turn acidifies the vesicle contents and alters BoNT structure so that the H_N domain is incorporated into the vesicle's membrane and L region is translocated from the endosome into the neuronal cytoplasm. The L region then catalyzes proteolysis of different SNARE proteins which stands for "soluble NSF (*N*-ethylmaleimide-sensitive factor) attachment protein receptor." As SNAREs are protein isoforms that are responsible for vesicle docking, fusion, and release through the cell membrane, BoNT effectively prevents presynaptic release of vesicle contents. The L domain for each toxin contains a highly specific zinc-dependent endopeptidase which cleaves a single target protein isoform at a particular location. For example, BoNT-A and BoNT-E cleave SNAP-25; BoNT-B, BoNT-D, BoNT-F, and BoNT-G cleave synaptobrevin (VAMP); and BoNT-C cleaves SNAP-25 and syntaxin [19]. This causes inhibition of presynaptic acetylcholine release. Following chemodenervation, the affected neuron undergoes resprouting in an attempt to reestablish functional contact with the postsynaptic neuron. However, this process is not physiologically significant with BoNT-A, and as the original synapse eventually reestablishes a functional connection at the original nerve terminals, there is accompanying elimination of the dispensable sprouts.

Part Ic: Contraindications to Use of Botulinum Toxin

Treatment with BoNT is contraindicated during pregnancy and lactation due to the lack of direct studies, and the US FDA lists it as a category C drug. Relative contraindications include patients with neuromuscular disease (i.e., myasthenia gravis, Eaton-Lambert syndrome, amyotrophic lateral sclerosis) as BoNT produces a defect at the neuromuscular junction. A theoretical contraindication exists with the administration of aminoglycosides and calcium channel blockers as these can impair neuromuscular transmission.

Part II: Headache and Migraine

Part IIa: Extracranial Etiology of Headache

As migraine headaches can be preceded by several hours of neck tenderness and visual aura, this led some to postulate that the intracranial meninges and extracranial periosteum (and pericranial muscles) have anatomic connections [20]. The involvement of extracranial pathways in the pathophysiology of certain migraine patients was proposed seven decades ago [21, 22] but has only recently gained traction. Indeed, a network of sensory and pain fibers were found to traverse the calvarial bones inside and outside the suture lines of young mice. As the mice aged and the calvarial bone became fully calcified, these connections degenerated except within the suture lines where they remained intact [23]. These unique sensory/pain fibers were found to bifurcate into three directions with paths leading to the dura, across the subarachnoid space to the pia, and through the suture line to the extracranial periosteum. Studies in humans similarly found the existence of sensory/pain fibers of intracranial origin that traversed and connected the intracranial dura, cranial sutures, extracranial periosteum, and pericranial muscles [23–25]. The identification of sensory and pain fiber network provides a theoretical construct in which muscle tenderness or local pericranial irritation could trigger migraine headaches. This theory assumes that the trigeminal sensory fibers are capable of conducting action potentials in ortho- and antidromic directions and that the pain signals reach the spinal trigeminal nucleus through the before-mentioned pathway and through additional extracranial sensory nerves.

Inflammation may play a role as well; investigations into the presence of inflammatory markers in human calvarial periosteum found upregulation of inflammatory genes in chronic migraineurs with bilateral occipital imploding headaches and associated chronic muscle tenderness [26]. The authors concluded that migraine attacks can originate in extracranial tissues that are sensitive to painful stimuli due to upregulation of inflammatory processes. Furthermore, the reduction in migraine frequency following nerve decompression surgeries [27–29], occipital nerve stimulation [30, 31], and nerve blocks [32, 33] lends credence to the concept of an extracranial source in some headaches/migraines [20]. Overall, the finding of extracranial sources for chronic migraine headaches has vast implications in the treatment and prophylaxis of these disorders.

Part IIb: Botulinum Toxin Prophylaxis for Migraine

The migraine pain pathway is thought to be generated in the brain stem, the cortex, or the pons. Subsequent to various provoking stimuli, there are vasodilation of the intracranial blood vessels and rapid neurogenic inflammation in the perivascular area. Migraine can also be subcategorized as either imploding or exploding dependent on whether the headache is perceived as being inflicted from the outside or as a pressure buildup inside the head, respectively. Therapeutic approaches for migraines can either be abortive (halting progression and enabling resolution of an active migraine) or prophylactic (with the aim to reduce attack frequency). Seminal reports that utilized BoNT-A as a prophylactic medication for headaches found that for some patients, BoNT-A would have great effectiveness, while in others, it was not beneficial [34–39]. As such, Jakubowski et al. performed both a prospective and a triple-blind retrospective analysis of neurological markers to distinguish BoNT-A responders and found that patient response to BoNT-A (defined as a >80% drop in migraine days) was solely related to headache type; patients with imploding or ocular headaches enjoyed a 94% and 100% response rate, respectively, while patients with exploding headaches experienced a meager 19% response rate [40]. The authors attributed this stratification due to the suggested view that exploding headache is mediated by intracranial innervations, whereas imploding and ocular headaches may involve extracranial innervation.

Similarly, it has been proposed that BoNT may act through inhibition of peripheral sensory neurons [41] as it was observed that pain improvement following BoNT-A treatment did not always correspond to the region of neuromuscular effects [42]. For example, in response to trigeminal nerve activation, several neuropeptides and neurotransmitters are released including neurokinin A, substance P, and calcitonin gene-related peptide (CGRP). The release of these substances is thought to contribute to the trigeminal sensory activation and result in allodynia and hyperalgia [43]. Conversely, BoNT is known to inhibit substance P release from embryonic dorsal root ganglion neurons [44], CGRP release from trigeminal ganglion neurons [45], and glutamate release from peripheral nociceptors in the dorsal horn [46]. BoNT is able to affect the release of these inflammatory mediators because they are regulated by SNARE docking proteins. Although BoNT affects pain processing, it does not affect A-delta or A-beta fibers which mediate acute pain as well as touch and pressure, respectively. This is because these sensory fibers are not mediated by neuropeptide release and thus are unaffected by BoNT. This is important as the underlying mechanism why BoNT does not inhibit the sensation of acute pain or result in local anesthesia.

Part IIc: Dosing and Administration of Botulinum Toxin for Migraine Prophylaxis

Botulinum toxin can be diluted to various concentrations. We generally dilute to a concentration of 2.5 U per 0.1 cm^3 of fluid. This is usually accomplished by instilling 4 cm^3 of sterile saline into a vial containing 100 U of botulinum toxin. Anatomical areas typically injected are based on the location of the headache as described by the patient and in our experience can include the following regions: glabella, temporal, frontal, suboccipital, and trapezius. It is imperative to note that injection sites are extramuscular especially in the occipital region and in the base of the neck and follow the distribution of superficial sensory nerves [47] (see Fig. 14.3). In terms of the frontalis injection sites, we find that following the course of the supratrochlear nerve (a branch of the frontal nerve which itself is from the ophthalmic division of the trigeminal cranial nerve) portends the best results. As such, the injections are distributed centrally over the frontalis muscle and divided into four to eight injection sites for each side in order to cover the entire central and lateral forehead areas. The BoNT will diffuse approximately 1–2 cm in diameter and deep into the frontalis muscle itself. When injecting the temporalis or temple region, there are four general areas of injection that align with the anterior, superior, inferior, and posterior quadrants of the temporalis muscle. In total, an average dose of 20–25 U of BoNT-A is used per side with an estimated 5 U per injection site. When injecting the posterior neck, the injections should be along the occipitalis and follow the distribution of the greater and lesser auricular nerves instead of a specific muscle path. BoNT can be injected into the splenius capitis and trapezius muscles in tender areas that usually localize to just below the nuchal ridge between the trapezius and sternocleidomastoid muscle. One to four sites can be injected with an average of 5–20 U of BoNT-A per site. Finally, for occipital/occipitalis muscle injections, the needle is placed just above the nuchal ridge. Usually 1–2 injection sites of 5–7.5 U per side are sufficient.

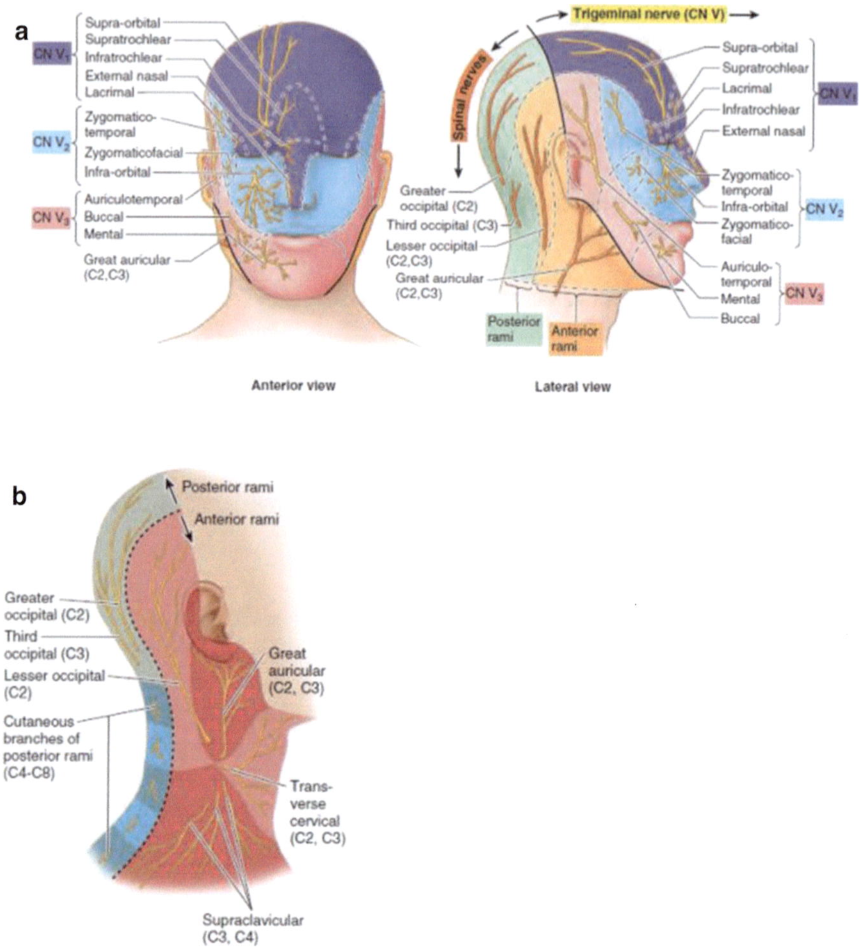

Fig. 14.3 Distribution of peripheral cutaneous nerves of the face and scalp. (**a**) Anterior and lateral views of the distribution of the trigeminal (CN V) and occipital (C2, C3) sensory nerves. (**b**) Cervical plexus of sensory nerves (C2, C3). Reproduced with permission from Moore, K. L., Dalley, A. F., and Agur, A. M. R., *Clinically Oriented Anatomy*, 7th edition, Philadelphia, PA: Wolters Kluwer/Lippincott, Williams & Wilkins, 2014

Adverse effects are usually mild or transient and are usually related to diffusion of BoNT to untargeted (but nearby) muscles and can result in cosmetic changes. Typical adverse effects during the treatment of headaches due to overzealous diffusion (with large volume injections) or improper placement can include blepharoptosis, brow ptosis, diplopia, and muscle weakness at the injection site [36].

In general, pain relief from BoNT may take several weeks to exhibit its maximal effect—as such, patients should continue to maintain a headache diary and should return for reevaluation as the BoNT effect subsides. There is significant variability in the optimal dosing frequency between patients as some experience effect well beyond the predicted pharmacokinetic duration of the medication. This lends credence to the theory that BoNT has a neuromodulating effect as well, and indeed some patients report a greater therapeutic effect with repeat injections [48].

Part III: Trigeminal Neuralgia

Part IIIa: Trigeminal Neuralgia Pathophysiology and Conventional Management

Trigeminal neuralgia (TN) produces characteristic pain along the distribution of one or more divisions of the trigeminal nerve. The pathogenesis is currently incompletely understood and controversial; however, the most common hypothesis involves microvascular compression [49, 50]. Compression by a vessel or tumoral growth on the trigeminal nerve, as well as inflammatory neuropathy (secondary to multiple sclerosis, diabetes, or Lyme disease), has also been identified as etiologies [51, 52].

Management consists of both therapeutics and surgery that aim to alleviate the neuropathic pain and improve quality of life. Oral antiepileptic drugs are the classic first line of treatment [53], although these are not well tolerated and produce central nervous system adverse events in a significant number of patients [54]. Furthermore, approximately 25–50% of patients eventually become tolerant and unresponsive to drug therapy [55]. As such, surgical and invasive options were developed for use in intractable cases and include neurovascular decompression, gamma knife radiosurgery, partial sensory rhizotomy, and percutaneous radiofrequency thermocoagulation [56]. Although marked improvement can be initially achieved in 63–94% of cases, invasive procedures are plagued by the possibility of severe complications (such as aseptic meningitis or hearing loss) [57] and of eventual pain recurrence. Furthermore, the anesthesia produced by destroying parts of the trigeminal nerve can be at times worse than the pain of TN for some patients. Indeed, approximately half of patients who underwent percutaneous radiofrequency rhizotomy developed recurrent pain within 2 years following the procedure [58]. Given these inherent risks, there was a need to develop a safer and better tolerated treatment plan. As BoNT-A was found to be efficacious in pain relief for other pain syndromes, it was a natural candidate when considering alternative options for TN.

Part IIIb: Treatment Mechanism of Botulinum Toxin on Trigeminal Neuralgia

As mentioned earlier, the mechanism by which BoNT relieves pain is controversial, and various hypotheses have been described. Some believe that it acts locally or on the trigeminal ganglia [46, 59], whereas others believe in a central antinociceptive effect. Matak et al. reported a central antinociceptive effect in rat models [60, 61], and

Wu et al. showed that peripherally applied BoNT-A reduces central sensitization and inhibits nociceptor expression [62]. Specifically, substance P is released primary by nociceptive afferents (C fibers), while CGRP is an inflammatory neuropeptide that is often found with substance P in many trigeminal and other sensory ganglia neurons. BoNT reduces the release of both of these neuromodulators. Finally, a recent animal study by Shimizu et al. showed that BoNT decreases the expression of the transient receptor potential vanilloid subfamily member 1 (TRPV1) in rats. As TRPV1 is integral to nociception in the trigeminal system, the investigators concluded that this molecular mechanism could explain how BoNT ameliorates craniofacial pain [63].

BoNT-A was first incorporated with TN treatment by studying its effect on TN-associated hemifacial spasm in 2002 where it was reported to successfully relieve twitching and pain [64]. Since then, multiple clinical trials have investigated its safety and efficacy in treating TN with many reporting favorable effects despite small sample sizes. A recent meta-analysis of randomized controlled trials showed a significant positive symptom relief in terms of the proportion of responders, mean paroxysm frequency, and visual analog scale score [56]. They also reported only transitory and well-tolerated adverse effects: facial asymmetry (14%) and local edema/hematoma (7%) [56]. Furthermore, an open-label trial used lower doses (6.45–9.11 U) of BoNT-A and reported significant pain relief and reduction in medication use that lasted for 60 days [65].

Part IIIc: Dosing and Administration of Botulinum Toxin for Trigeminal Neuralgia

Patients are deemed adequate candidates for injection if they are able to localize the allodynia and hyperesthesia to a specific facial distribution. A grid of the facial pain (including mucosal surfaces) can be mapped with a touch of cotton (for hyperesthesia) or pinprick (for allodynia) (Fig. 14.4). Once the map is drawn, grid lines are placed 1cm apart due to the usual dispersion of botulinum toxin of 1–2 cm per injection site. BoNT-A can then be injected intradermally as close to receptors as possible, at each crosshatch. The senior author's preferred starting dose is 2.5 units of BoNT-A per injection site (concentration of 2.5 units/0.1 cm^3). If this dosage does not result in significant (>50%) pain relief after 4 weeks, then a booster dosage of 2.5 units per injection site can be given at that time. If the patient receives benefit from this booster dose, then 5 units per injection site can be used in future visits once the effect has worn off. If the patient does not receive a significant pain relief after a booster dose, they are considered a nonresponder. These dose calculations are based on a study by the senior author [66].

As facial paresis is expected when administering chemodenervation to the face, especially with higher doses, patients should be properly advised that this is temporary and that contralateral BoNT-A can be administered to achieve symmetry if desired. As mentioned earlier, facial edema or hematoma is also a potential adverse effect of BoNT-A injection, although this is less common (significantly less common with proper technique) and typically resolves within 5–7 days.

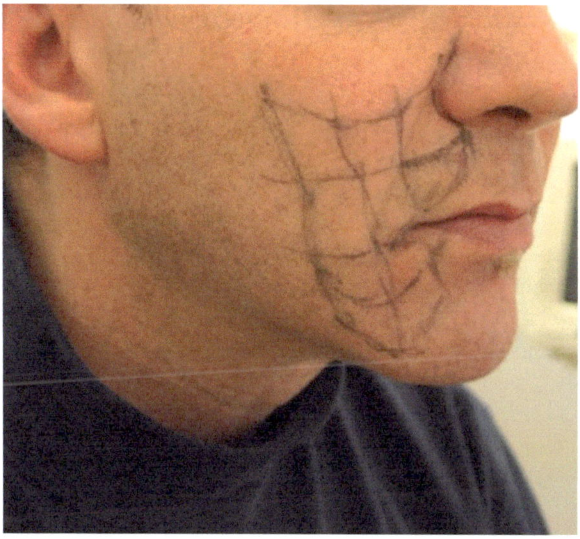

Fig. 14.4 Grid for trigeminal neuralgia injection. Photograph highlighting the grid pattern drawn to represent the location of the patient's allodynia and/or hypesthesia. Crosshatches are made every 1 cm to allow for the typical 1 cm circumferential area of diffusion following injection

Part IV: Temporomandibular Disorder

Part IVa: Current Management of Temporomandibular Disorder

Temporomandibular disorder (TMD) is a nonspecific term that describes a group of temporomandibular joint and muscle disorders that affects the masticatory system due to inflammation of the temporomandibular joint. It can be further subdivided into myofascial or arthrogenic depending on the proposed etiology [67]. Myofascial TMD results from hyperfunctional muscles of mastication that results in a chronic myositis and can be due to spasm of the masseter, temporalis, and/or pterygoid musculature. Arthrogenic TMD is secondary to intracapsular pathology [68], and as such, these patients are not treated with BoNT. In general, TMD pain is typically localized to the joint, and symptoms can include referred otalgia, headache, transmitted neck pain, decreased jaw mobility, difficult or painful mastication, and crepitus of the joint with movement. Current treatments include physiotherapy, acupuncture, massage, systemic anti-inflammatory medications, muscle relaxants, tranquilizers, and dental/occlusal appliances. Rarely is a surgical intervention (arthrocentesis, intra-articular steroid injection, arthroscopy, and open arthrotomy) undertaken [69]. Despite the plethora of available treatment strategies, there is currently no gold standard treatment due to the lack of high-level systematic reviews or direct comparison studies [70]. Arguments for the use of BoNT in alleviating TMD pain rest on the tenet that BoNT affects afferent nerves and decreases inflammatory mediatory release as mentioned in previous sections above.

Part IVb: Botulinum Toxin for Temporomandibular Disorder

The application of BoNT for TMD is principally based on local musculoskeletal effects and/or its neuromodulating effects on afferent nerves. It is thought that hyperfunctional or spastic contractions of the masticatory muscles (masseter, temporalis, and pterygoid) produce excess strain on the temporomandibular joint and produce chronic myositis. By weakening these muscles with BoNT, less strain is produced, and therefore, the patient experiences pain relief. Furthermore, chronic local muscle contraction has been shown to cause inflammation and localized hypoxia which produces chronic myofascial pain [71]; by reducing hyperfunctional muscle contraction, the local damage and inflammation can be reduced, and central pain thresholds elevated. Additionally, the ability of BoNT to decrease the release of inflammatory mediators (substance P, CGRP, glutamate) may play an important role in pain reduction [72].

Numerous studies have investigated the role of BoNT in long-term relief of myofascial TMD pain; however, there is considerable variation in trial design. Freund et al. reported the utility of BoNT in 46 TMD patients by injecting 150 units of BoNT-A to the masseters and temporalis muscles and found significant pain reduction, function improvement, greater mouth opening, and decreased tenderness [73]. Later, Freund and Schwartz reported successful alleviation of a variety of disorders that fall under the general category of TMD including bruxism and clenching, oromandibular dystonias, myofascial pain, trismus, hypermobility, masseter and temporalis hypertrophy, and headaches [74]. An unpublished open-label study by the senior author of 100 TMD patients found a 70% response rate (≥50% reduction in pain severity or frequency) to BoNT-A injections.

In a recent double-blinded trial comparing incobotulinumtoxinA to placebo injections into the masseter, temporalis, and lateral pterygoid muscles, those patients who received incobotulinumtoxinA reported a significant 76–83% reduction in pain over a 3-month period, while placebo resulted in a 30% reduction in pain in the first month following the injection. The patients injected with saline were then given a crossover injection of incobotulinumtoxinA, and they approached the pain relief values as reported by those patients who had originally received incobotulinumtoxinA [70].

Part IVc: Dosing and Administration of Botulinum Toxin for Temporomandibular Disorder

Masticatory muscles are typically targeted for BoNT injection in a fixed-position technique that is individualized by tailoring the dose or constellation of muscle groups based on physical examination and patient symptoms. This is mainly performed by careful analysis of the amount and location of muscle tenderness and pain. That being said, the temporalis and masseter muscles are almost always affected and are usually injected at an average dose range of 10–25 U for each temporalis and 25–50 U for each masseter muscle with a concentration of 2.5–5.0 units per 0.1 mL of BoNT-A. Having patients clench their teeth aids in localization of transcutaneous injection into both the masseter and temporalis muscles. The decision to also inject the lateral pterygoids rests on the presence of significant lateral jaw deviation, pain localized to under the cheeks, or bruxism, and average doses are 7.5–10 U to each muscle. We inject the lateral pterygoid muscles intraorally by placing the EMG-guided needle between the pterygoid plate and the coronoid process of the mandible at an angle parallel to the length of the muscle. This allows for injection along the length of the muscle, whereas transcutaneous injection would instill the BoNT only along the width of the muscle. Proper placement is confirmed by having the patient produce lateral jaw excursion that results in robust EMG signaling.

Adverse effects are uncommon and often mild. Difficult mastication is the most common adverse effect due to masticatory muscle weakness and is dose-dependent. With chronic injections, muscle atrophy may cause cosmetic alterations and should be discussed with the patient. Higher volume BoNT injections increase the undesired excess diffusion, resulting in brow ptosis, blepharoptosis, or diplopia. This can also occur if the temporalis muscle is injected too close to the orbit. If the masseter muscle is injected in close proximity to the zygomaticus major, facial asymmetry can result as well. To avoid this, we direct the EMG needle laterally to minimize the diffusion of BoNT. Although infrequent, if masseter injections diffuse to the parotid gland, dry mouth can occur as well [68].

Part V: Conclusion

The action of BoNT on docking proteins to inhibit vesicle release has advantages beyond simple neuromuscular blockade. BoNT has clinical utility in myofascial and inflammatory syndromes that include chronic migraine, trigeminal neuralgia, and temporomandibular disorders with many patients who were previously recalcitrant or suboptimal responders to treatment experiencing significant relief. BoNT has been shown to act both centrally and peripherally, affecting neuromodulators to decrease nociception and inflammatory signals. Although significant strides have been made to elucidate the pathophysiology behind these syndromes and the effects of BoNT, further research is imperative to advance our understanding. Furthermore, the adverse effects of BoNT are infrequent, usually mild, and temporary in nature. In conclusion, BoNT is a safe alternative treatment for many myofascial and inflammatory syndromes and boasts a good safety profile.

References

1. Erbguth FJ. Historical notes on botulism, Clostridium botulinum, botulinum toxin, and the idea of the therapeutic use of the toxin. Mov Disord. 2004;19(Suppl 8):S2–6.
2. Kerner J. Vergiftung durch verdorbene Wü rste. Tübinger Blätter fur Naturwissenschaften und Arzneykunde. 1817;3:1–25.

3. Kerner J. Neue Beobachtungen uber die in Wurttemberg so haufig vorfallenden todlichen Vergiftungen durch den Genuss geraucherter Wurste. Osiander: Tubingen; 1820.
4. Kerner J. Das Fettgift oder die Fettsaure und ihre Wirkungen auf den thierischen Organismus, ein Beytrag zur Untersuchung des in verdorbenen Wursten giftig wirkenden Stoffes. Cotta: Stuttgart; 1822.
5. Erbguth FJ, Naumann M. On the first systematic descriptions of botulism and botulinum toxin by Justinus Kerner (1786-1862). J Hist Neurosci. 2000;9(2):218–20.
6. Van Ermengem E. Uber einen neuen anaeroben Bacillus und seine Beziehung zum Botulismus. Z Hyg Infektionskr. 1897;26:1–56.
7. Leuchs J. Beitrage zur Kenntnis des Toxins und Antitoxins des Bacillus botulinus. Z Hyg Infektionskr. 1920;65:55–84.
8. Tchitchikine A. Essai d'immunisation par la voie gastrointestinal contre la toxine botulique. Ann Inst Pasteur. 1905;xix:335.
9. Burke GS. The occurrence of Bacillus botulinus in nature. J Bacteriol. 1919;4(5):541–53.
10. Scott AB, Rosenbaum A, Collins CC. Pharmacologic weakening of extraocular muscles. Invest Ophthalmol. 1973;12(12):924–7.
11. Scott AB. Botulinum toxin injection of eye muscles to correct strabismus. Trans Am Ophthalmol Soc. 1981;79:734–70.
12. Ting PT, Freiman A. The story of Clostridium botulinum: from food poisoning to Botox. Clin Med (Lond). 2004;4(3):258–61.
13. Lew MF, Brashear A, Factor S. The safety and efficacy of botulinum toxin type B in the treatment of patients with cervical dystonia: summary of three controlled clinical trials. Neurology. 2000;55(12 Suppl 5):S29–35.
14. Benecke R, et al. A new botulinum toxin type A free of complexing proteins for treatment of cervical dystonia. Neurology. 2005;64(11):1949–51.
15. Gimenez DF, Gimenez JA. The typing of botulinal neurotoxins. Int J Food Microbiol. 1995;27(1):1–9.
16. Arndt JW, et al. A structural perspective of the sequence variability within botulinum neurotoxin subtypes A1-A4. J Mol Biol. 2006;362(4):733–42.
17. Whitemarsh RC, et al. Characterization of botulinum neurotoxin A subtypes 1 through 5 by investigation of activities in mice, in neuronal cell cultures, and in vitro. Infect Immun. 2013;81(10):3894–902.
18. Aoki KR. Physiology and pharmacology of therapeutic botulinum neurotoxins. Curr Probl Dermatol. 2002;30:107–16.
19. Sutton RB, et al. Crystal structure of a SNARE complex involved in synaptic exocytosis at 2.4 A resolution. Nature. 1998;395(6700):347–53.
20. Burstein R, et al. Extracranial origin of headache. Curr Opin Neurol. 2017;30(3):263–71.
21. Wolff HG, Tunis MM, Goodell H. Studies on headache; evidence of damage and changes in pain sensitivity in subjects with vascular headaches of the migraine type. AMA Arch Intern Med. 1953;92(4):478–84.
22. Selby G, Lance JW. Observations on 500 cases of migraine and allied vascular headache. J Neurol Neurosurg Psychiatry. 1960;23:23–32.
23. Kosaras B, et al. Sensory innervation of the calvarial bones of the mouse. J Comp Neurol. 2009;515(3):331–48.
24. Schueler M, et al. Extracranial projections of meningeal afferents and their impact on meningeal nociception and headache. Pain. 2013;154(9):1622–31.
25. Schueler M, et al. Innervation of rat and human dura mater and pericranial tissues in the parieto-temporal region by meningeal afferents. Headache. 2014;54(6):996–1009.
26. Perry CJ, et al. Upregulation of inflammatory gene transcripts in periosteum of chronic migraineurs: implications for extracranial origin of headache. Ann Neurol. 2016;79(6):1000–13.
27. Janis JE, et al. A review of current evidence in the surgical treatment of migraine headaches. Plast Reconstr Surg. 2014;134(4 Suppl 2):131S–41S.

28. Chepla KJ, Oh E, Guyuron B. Clinical outcomes following supraorbital foraminotomy for treatment of frontal migraine headache. Plast Reconstr Surg. 2012;129(4):656e–62e.
29. Guyuron B, et al. A placebo-controlled surgical trial of the treatment of migraine headaches. Plast Reconstr Surg. 2009;124(2):461–8.
30. Saper JR, et al. Occipital nerve stimulation for the treatment of intractable chronic migraine headache: ONSTIM feasibility study. Cephalalgia. 2011;31(3):271–85.
31. Young WB. Occipital nerve stimulation for chronic migraine. Curr Pain Headache Rep. 2014;18(2):396.
32. Dach F, et al. Nerve block for the treatment of headaches and cranial neuralgias—a practical approach. Headache. 2015;55 Suppl 1:59–71.
33. Blumenfeld A, Ashkenazi A, Evans RW. Occipital and trigeminal nerve blocks for migraine. Headache. 2015;55(5):682–9.
34. Binder WJ, et al. Botulinum toxin type A (BOTOX) for treatment of migraine headaches: an open-label study. Otolaryngol Head Neck Surg. 2000;123(6):669–76.
35. Ondo WG, Vuong KD, Derman HS. Botulinum toxin A for chronic daily headache: a randomized, placebo-controlled, parallel design study. Cephalalgia. 2004;24(1):60–5.
36. Silberstein S, et al. Botulinum toxin type A as a migraine preventive treatment. For the BOTOX Migraine Clinical Research Group. Headache. 2000;40(6):445–50.
37. Tepper SJ, et al. Botulinum neurotoxin type A in the preventive treatment of refractory headache: a review of 100 consecutive cases. Headache. 2004;44(8):794–800.
38. Dodick DW, et al. Botulinum toxin type a for the prophylaxis of chronic daily headache: subgroup analysis of patients not receiving other prophylactic medications: a randomized double-blind, placebo-controlled study. Headache. 2005;45(4):315–24.
39. Evers S, et al. Botulinum toxin A in the prophylactic treatment of migraine—a randomized, double-blind, placebo-controlled study. Cephalalgia. 2004;24(10):838–43.
40. Jakubowski M, et al. Exploding vs. imploding headache in migraine prophylaxis with botulinum toxin A. Pain. 2006;125(3):286–95.
41. Aoki KR. Review of a proposed mechanism for the antinociceptive action of botulinum toxin type A. Neurotoxicology. 2005;26(5):785–93.
42. Brin MF, et al. Localized injections of botulinum toxin for the treatment of focal dystonia and hemifacial spasm. Mov Disord. 1987;2(4):237–54.
43. Silberstein SD, Lipton RB, Goadsby PJ. Headache in clinical practice. Oxford: Isis Medical Media; 1998.
44. Welch MJ, Purkiss JR, Foster KA. Sensitivity of embryonic rat dorsal root ganglia neurons to Clostridium botulinum neurotoxins. Toxicon. 2000;38(2):245–58.
45. Durham PL, Cady R, Cady R. Regulation of calcitonin gene-related peptide secretion from trigeminal nerve cells by botulinum toxin type A: implications for migraine therapy. Headache. 2004;44(1):35–42; discussion 42–3.
46. Cui M, et al. Subcutaneous administration of botulinum toxin A reduces formalin-induced pain. Pain. 2004;107(1–2):125–33.
47. Blumenfeld AM, et al. Insights into the functional anatomy behind the PREEMPT injection paradigm: guidance on achieving optimal outcomes. Headache. 2017;57(5):766–77.
48. Mathew NT, Kaup AO. The use of botulinum toxin type A in headache treatment. Curr Treat Options Neurol. 2002;4(5):365–73.
49. Obermann M, Holle D, Katsarava Z. Trigeminal neuralgia and persistent idiopathic facial pain. Expert Rev Neurother. 2011;11(11):1619–29.
50. Jia DZ, Li G. Bioresonance hypothesis: a new mechanism on the pathogenesis of trigeminal neuralgia. Med Hypotheses. 2010;74(3):505–7.
51. Garza I, et al. Headache and other craniofacial pain. In: Daroff R, et al., editors. Bradley's neurology in clinical practice. 6th ed. Philadelphia: Elsevier; 2012. p. 1703–44.
52. Guardiani E, et al. A new treatment paradigm for trigeminal neuralgia using Botulinum toxin type A. Laryngoscope. 2014;124(2):413–7.

53. Cruccu G, et al. AAN-EFNS guidelines on trigeminal neuralgia management. Eur J Neurol. 2008;15(10):1013–28.
54. Zakrzewska JM. Medical management of trigeminal neuropathic pains. Expert Opin Pharmacother. 2010;11(8):1239–54.
55. Cruccu G, Truini A. Refractory trigeminal neuralgia. Non-surgical treatment options. CNS Drugs. 2013;27(2):91–6.
56. Morra ME, et al. Therapeutic efficacy and safety of Botulinum Toxin A Therapy in Trigeminal Neuralgia: a systematic review and meta-analysis of randomized controlled trials. J Headache Pain. 2016;17(1):63.
57. Bond AE, et al. Operative strategies for minimizing hearing loss and other major complications associated with microvascular decompression for trigeminal neuralgia. World Neurosurg. 2010;74(1):172–7.
58. Taha JM, Tew JM Jr. Treatment of trigeminal neuralgia by percutaneous radiofrequency rhizotomy. Neurosurg Clin N Am. 1997;8(1):31–9.
59. Xiao L, et al. Botulinum toxin type A reduces hyperalgesia and TRPV1 expression in rats with neuropathic pain. Pain Med. 2013;14(2):276–86.
60. Matak I, et al. Behavioral and immunohistochemical evidence for central antinociceptive activity of botulinum toxin A. Neuroscience. 2011;186:201–7.
61. Matak I, Riederer P, Lackovic Z. Botulinum toxin's axonal transport from periphery to the spinal cord. Neurochem Int. 2012;61(2):236–9.
62. Wu C, et al. Central antinociceptive activity of peripherally applied botulinum toxin type A in lab rat model of trigeminal neuralgia. Springerplus. 2016;5:431.
63. Shimizu T, et al. Reduction of TRPV1 expression in the trigeminal system by botulinum neurotoxin type-A. Neurobiol Dis. 2012;48(3):367–78.
64. Micheli F, Scorticati MC, Raina G. Beneficial effects of botulinum toxin type a for patients with painful tic convulsif. Clin Neuropharmacol. 2002;25(5):260–2.
65. Piovesan EJ, et al. An open study of botulinum-A toxin treatment of trigeminal neuralgia. Neurology. 2005;65(8):1306–8.
66. Sirois D, et al. Botulinum toxin A in trigeminal neuralgia: outcome of placebo-controlled RCT. Oral Surg ORal Med Oral Pathol Oral Radiol Endod. 2011;112:e130.
67. Ohrbach R, Stohler C. Diagnosis of temporomandibular disorders: a critical review of current diagnostic systems. J Cranio Disord Fac Oral Pain. 1992;6(4):307–17.
68. Mor N, Tang C, Blitzer A. Temporomandibular myofacial pain treated with botulinum toxin injection. Toxins (Basel). 2015;7(8):2791–800.
69. Song PC, Schwartz J, Blitzer A. The emerging role of botulinum toxin in the treatment of temporomandibular disorders. Oral Dis. 2007;13(3):253–60.
70. Patel AA, Lerner MZ, Blitzer A. IncobotulinumtoxinA injection for temporomandibular joint disorder. Ann Otol Rhinol Laryngol. 2017;126(4):328–33.
71. Shilpa PS, et al. Botulinum toxin: The Midas touch. J Nat Sci Biol Med. 2014;5(1):8–14.
72. Bossowska A, et al. Botulinum toxin type A induces changes in the chemical coding of substance P-immunoreactive dorsal root ganglia sensory neurons supplying the porcine urinary bladder. Toxins (Basel). 2015;7(11):4797–816.
73. Freund BJ, Schwartz M. Relief of tension-type headache symptoms in subjects with temporomandibular disorders treated with botulinum toxin-A. Headache. 2002;42(10):1033–7.
74. Schwartz M, Freund B. Treatment of temporomandibular disorders with botulinum toxin. Clin J Pain. 2002;18(6 Suppl):S198–203.

Chapter 15
Psychological and Psychiatric Treatment of Chronic Head and Face Pain

Taylor E. Rush and Harold W. Goforth

Introduction

Head and facial pain can affect many aspects of a patient's daily life. Chronic pain can affect a variety of ways in which people function, including sleep behaviors, activity patterns, and emotional experiences. As a result, they often require a multidisciplinary approach for successful comprehensive management. Behavioral interventions and psychotropic medication can serve as effective adjuncts to treatment in order to help meet this need and to enhance quality of life. Cognitive-behavioral strategies, relaxation techniques, biofeedback, and operant learning interventions have all been shown to be helpful techniques for behavioral headache management. This chapter will review the central theoretical tenets of cognitive and behavioral interventions, the research that supports their use, as well as a review of psychotropic modalities of treatment for headache prevention and mood management.

T. E. Rush (✉)
Center for Neurological Restoration, Neurological Institute, Cleveland Clinic, Cleveland, OH, USA
e-mail: rusht@ccf.org

H. W. Goforth
Center for Neurological Restoration, Neurological Institute, Cleveland Clinic, Cleveland, OH, USA

Lerner College of Medicine, Cleveland Clinic Foundation, Center for Neurological Restoration, Section of Headache Medicine, Cleveland, OH, USA
e-mail: goforth@ccf.org

J. Y. Suen, E. Petersen (eds.), *Diagnosis and Management of Head and Face Pain*, https://doi.org/10.1007/978-3-319-90999-8_15

Non-pharmacological Headache Interventions

Cognitive and Behavioral Therapy Interventions

Cognitive-Behavioral Therapy Model Cognitive-behavioral therapy (CBT) has been considered a gold standard psychological intervention for a wide variety of conditions, including depression, anxiety, as well as pain. Psychiatric comorbidities are fairly common in headache disorders. For instance, those with migraine headaches have a 2–4 times higher likelihood of exhibiting co-occurring depression, a 2–7 times higher likelihood of exhibiting anxiety symptoms, and a 3–4 times higher likelihood of experiencing panic episodes [1]. This makes CBT interventions an ideal choice to help successfully manage the behavioral and affective components of patients' pain experiences.

The underlying assumption of CBT is that a person's thoughts, feelings, and emotions are strongly connected and maladaptive appraisals of situations can contribute to dysfunctional coping styles. Over time, this can lead to entrenched patterns of poor coping which can negatively affect a person's mood, relationships, and overall quality of life. For those with chronic head pain, these symptoms may also have deleterious effects on health-promoting behaviors (e.g., exercise, stress-reducing activities, healthy eating, adequate sleep), which can then increase the likelihood of more frequent and/or severe headache episodes.

The research on CBT for headache has provided strong evidence of treatment efficacy. It has been associated with decreased headache frequency by up to 50%, higher reported self-efficacy and internal locus of control, less pain-focused cognitions, improved mood, and increased medical treatment adherence [2]. In addition, CBT has been shown to be cost-effective and can reduce health-care utilization in chronic pain populations [3].

Physiologically, CBT appears to help activate parasympathetic nervous system activity, which can include normalized heart rate and blood pressure, increased peripheral blood flow, and decreased muscle tension. In addition, it can assist with HPA axis and nociceptive regulation by decreasing activity of pro-inflammatory cytokines [4].

Common Negative Thought Patterns Part of CBT treatment involves having patients identify maladaptive appraisals and thought patterns in order to challenge and reframe them in a more realistic, helpful way. This can help to attenuate strong negative emotional reactions that can also feed into poor behavioral coping reactions. When patients can identify negative thought patterns, it becomes easier for them to dispute them and minimize the associated threat.

Catastrophizing is a common negative thought pattern observed in chronic pain conditions. Pain is appraised as a high-level threat and often associated with feelings of helplessness and the inability to stop thinking about pain sensations [5]. The experience of pain is often associated with the belief that physical harm or damage to the body may occur, which can deter a person from engaging in normal activity. Instead, they will pursue safety behaviors, such as rest, isolation, avoidance of potential triggers (e.g., loud noises, bright lights, etc.), and excessive or inappropriate medication use.

Another common negative thought patterns include fear-avoidance cognitions, characterized by strong beliefs that activity will cause pain to worsen [6]. Threatening activities can range from high-impact physical activity, such as rigorous exercise, to minimal impact daily activities such as sitting in front of a computer or driving. This can result in specious reasoning that safety behaviors such as rest and activity avoidance will keep head pain at bay. However, this pattern of activity avoidance can lead to physical deconditioning, which can then cause pain to worsen.

[Example starts] Jane experiences chronic migraines. When pain becomes severe, she thinks, "Here we go again- my day is ruined! This headache is only going to get worse, so I need to cancel my plans." Resultantly, she feels stressed, frustrated, irritable, and out of control of her situation. In reaction to these thoughts and emotions, she withdraws from planned activity, lies down, and takes medication. She may also possibly seek emergent medical help. Over time, Jane develops anticipatory anxiety about her headache episodes (e.g., "If I go somewhere with bright lights or loud noises it will make my headaches worse") and therefore avoids activities that she thinks may induce headaches. This can lead to an overall decrease in activity and functioning and increase in stress due to low quality of life and fear of worsening pain. Additionally, Jane may experience an increase in migraines despite all of her safety behaviors to avoid them [example ends].

Cognitive Restructuring CBT targets changing maladaptive cognitive and behavioral coping patterns in order to enhance adaptive coping and minimize mood and anxiety symptoms that may be comorbid with pain. This involves learning how to identify negative thought patterns and challenging them with more adaptive, realistic thoughts (see Table 15.1). Patients are also taught to acknowledge that pain is not harmful and accept that, while it may not be curable, it is manageable. Setting this expectation at the beginning of treatment is very important so that the patient understands that CBT is not a curative intervention for pain. If realistic expectations are not discussed at the beginning of treatment, successful outcomes are less likely.

Activity Pacing Another key component to effective behavioral management of headaches is moderating activity levels and including activities that promote health. Often, those experiencing chronic pain will demonstrate a boom-bust activity

Table 15.1 Examples of cognitive restructuring

Maladaptive cognition	Restructured cognition
This pain is going to get worse	The pain may get worse, but it will not stay that way forever
There is nothing I can do to stop it	I have tools that can help me manage this
I need to cancel my plans	I can continue to function despite the presence of pain
I need to go to the emergency room	I can manage this without acute medical intervention
Medication is the only thing that helps	I have other strategies that can be just as, if not more, helpful than medication
Activity will worsen my pain	Activity can help me cope more effectively and will not harm me

pattern, where they will overextend themselves on less severe pain days and then rest extensively on more severe days. Engaging in this pattern can result in worsening pain and lower functioning over time. Additionally, as their number of functional days decrease, patients will often begin to exclude pleasant activities, such as hobbies and socializing, and health-promoting activities, such as exercise and self-care.

Learning how to appropriately pace activity and incorporate salutatory behaviors can be a trial and error process. Patients are often asked to log their daily activity and keep their hours of activity per day equitable across high and low pain days. They are encouraged to break up activities that may have historically exacerbated pain, such as exercise, long drives, and computer work, into manageable stretches of time punctuated by breaks. Patients can determine what constitutes a manageable stretch by timing how long they can do an activity before pain begins to worsen. The next time they engage in the activity, they are advised to take a break prior to the point of pain exacerbation. Over time, patients are encouraged to slowly increase the intensity or duration of activity to improve overall functional capacity.

Sleep Hygiene Sleep dysregulation is often an associated symptom of chronic head pain. Insomnia issues are reported in up to two-thirds of chronic headache patients and sleep apnea reportedly co-occurs in up to 60% of this population [7]. For many, problematic sleep can then contribute to significant daytime fatigue, difficulties with concentration, mood dysregulation, and poor performance on daily activities. Behavioral strategies for improving sleep have been found to be more efficacious than medications [8] and therefore play an important role in the successful behavioral management of headaches.

Behavioral strategies for insomnia can fall into three categories: sleep hygiene, stimulus control, and sleep restriction. Table 15.2 below gives a brief description of some of the techniques for each of these strategies.

Relaxation Strategies/Biofeedback Stress has been identified as a potential predisposing and exacerbating factor for chronic head and facial pain. Psychologically, stress typically occurs when the perceived demands of a situation exceed a person's perceived ability to meet those demands. If a stressor is appraised as uncontrollable and the person has few resources to help manage the stressor, physiological as well as psychological stress will likely result. Research has shown that the intensity of stress is correlated with headache frequency [9]. Additionally, pain can contribute to significant daily stress, as it can enhance normal stressors in addition to being a stressor itself. When the body is exposed to prolonged discomfort, it can lead to chronic activation of the sympathetic nervous system's "fight-or-flight" response. This can have a cascading effect on autonomic functioning, including rising blood pressure, heart rate, cortisol levels, immune and inflammatory responses, and muscle tension. Behaviorally, stress can lead to poor self-care; infrequent health-promoting activities, such as healthy eating, adequate hydration, and physical activity; and disengagement from adaptive coping strategies. Together, these biological and behavioral factors can exacerbate the experience of pain.

Table 15.2 Behavioral sleep interventions

Behavioral intervention	Techniques
Sleep hygiene	– Keep consistent bedtimes and wake times – Avoid caffeine, alcohol, nicotine, and spicy foods in the hours leading up to bedtime – Exercise daily – Create a bedtime routine to help wind down – Avoid naps – Increase exposure to natural light during day – Avoid screens (TV, tablets, phones) in the hour leading up to bed
Stimulus control	– Restrict activity in the bedroom (sleep and sex only) – Go to bed only when tired – Get out of bed if not asleep within 15 min; proceed to engage in boring, sedentary activity outside of bedroom – Avoid clock watching
Sleep restriction	– Keep a sleep journal logging total sleep time and actual time spent asleep, and calculate sleep efficiency (SE = time asleep/time in bed) – If SE ≤ 80–85%, reduce time in bed by 15 min increments each week SE stays ≤80% – Once SE > 85%, can slowly add 15 min to time in bed each week until normative bed and wake times are obtained

Lipton and colleagues [10] have examined how the dissipation of stress can specifically contribute to the development of migraine, described as the "let-down" hypothesis. The let-down hypothesis was tested in a small study, which interestingly showed that, while stress level was not associated with migraine frequency, a quick decline in stress over a 24 h period almost doubled the odds of migraine onset in the following 6–18 h. Physiologically, this may be due to lowered HPA activation and reduced glucocorticoid production, which can subsequently trigger a migraine.

Given how stress can potentially precipitate and exacerbate pain, learning how to successfully manage stress can be a critical skill set for effective pain management. By engaging in relaxation strategies, the body's stress response can be better regulated and allow restorative processes to work more effectively, including activating the body's parasympathetic or "rest and digest" response. Cognitively, relaxation techniques help to provide distraction from pain, increase awareness of emotional states, as well as understand the physiological signs of stress and tension on the body. Over time, this information can be used to better manage stress as well as pain sensations. A summary of common relaxation strategies for pain management can be found in Table 15.3.

Biofeedback is considered an objective way in which to monitor the body's response to various relaxation techniques. By receiving real-time feedback on their physiological functioning, such as heart rate, body temperature, muscle tension, and galvanic skin response, patients can become aware of physical responses to pain and stress. They can then use that information to target relaxation strategies to enhance physiological self-regulation. Biofeedback has been shown to be an effective behavioral strategy for head and facial pain management. Specifically, electromyographic

Table 15.3 Summary of relaxation strategies

Relaxation strategy	Description	Mechanism of action
Diaphragmatic breathing	Engaging the diaphragm to breath, allowing the lungs to fill more effectively. Using the diaphragm to breath causes the belly to expand on the inhale, hence the nickname "belly breathing"	Slows the breath rate, allowing better oxygen intake
Progressive muscle relaxation	Systematically tensing and releasing different muscle groups in the body, anywhere from 8 to 32 groups in total	Increases awareness of areas of the body that tend to hold chronic tension and gives an opportunity to relax them, facilitating better awareness of tense and relax states
Autogenic relaxation	Systematically focusing on different areas of the body and imagining them becoming heavy and warm. This can be paired with an image that helps to enhance sensations of heaviness and warmth (e.g., immersing into a warm bath)	Can help to increase peripheral blood flow and decrease chronic muscle tension
Guided imagery	Creating a relaxing mental scene using all five senses	Can serve as a cognitive distraction from pain stimuli

(EMG) for tension-type headaches and thermal biofeedback for migraine have demonstrated efficacy in reducing pain severity and frequency [11]. It has also been found to help reduce medication overuse [12]. When compared to other behavioral interventions for headache, biofeedback and relaxation training has demonstrated to be as effective as CBT-based strategies and more effective than placebo [11].

Operant Behavioral Conditioning

In addition to the above described interventions, operant behavioral therapy has long been established as a way to help decrease pain experiences by targeting reduction of pain behaviors (e.g., talking about pain, grimacing, abnormal posturing, excessive rest). It was first introduced by Fordyce [13], who applied operant learning theory (which posits that learned behavior is a direct result of reinforcement and/or punishment) to pain. He believed that positive reinforcement (positive attention, caregiving) as well as negative reinforcement (e.g., encouraging medication use or utilization of emergency services to abate symptoms, making the environment dark and quiet, encouraging rest) in response to pain behaviors would increase them over time. Therefore, Fordyce recommended that pain behaviors be ignored, while more adaptive and functional behaviors be reinforced via verbal cues and positive attention. Various studies testing this theory have shown that participants who underwent interventions where these principles were applied exhibited less pain behavior, increases in activity, and lower pain ratings [14].

Role of Family Support

Relationship dynamics and interactions can play a significant role in whether a person is able to adaptively manage chronic pain. Research shows that if family members preferentially give attention and support in response to pain behaviors, those behaviors become more frequent and pain ratings are higher [15]. Conversely, family members who invalidate their loved one's experience with chronic pain can lead to increased risk of mood dysregulation and maladaptive coping [16]. There can be significant benefit from incorporating family into behavioral interventions. This can provide an opportunity for loved ones to learn ways in which they can be supportive without reinforcing pain behavior or minimizing their family member's struggle. These family-based interventions can focus on facilitating assertive communication, including verbalizing and acknowledging how pain has affected their respective roles in their relationship. It can also be helpful for family members to elucidate expectations moving forward for how to appropriately handle pain crises, so all involved understand how they can show support without being enabling or withholding.

Pharmacological Interventions

The use of psychotropic medication for headache prevention in addition to mood management has been more commonly accepted through the past several decades. These medications can be an effective way to address headache pain directly as well as any comorbid mood or anxiety symptoms. The following paragraphs will provide a brief overview of various medication classes and the research supporting their use.

MAOI Therapies

The monoamine oxidase inhibitor theory of migraines states that alterations of monoamines in the central nervous system produce dysregulated responses in the cerebral vasculature to produce migrainous headaches. An early study looking at the effect of treating migraine with beta-blockers and nonselective monoamine oxidase inhibitors (phenelzine) demonstrated a significant improvement in frequency and severity of migraine attacks. Anxiety and depression were also improved in both the phenelzine monotherapy group and the group receiving dual therapy with beta-blockers (atenolol) [17]. Other data looking at selective MAOIs have not been supportive of their use in the prevention of migraine headaches. Selegiline in particular failed to demonstrate improvement upon migraine without aura; however, the doses of oral selegiline used in the study did not reach therapeutic levels to allow the inhibition of MAO-A in this group. It may be more accurate with regard to this study to note that selective MAO-B inhibitors are ineffective in the prevention of migraine rather than interpret this as a failure of MAOIs in general [18].

Tricyclic Therapies

Following the advent of tricyclic antidepressants, these became one of the most widespread groups of medications used for migraine prevention in both pediatric and adult patients. While tricyclics are one of the most common medication classes prescribed for the prevention of migraine headache, there is a paucity of large-scale or randomized trials with respect to this class of agents. Amitriptyline is the most common of the tricyclics that are prescribed for migraines, although nortriptyline and desipramine are other potential agents that may have improved side effect profiles.

One large-scale trial of amitriptyline that was performed between 1976 and 1979 was not fully reported until 2011 but involved a placebo-controlled trial of amitriptyline of 20-week duration. Study participants included both intermittent migraine patients and chronic daily headache. Dropout rates were significant across the study with only 48% completing week 20. There was a significant improvement in headache frequency for amitriptyline over placebo at 8 weeks, but not at 12, 16, or 20 weeks. The amitriptyline effect was more pronounced for those subjects with chronic daily headache where superiority of amitriptyline was evident at 8 weeks and 16 weeks, but not 20 weeks.

A retrospective cohort study examining amitriptyline dose and treatment outcomes demonstrated that there is a significant range of amitriptyline dosing from 2.5 to 100 mg daily, which are considered lower doses in the dosing spectrum of amitriptyline. Interestingly, amitriptyline was well tolerated and approximately three-fourths of patients were found to derive significant clinical benefit in the reduction of migraine frequency [19].

Amitriptyline has also been demonstrated to be cost-effective in the prevention of migraine headaches among low- and middle-income countries. Amitriptyline was considered more cost-effective than either topiramate or propranolol [20]. Amitriptyline has also been combined with cognitive-behavioral therapy (CBT) for chronic migraines in adolescents and children. The data demonstrated a robust marginal reduction in headache frequency when CBT was added to amitriptyline treatment over amitriptyline treatment alone. These benefits were sustained at 12 months [21].

Amitriptyline has shown to be comparably efficacious to other well-established and FDA-approved medications for migraine such as divalproate over a 6-month period. Divalproex was more effective at 3 months with respect to headache frequency and visual analog scale of severity. However, the significant differences between the two treatment groups had dissipated by 6 months when no significance was found between the two groups. Hair loss, menstrual irregularities, polycystic ovaries, and weight gain were all more common in the divalproex group [22].

The Canadian Headache Society produced a set of guidelines that stratified available medications for migraine prevention according to available data. Amitriptyline received strong recommendation for use [23].

Other tricyclic depressants have also been identified as effective choices for migraine prophylaxis. Monotherapy with any one migraine preventative agent has been noted to improve only a minority of individuals. However, dual therapy with different classes of migraine preventatives has been shown to be more effective than monotherapy alone. One study examined the role of additive nortriptyline 30 mg daily to topiramate 100 mg daily in monotherapy nonresponders. Seventy-eight percent of patients receiving polytherapy demonstrated at least a 50% reduction in headache frequency compared to 37% of those assigned to the monotherapy groups. Combination therapy of topiramate and nortriptyline was effective in patients with inadequate improvement on monotherapy of either agent alone [24].

Beta-Blocker Therapies

A randomized double-blind controlled trial examined the efficacy of low-dose propranolol 40 mg daily, nortriptyline 20 mg daily, and combination therapy of the two agents. The period of treatment was 2 months. Treatment with propranolol alone or in combination was effective, but monotherapy with nortriptyline was not effective. This study was limited by a very small sample size that was underpowered for the number of groups and possible outcomes [25]. Another open-label study examining the role of amitriptyline in 25 and 50 mg dosages over a 2-month period also demonstrated a weak effect upon migraine prevention and reduced the number of monthly migraines from an average of 7 to 6 per month [26]. Thus, while most treatment algorithms embrace amitriptyline or other tricyclics in the prevention of migraine headaches, the data supporting this use is not uniformly consistent.

SSRIs and SNRIs

Other antidepressant classes of medications have been examined for migraine prevention and treatment of depression in migraine populations. A review of selective serotonin reuptake inhibitors (SSRI) for preventing migraine and tension headaches identified 13 studies utilizing 5 different SSRIs. SSRIs did not significantly lower headache index score in patient with migraine when compared to placebo after 2 months. SSRIs were more tolerable than tricyclic compounds [27].

A prospective study comparing venlafaxine to escitalopram demonstrated a clear advantage of venlafaxine over escitalopram in terms of headache frequency, duration, and severity. Daily work performance also improved in the venlafaxine group. The escitalopram group also showed reductions in frequency, duration, and severity, but the reductions were less robust than in the venlafaxine group. These effects were independent of mood disorders. [28]. Other SSRI studies examining the role of fluoxetine have demonstrated small but significant effect sizes with respect to migraine frequency while improving mood in these populations [29, 30].

A randomized, double-blind, crossover study examining venlafaxine versus amitriptyline in the preventative treatment of migraine demonstrated that both drugs have benefits in pain parameters. Venlafaxine was more tolerable than amitriptyline in this study, and fewer patients dropped out of the venlafaxine arm. The study was limited by a small sample size ($n = 52$) [31].

Duloxetine is a selective serotonin-norepinephrine reuptake inhibitor that has received considerable attention for its use in pain syndromes. One recent prospective study examined the role of duloxetine 60–120 mg daily in the prevention of episodic migraine in persons without depression. The study was limited by a small sample size, but greater than 50% of participants receiving duloxetine (mean dose 110 mg daily) had a 50% or greater improvement in number of monthly headache days [32]. An older 8-week open-label trial of duloxetine 60 mg daily for comorbid major depressive disorder and chronic headache noted significant improvements in both depression scores and headache frequency [33]. Duloxetine appears well tolerated across both studies.

In summary, there appears to be generally good but not uniformly agreeable data for the use of antidepressant therapies in the prevention of migraine headaches as well as mood management. Data appear more robust for lower-dose tricyclic compounds and dual serotonin-norepinephrine reuptake inhibitors than for selective serotonin reuptake inhibitors. Amitriptyline appears to be the compound most commonly prescribed for migraine prevention, although more recent data suggest a growing role for venlafaxine and duloxetine as alternatives.

Placebo Effects

Placebo effects in headache treatment have demonstrated that patient expectations, as well as provider proclamations and attitude regarding the treatment, can play a role in pharmacological and behavioral treatment efficacy. In RCTs of acute headache medication that had treatment and placebo groups, reported pain improvements in placebo groups have been upward of 28% versus 58% in active treatment [34]. Unfortunately, no studies have been conducted that assign patients to a wait-list control as well as placebo and active treatment groups. For preventative pharmacotherapies, RCT meta-analyses show that 21% of those in placebo groups report a ≥50% reduction in number of headache days, in comparison to 41% in active treatment. Few RCTs of behavioral therapies have been conducted, and many studies are confounded by selection bias as well as facilitator variability. This makes replication of some interventions difficult, especially since level of engagement in therapeutic providers as well as patients can affect treatment gains and placebo effects. However, the research that has been done has shown that participants who underwent true biofeedback reported better symptom improvement than those who participated in sham behavioral therapies. This has also shown to be true with relaxation training and cognitive-behavioral interventions.

Conclusion

Psychological and psychiatric treatment can be integral aspects of comprehensive head and facial pain management. Behavioral interventions can help equip patients with self-regulatory skills necessary to manage mood, pain exacerbations, physiological stress, activity levels, and social engagement. This can help to enhance a sense of control over symptom management and contribute to a higher quality of life. Psychotropic medications can be used in concert with behavioral strategies in order to help with headache prevention as well as mood dysregulation.

References

1. Hamelsky SW, Lipton RB. Psychiatric comorbidities of migraine. Headache. 2006;46:1327–33. https://doi.org/10.1111/j.1526-4610.2006.00576.x.
2. Harris P, Loveman E, Clegg A, et al. Systematic review of cognitive behavioral therapy for the management of headaches and migraines in adults. Br J Pain. 2015;9(4):213–24. https://doi.org/10.1177/2049463715578291.
3. Ehde DM, Dillworth TM, Turner JA. Cognitive-behavioral therapy for individuals with chronic pain: efficacy, innovations, and directions for research. Am Psychol. 2014;69(2):153–66. https://doi.org/10.1037/a0035747.
4. Moreira FP, Cardoso TA, Mondin TC, et al. The effect of proinflammatory cytokines in cognitive behavioral therapy. J Neuroimmunol. 2015;285:143–6.
5. Quartana PJ, Campbell CM, Edwards RR. Pain catastrophizing: a critical review. Expert Rev Neurother. 2009;9(5):745–58. https://doi.org/10.1586/ERN.09.34.
6. Borkum JM. Maladaptive cognitions and chronic pain: epidemiology, neurobiology, and treatment. J Ration Emot Cogn Behav Ther. 2010;28:4–24. https://doi.org/10.1007/s10942-010-0109-x.
7. Singh NN, Sahota P. Sleep-related headache and its management. Curr Treat Options Neurol. 2013;15:704–22. https://doi.org/10.1007/s11940-013-0258-1.
8. Mitchell MD, Gehrman P, Umschied CA. Comparative effectiveness of cognitive behavioral therapy for insomnia: a systematic review. BMC Fam Pract. 2012;13:40–51. http://www.biomedcentral.com/1471-2296/13/40
9. Schramm SH, Moebus S, Lehmann N, et al. The association between stress and headache: a longitudinal population-based study. Cephalalgia. 2015;35(10):853–63. https://doi.org/10.1177/0333102414563087.
10. Lipton RB, Buse DC, Hall CB, et al. Reduction in perceived stress as a migraine trigger: testing the "let-down headache" hypothesis. Neurology. 2014;82:1395–401.
11. McGrady AV, Andrasik F, Davies T, et al. Psychophysiologic therapy for chronic headache in primary care. J Clin Psychiatry. 1999;1(4):96–102.
12. Rausa M, Palomba D, Cevoli S. Biofeedback in the prophylactic treatment of medication overuse headache: a pilot randomized controlled trial. J Headache Pain. 2016;17:87–95. https://doi.org/10.1186/s10194-016-0679-9.
13. Fordyce WE. Behavioral methods for chronic pain and illness. St Louis: C.V. Mosby; 1976.

14. Gatzounis R, Schrooten MGS, Crombez G, et al. Operant learning theory in pain and chronic pain rehabilitation. Curr Pain Headache Rep. 2012;16:117–26. https://doi.org/10.1007/s11916-012-0247-1.
15. Block AR, Kremer EF, Gaylor M. Behavioral treatment of chronic pain: the spouse as a discriminative cue for pain behavior. Pain. 1980;9:243–52.
16. Kerns RD, Haythornwaithe J, Southwick S, et al. The role of marital interaction in chronic pain and depressive symptom severity. J Psychosom Res. 1990;34(4):401–8.
17. Merikangas KR, Merikangas JR. Combination monoamine oxidase inhibitor and beta-blocker treatment of migraine, with anxiety and depression. Biol Psychiatry. 1995;38(9):603–10.
18. Kuritzky A, Zoldan Y, Melamed E. MAO B inhibitor, is not effective in the prophylaxis of migraine without aura: an open study. Headache. 1992;32(8):416.
19. Doyle Strauss L, Weizenbaum E, Loder EW, et al. Amitriptyline dose and treatment outcomes in specialty headache practice: a retrospective cohort study. Headache. 2016;56(10):1626–34.
20. Linde M, Steiner TJ, Chisholm D. Cost-effectiveness analysis of interventions for migraine in four low- and middle-income countries. J Headache Pain. 2015;16:15.
21. Powers SW, Kashikar-Zuck SM, Allen JR. Cognitive behavioral therapy plus amitriptyline for chronic migraine in children and adolescents: a randomized clinical trial. JAMA. 2013;310(24):2622–30.
22. Kalita J, Bhoi SK, Misra UK. Amitriptyline vs divalproate in migraine prophylaxis: a randomized controlled trial. Acta Neurol Scand. 2013;128(1):65–72.
23. Pringsheim T, Davenport W, Mackie G, et al. Canadian Headache Society guideline for migraine prophylaxis. Can J Neurol Sci. 2012;39(2 Suppl 2):S1–59.
24. Krymchantowski AV, da Cunha Jevoux C, Bigal ME. Topiramate plus nortriptyline in the preventive treatment of migraine: a controlled study for nonresponders. J Headache Pain. 2012;13(1):53–9.
25. Domingues RB, Silva AL, Domingues SA, et al. A double-blind randomized controlled trial of low doses of propranolol, nortriptyline, and the combination of propranolol and nortriptyline for the preventive treatment of migraine. Arq Neuropsiquiatr. 2009;67(4):973–7.
26. Lampl C, Huber G, Adl J, Luthringshausen G, et al. Two different doses of amitriptyline ER in the prophylaxis of migraine: long-term results and predictive factors. Eur J Neurol. 2009;16(8):943–8.
27. Moja PL, Cusi C, Sterzi RR, Canepari C. Selective serotonin re-uptake inhibitors (SSRIs) for preventing migraine and tension-type headaches. Cochrane Database Syst Rev. 2005;20(3):CD002919.
28. Tarlaci S. Escitalopram and venlafaxine for the prophylaxis of migraine headache without mood disorders. Clin Neuropharmacol. 2009;32(5):254–8.
29. Adly C, Straumanis J, Chesson A. Fluoxetine prophylaxis of migraine. Headache. 1992;32(2):101–4.
30. Saper JR, Silberstein SD, Lake AE, et al. Double-blind trial of fluoxetine: chronic daily headache and migraine. Headache. 1994;34(9):497–502.
31. Bulut S, Berilgen MS, Baran A, et al. Venlafaxine versus amitriptyline in the prophylactic treatment of migraine: randomized, double-blind, crossover study. Clin Neurol Neurosurg. 2004;107(1):44–8.
32. Young WB, Bradley KC, Anjum MW, et al. Duloxetine prophylaxis for episodic migraine in persons without depression: a prospective study. Headache. 2013;53(9):1430–7.
33. Volpe FM. An 8-week, open-label trial of duloxetine for comorbid major depressive disorder and chronic headache. J Clin Psychiatry. 2008;69(9):1449–54.
34. Autret A, Valade D, Debiais S. Placebo and other psychological interactions in headache treatment. J Headache Pain. 2012;13:191–8. https://doi.org/10.1007/s10194-012-0422-0.

Chapter 16
Acupuncture in the Management of Head and Neck Pain: An Introduction

Anthony F. Jahn

Introduction

The treatment of medical disorders with the insertion of needles into various parts of the body originated thousands of years ago. The earliest acupuncture needles, small shards of stone, date to Neolithic times (8000–3500 BC). An ice age mummy discovered in Southern Tyrol in 1988, and estimated to have lived around 3200 BC, was found to bear numerous tattoo scars, many corresponding to known acupuncture points [1] . By contrast, the earliest Western medical document, the Edwin Smith Papyrus from Egypt, dates to 1600 BC, and the works attributed to Hippocrates were written even more recently, around 470–360 BC.

Given the current emphasis on evidence-based medicine, it is interesting to consider that acupuncture may well be the oldest outcome-based therapeutic modality. Based on thousands of years of careful observation and detailed documentation, acupuncture began at a time when scientific methods and instruments, and the resultant body of knowledge pertaining to human anatomy, physiology, and pathology, did not exist.

Although practically based, acupuncture later became incorporated into a theoretical construct, which helped not only to organize and explain clinical findings but also to direct therapy and predict results. These features are of course the features of any useful medical hypothesis. Hypotheses are the grasping tools of knowledge, and their value derives from the ability to explain, organize, and predict clinical effects. In the case of acupuncture, the theoretical framework was that of Taoism, a philosophy originating around the fourth or third century BC with the Chinese sage Lao-Tze. While Taoist concepts continue to organize and even guide Traditional Chinese Medicine (TCM), it is important to realize that the practice of acupuncture preceded Taoism by centuries.

A. F. Jahn
Professor of Clinical Otolaryngology, Icahn School of Medicine at Mount Sinai, New York, NY, USA

J. Y. Suen, E. Petersen (eds.), *Diagnosis and Management of Head and Face Pain*, https://doi.org/10.1007/978-3-319-90999-8_16

With the application of Western scientific methods, acupuncture continues to develop—new points are identified, clinical effects are validated, and new effects of established points are established. Acupuncture today is a vital and contemporary treatment modality which is increasingly becoming a part of Western medical therapy.

Basic Concepts of Chinese Medicine

The Chinese and Western approaches to health and disease are fundamentally different. Chinese medicine rejects the mind/body dualism of Western medicine and considers seeming opposites, such as structure and function, as both manifestations of the same energy. This concept, of Yin and Yang, pairs apparently contrasting phenomena and unifies them through the ceaseless flow of energy, one seamlessly becoming the other. Yin and Yang are not absolute designations, but relative and interdefining, referring more to their comparative nature and behavior than absolute physical characteristics. As an example, the ventral surface of the body is considered Yin when compared to the back (dorsal being Yang and ventral Yin) but Yang when compared to the abdominal contents (superficial is Yang and internal is Yin). Also, since phenomena are in a constant state of transition, they typically contain elements of both Yin and Yang, as illustrated by the familiar Tao symbol (Fig. 16.1). This applies not only of the human body but also to the physical world around us. So, while noontime is considered Yang and midnight as Yin, dawn is "Yang in Yin" (day entering night), while dusk is "Yin in Yang" (night entering day).

A ceaseless flow of energy, called *qi* (chee), animates every aspect of life regardless of its momentary manifestation and exists as a continuous process of transformation between apparent opposites such as structure and function. Health is the result of this constant and unimpeded flow of energy.

While Western medicine is historically based on structure (anatomy), in Chinese medicine, the organs of the body are defined primarily in terms of their function. For example, the Chinese concept of the functional "kidney" is not just an excretory organ but also includes the adrenal and reproductive glands and is therefore considered a storehouse of energy. Chinese medicine recognizes that while structure (Yin) gives rise to function (Yang), function also determines structure and emphasizes the incessant process of energy interchange between these two states. The only thing constant, in fact, is change.

Further, Chinese medicine considers that health results not only from an unimpeded and healthy flow of energy within the body but also within the larger context of our natural environment, including the weather, the seasons, and our diet. Environmental influences, such as cold, damp, or wind, are often identified as pathogenic factors with a potential to "invade" the body, and the body's defenses against such "external ills" need to be shored up and maintained. Internal noxious factors are also identified and then rectified by adjusting the flow of energy. Chinese diagnosis typically does not end with a specific disease but is couched in terms of the noxious agent (external and internal) and the body's response patterns. For example, vertigo may be found to be due to insufficient kidney energy or excessive

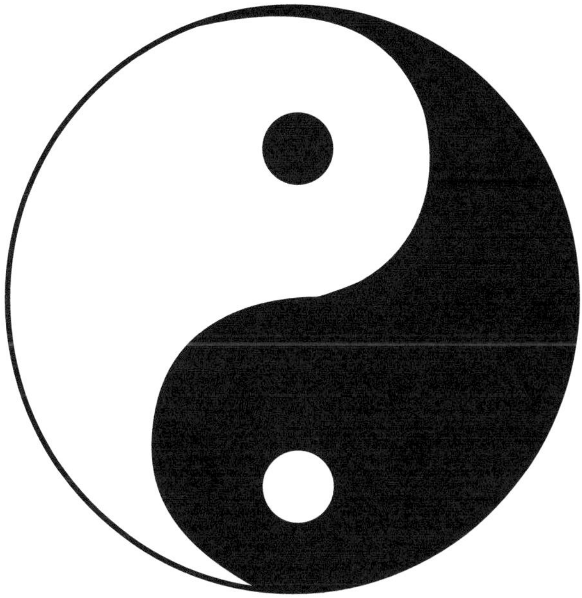

Fig. 16.1 The traditional symbol of Tao, illustrating the interrelationship of opposites, Yin (white) and Yang (black). The symbol conveys the constant movement of energy and the gradual and ceaseless transition of apparent opposites, whether light and dark, hot and cold, or structure and function. The small circular inserts suggest that even in complete Yin there is always some Yang and vice versa

liver "wind," depending on other clinical manifestations. It is of interest in this regard to note the gradual redefinition of our Western concepts of pathogenesis, which is no longer focused just on a pathogenic microbe but also considers the body's immune response and reserves, as well as its resident microbiome.

Disease then is the result of unbalanced energy flow in the body, a flow that is either deficient, excessive, or impeded. The purpose of acupuncture (and other modalities of traditional Chinese medicine) is to optimize this flow of energy and to allow the body to heal itself by optimizing the flow of qi energy. This is achieved by increasing deficient flow and decreasing excessive flow, as well as by opening up blocked energy pathways in the body.

At the risk of oversimplifying, we might sum up the difference between Chinese and Western thinking by saying that Western medicine considers health to be the absence of disease, while Chinese medicine considers disease to be the absence of health.

Meridians

Qi energy circulates through the body along specific pathways, called meridians. Meridians form a three-dimensional network which connects the entire body, both the surface and the organs, and they also interconnect with one another. The main meridians are named after the internal organ where they terminate. The needling of discrete acupoints along the meridians has been found to be effective for treatment of disorders which are often distant from the area of needle insertion. For example, inserting a needle into the hypothenar eminence of the hand (Small Intestine 3) can effectively relieve a neck spasm, since the lateral neck is in the territory of the small intestine meridian. Similarly, a needle in the thenar eminence (Lung 10) can markedly reduce pain from pharyngitis or tonsillitis.

In the context of this book, it should be pointed out that many meridians traversing the body extend to the head and neck, accounting for the observation that distal stimulation of the limbs or torso can bring about therapeutic effects in the head, neck, and face (Fig. 16.2). Further, not only are distant points effective, but they are often more potent in the treatment than local stimulation, suggesting that, by recruit-

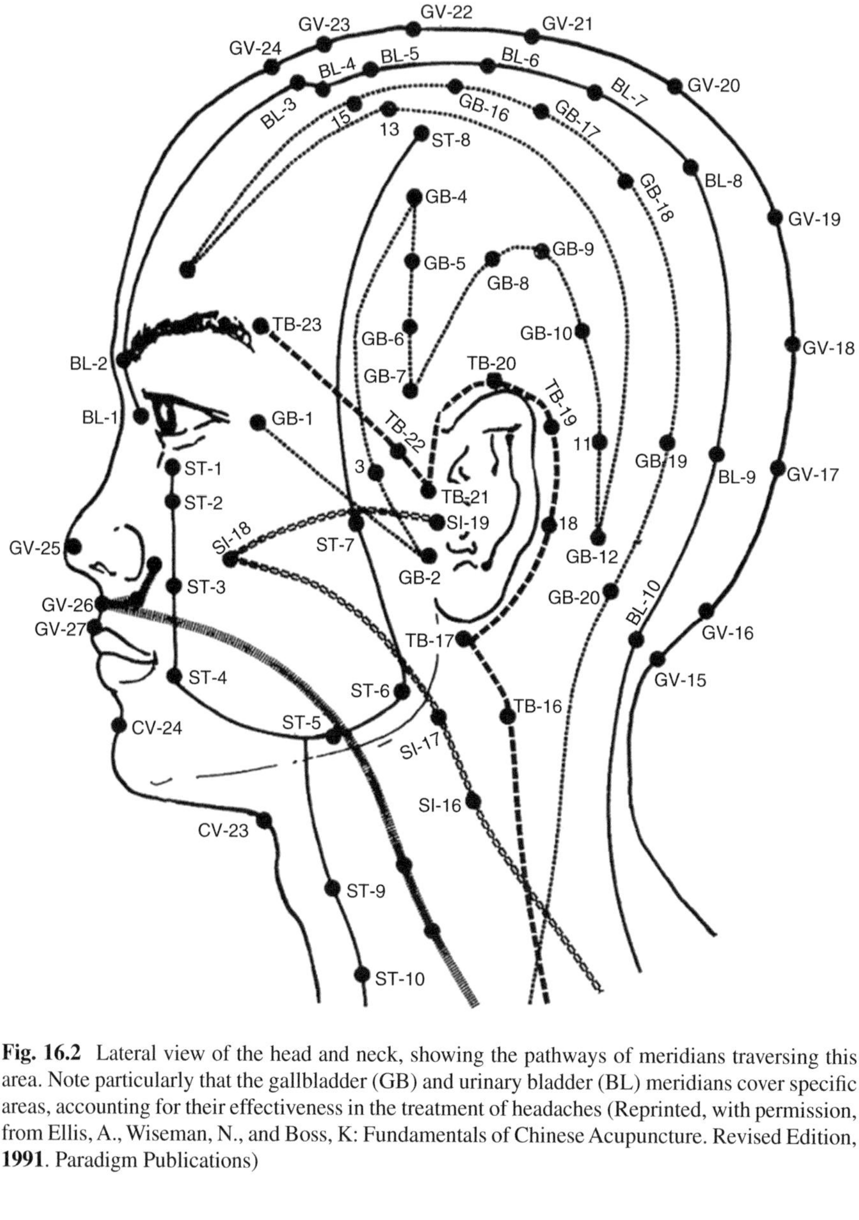

Fig. 16.2 Lateral view of the head and neck, showing the pathways of meridians traversing this area. Note particularly that the gallbladder (GB) and urinary bladder (BL) meridians cover specific areas, accounting for their effectiveness in the treatment of headaches (Reprinted, with permission, from Ellis, A., Wiseman, N., and Boss, K: Fundamentals of Chinese Acupuncture. Revised Edition, **1991**. Paradigm Publications)

ing and marshalling qi from more distant areas, a greater amount of energy flow might arrive at the treated area.

It appears most likely that acupuncture involves bioelectricity. It is known that the skin layer is an electric dipole, exhibiting a potential difference between its surface and deep layer. It has also been shown that at least some active acupoints show decreased electrical resistance. These sharply demarcated loci, measuring 1–2 mm in diameter, demonstrate resistances as low as 10 kilo-ohms, compared to 3 megaohms in the surrounding skin [2]. Piercing the skin in effect shorts this "battery" and creates a localized flow of electricity, known as a "current of injury." The current of injury has been implicated in healing and may be the triggering electrical event in acupuncture treatment. The intensity of this effect can be increased by the use of electric current applied through the acupuncture needle. By increasing the duration and intensity of electric stimulation over time, remarkable degrees of analgesia can be attained.

Despite several interesting and suggestive studies, the structural correlates of acupoints and especially of meridians are not clear. Some acupoints correspond to areas where neurovascular bundles penetrate the deep fascia. Others have shown decreased electrical resistance at point of insertion into the skin. Some dye studies have identified meridians, but a comprehensive explanation for meridians and acupoints is still lacking.

One intriguing proposal, by Dr. Daniel Keown [2], is that the collagen in connective tissue might be the common pathway by which acupuncture impulses propagate. Collagen is ubiquitous in the body and is found not only in the fascia, vessels, tendons, and bones but also in the internal framework and parenchymatous capsules of organs (e.g., pericardium, Glisson's capsule, Gerota's fascia) as well as in structures as diverse as the dura and the sclera. Collagen is electroconductive and also has piezoelectric properties [2], a phenomenon which has been extensively studied for its role in bone healing. Deformation of collagen, either from pathology or from needle insertion, can alter the local electric field, modifying cellular resonance, with distant consequences. Keown suggests that "the connective fabric of our body, the tissue that wraps and joins our entire body, is in effect an interconnected, living electrical web."

But narrowly focusing on specific structural pathways overlooks the constant and complex extra-neuronal electric activity which occurs within and around every cell of the body. It has been suggested [3] that every cell undergoes, on average, 100,000 chemical reactions per second, many involving exchange of ions and the generation of micro-electric currents. In fact, electric flow on the ionic level is how cells communicate, grow, differentiate, and organize. In the central nervous system, complex and synchronized activities such as pattern recognition occur faster and over larger areas of the brain than neuronal-synaptic transmission would permit and have been attributed not to the generation of electrical impulses but rather modulation of a constant baseline bioelectric activity.

The apparent absence of anatomically identifiable meridians is puzzling, but it should not lead to skepticism. Our inability to satisfactorily explain clinically observed phenomena does not negate their reality and may reflect nothing more than current methodological limitations. In the case of acupuncture, our state of uncertainty may be due in part to our inability to measure and experimentally model bioelectric activity on the molecular and cellular level and should not prevent the acceptance of the effectiveness of acupuncture therapy. A large and growing Western literature suggests that acupuncture is effective and should be integrated into our management of patients.

Acupuncture Analgesia

The nature of acupuncture analgesia (AA) is an area of extensive basic and clinical research. The interested reader is referred to a more detailed overview by Dr. Bruce Pomeranz, whose work has been synopsized for this section [4]. Pomeranz has found that the stimulation of small diameter nerves in muscles sends impulses to the spinal cord, and then three centers (spinal cord, midbrain, and pituitary) are activated to release endorphins and monoamines, which block pain messages.

An injury to the skin activates the sensory receptors of small afferent nerve fibers in underlying muscle. Depending on the type of neuron, the sensory fibers synapse either onto the spinothalamic tract in the spinal cord or directly onto the thalamus. From the thalamus, the impulse is carried to the primary somatosensory cortex. If there is no muscle at the site of needle insertion, an alternative pathway of afferent impulse propagation is proposed, involving a synapse onto the anterolateral tract of the spinal cord, which projects onto the spinal cord, the midbrain, and the pituitary-hypothalamic complex. The anterolateral tract of the spinal cord contains endorphinogenic cells, which release either enkephalin or dymorphin. These spinal cord endorphins block the proximal transmission of nerve signals for pain. Serotonin and norepinephrine, released by the midbrain, are also possibly implicated in the mechanism of AA, since the experimental ablation of this area blocks the analgesic effects of acupuncture.

Projections of peripheral nerve signals directly onto the hypothalamus-pituitary complex trigger the release of beta-endorphin into the blood and the CSF. It is of interest in this regard that naloxone, a morphine antagonist, will block analgesia induced by acupuncture, but will not block analgesia or hypalgesia induced by hypnosis [5]. Acupuncture non-responders, Pomeranz suggests, may be genetically deficient in opiate receptors.

The release of beta-endorphin from the pituitary is accompanied by an equimolar release of ACTH, triggering the release of adrenal corticosteroids, which can be measured peripherally as elevations in serum cortisol. This dual release may account for the combined analgesic and anti-inflammatory effect of acupuncture on conditions such as arthritis. Sham acupuncture (the stimulation of random, non-active skin points) appears to have no effect on serum cortisol. It is of interest that in ear acupuncture the main analgesia point (thalamus point) and the ACTH- releasing point have been found to be immediately adjacent to each other, in the floor of the concha, a clinical finding that seems to be explained by the experimental work cited above.

Chinese Diagnosis

Chinese diagnosis does not look for specific illnesses but rather syndromic patterns which identify pathogenic influences and reflect either excessive or insufficient energy flow along certain meridians. Since the meridians are named after the internal organs where they terminate, diagnoses such as "spleen deficiency" or "excessive liver heat" may be made. Different phases of a disease may be dominated by different noxious influences. For example, herpes zoster is associated with the liver and gallbladder meridians. The acute phase of herpes zoster is interpreted as wind-heat, the appearance of purulent vesicles as damp-heat, while postherpetic neuralgia is considered to be due to residual heat with wind [6].

The utility of such diagnoses is that they implicate not only the organ but also suggest the treatment. Excessive heat (or wind) in the liver, one cause of headache, might be treated either by reducing the energy flow in that channel or by reinforcing the flow of inhibiting energy from another meridian (in this case, lung), which controls the liver. The pattern of reinforcing and inhibiting influences among the meridians is known as Five Element theory and is beyond the scope of this chapter.

Clinical evaluation involves the usual Western paradigm of detailed history, followed by physical examination. In addition, the TCM physician also examines the tongue and palpates the radial pulse. The appearance of the tongue, its color, state of hydration, and surface, points to specific syndromes. For example, the presence of dentate impressions along the tongue margin suggests "deficiency in the spleen." Pulse diagnosis is more complex and involves palpating the left and right radial pulse separately, using three fingers laid along each pulse. The palpating fingers then compress the radial artery at three levels, superficially, at the midpoint, and then deeply, compressing the artery against the radius. The strength and quality of the pulse at each measurement is noted and again points to specific syndromic deficiencies and excesses.

For those practitioners who don't have the training or experience to make a Chinese diagnosis, acupuncture can still be used in a more limited but effective fashion. Even a simple understanding of the meridians, along with learning the specific effect of stimulating different acupoints, can lead to positive results in the treatment of many conditions, including pain.

Pain Syndromes and Their Treatment

While the optimal use of acupuncture requires years of study, Western practitioners with even limited knowledge can make use of this modality to augment conventional pain management methods. Once the appropriate points are identified, they can also be stimulated with local pressure (acupressure), transcutaneous electric nerve stimulation (TENS), and conventional acupuncture or by applying electric current to the inserted needle (electroacupuncture), to produce increasing levels of analgesia.

For head and neck pain, one universally applicable point is Hegu (Large Intestine 4), with the needle inserted into the first interosseous muscle of the hand, between the first and second metacarpal. Stimulation of this point has an analgesic effect on most kinds of head and neck pain, from headache to dental pain. Another generally effective pain point is Neiting (Stomach 44), located between the second and third metatarsal of the foot.

A general principle of acupuncture treatment is to needle points on the meridian which supplies the area of pain. While inserting needles at the site of the pain is helpful, the use of distant points appears to be more effective, so a knowledge of the location and distribution of meridians is important. Additional benefit can be derived by needling meridians and points that have a secondary effect on the affected meridians, as well as points that have generally tonifying or sedating effects.

Since pain is usually attributed to a blockage of energy flow along specific meridians, the treatment of headache often involves opening and energizing the channels which connect to specific areas of the head. For example, headache at the base of the head and above the eyebrows (Shao-Yang type) corresponds to the territory of the gallbladder meridian and is treated by needling points along this meridian, which is located along the lateral side of the body, beginning at the outer canthus of the eye and ending between the fourth and fifth toe. Temporal headache (Yang-Ming type) is in the territory of the stomach meridian, which begins above the infraorbital foramen and runs down along the ventral surface of the body to terminate between the second and third metatarsal of the foot. The long path of this meridian explains why needling the foot at this point (Stomach 44) can relieve headache and toothache. Similarly, headache in the territory of other meridians can be treated by needling distant points on that meridian, on the torso, or on the extremities.

Acupuncture has been especially successful for musculoskeletal pain in the head and neck area, such as temporomandibular dysfunction and neck pain due to cervical spine disease. It is also useful for pain related to infections, dental analgesia, as well as cancer pain. It has also been applied in the management of postoperative pain, as well as neuropathic pain, such as trigeminal neuralgia and postherpetic neuralgia. Specific discussion of these and other pain syndromes is available in the literature but beyond the scope of this introductory chapter.

Microsystem Acupuncture

Conventional acupuncture treats points all over the surface of the body. Additionally, it has been determined that points representing the entire body can be found in just one area, such as the hand, the foot, the ear, the scalp, or even the nose, and that needling points just in the one specific area can have a beneficial effect over the entire body. For Western physicians already struggling to make sense of how acupuncture works, this concept seems to defy all conventional explanation.

The most widely used microsystem involves the ear. The auricle has active points that correspond to every part of the body, and auricular acupuncture has been successfully used to treat not only pain but also other somatic disorders, as well as psychologic problems. The distinguishing advantages of auricular acupuncture for the Western physician are several. First, active points (usually demonstrating increased tenderness) develop, which are diagnostic, in that they signal which part of the body is dysfunctional. Second, there is no need to make a syndromic diagnosis. Third, the improvement occurs within minutes and may not require repeated treatments for a cumulative effect. Finally, auricular acupuncture is relatively easy to learn and can be easily incorporated into an office visit, with the patient fully dressed and sitting.

Placebo Effect in Acupuncture

Placebo is a significant component of any form of therapy and can be triggered by factors as innocuous as a white coat. It is more significant when the treatment is unpleasant (such as a bitter red-colored sugar pill or an injection) and may account for up to 50% of perceived improvement. Since acupuncture constitutes a noxious stimulus, there is a significant placebo benefit associated with needling [7]. The placebo effect has made it difficult to isolate the actual benefit of acupuncture; however studies comparing active acupuncture points with other acupoints not active for that condition or even random skin points which are not located on any meridian (sham points) suggest that there is a definite benefit to acupuncture beyond placebo [8]. Furthermore, the subjective nature of perceived pain reduction has made quantification of benefits difficult. This may account for the fact that many Western studies on the acupuncture treatment of pain have been inconclusive.

Incorporating Acupuncture into Pain Management

The purpose of this chapter has been to introduce physicians to some of the basic concepts of acupuncture therapy. It is necessarily limited: the mastery of acupuncture, like the mastery of Western medicine, is a complex and lifelong journey. Hopefully, the reader will come away with enough information to consider adding acupuncture to the current armamentarium of pain management for head and neck disorders. It is suggested that acupuncture, like other non-conventional treatment modalities, should be considered not as alternative but as complementary. Unlike pharmaceuticals, acupuncture is inexpensive, often effective, and has no significant side effects, such as habituation. Including an experienced acupuncturist in the management of difficult pain syndromes will bring a more comprehensive approach to these conditions which may enhance the ultimate outcome.

Acknowledgment The advice and support of my teacher, Prof. Dr. Gertrude Kubiena of Vienna, Austria, is gratefully acknowledged.

References

1. Samadelli M, Melis M, Miccoli M, et al. Complete mapping of the tattoos of the 5300 year old Tyrolean Iceman. J Cultural Heritage. 2015;16(5):753–8.
2. Keown D. The spark in the machine. 2014. London: Singing Dragon.
3. McTaggart L. The Field. London: Harper Collins; 2001.
4. Pomerantz B, Berman B. Scientific basis of acupuncture. In Stux G, Berman B, Pomeranz B, editors. Basics of acupuncture. 5th Revised ed. Berlin: Springer, 2002.
5. Mayer DJ, Price DD, Raffi A. Antagonism of acupuncture analgesia in man by the narcotic antagonist naloxone. Brain Res. 1977;121(2):368–72.
6. Kubiena G, Sommer B. Practice handbook of acupuncture. Edinburgh: Churchill Livingstone; 2010.
7. Dowson DI, Lewith GT, Machin D. The effects of acupuncture versus placebo in the treatment of headache. Pain. 1985;21(1):35–42.
8. Melchart D, Streng A, Hoppe A, Brinkhaus B, et al. Acupuncture in patients with tension-type headache: randomised controlled trial. BMJ. 2005;331:376.

Chapter 17
Gamma Knife Radiosurgery for Trigeminal Neuralgia

José A. Peñagarícano

Introduction

The treatment of medically refractory trigeminal neuralgia with radiosurgery technique was reported by Leksell in 1971 [1]. Multiple publications, some with hundreds of patients, have reported on the efficacy of radiosurgery in medically refractory cases of trigeminal neuralgia. The main advantages of radiosurgery over other invasive procedures are minimal invasiveness and low risk of complications. At our center, frame-based gamma knife radiosurgery uses a single 4mm shot to target the trigeminal nerve at the root entry zone, shaping the field to minimize radiation dose to the brainstem (Fig. 17.1). Although today the standard prescribed dose is between 80 and 90 Gy, there is variability across the literature. Similarly, there is some variation in the placement of the isocenter. The goal of the radiosurgeon is to find a balance between the success of the procedure and the risk of the patient in developing toxicity.

Gamma Knife Radiosurgery for Medically Refractory Trigeminal Neuralgia

Probability of significant pain relief results is presented on Table 17.1.

J. A. Peñagarícano
Department of Radiation Oncology, University of Arkansas for Medical Sciences, Little Rock, AR, USA
e-mail: penagaricanojosea@uams.edu

J. Y. Suen, E. Petersen (eds.), *Diagnosis and Management of Head and Face Pain*, https://doi.org/10.1007/978-3-319-90999-8_17

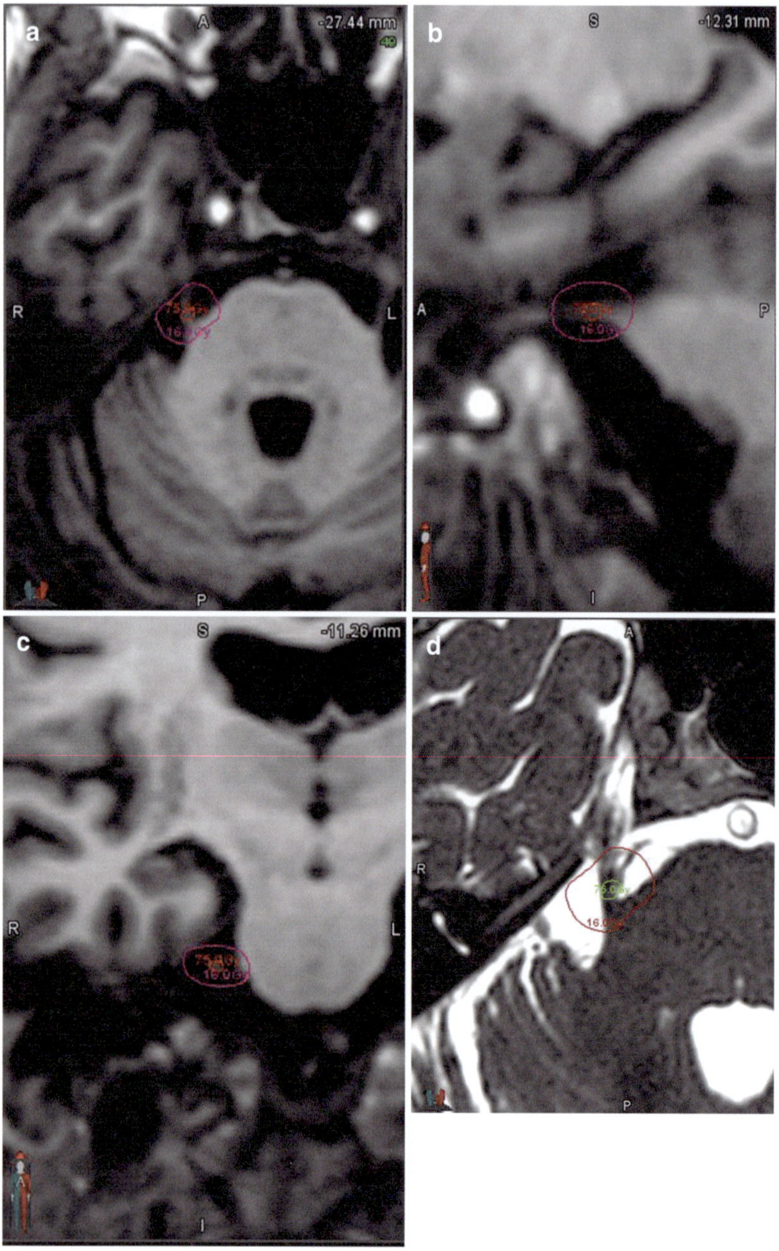

Fig. 17.1 T1 Axial (**a**), T1 sagittal (**b**), T1 coronal (**c**) and T2 axial (**d**) magnetic resonance imaging showing the radiosurgery target at the right trigeminal nerve in a patient with typical trigeminal neuralgia prescribed 80Gy. The red circle represents the 16Gy isodose line. Notice how this line is shaped to minimize brainstem volume. This was done by selective blocking of the radiation beam. The green line represents the 75Gy line. Note the relation of this line with the trigeminal nerve. The 80Gy line is not visible as it is a point within a voxel.

Table 17.1 Probability of significant pain relief in patients treated for medical refractory trigeminal neuralgia with Gamma Knife radiosurgery

Institution	Number of patients	Probability of significant pain relief	Most common prescribed dose
University of Pittsburgh [2]	503	73%, 65%, 41%, 26%[a]	80 Gy
University of Arkansas for Medical Sciences [4]	44	78%, 50%, 33%[b]	80 Gy
Ruber International Hospital [5]	117	85%, 81%, 76%[c]	90 Gy
Cleveland Clinic/Mid-Michigan Hospital [6]	870	79%, 82%, 92%[d]	≥90 Gy but ≤95 Gy

[a]Probability of significant pain relief at 1, 2, 5, and 10 years, respectively
[b]Initial, 2-, and 5-year rates of pain-free outcome, respectively
[c]BNI Class I rate at 3, 5, and 7 years, respectively
[d]4-year rate of excellent or good pain response for patients treated to ≤82 Gy, 83–86 Gy, and ≥90 Gy, respectively

University of Pittsburgh Series [2]

The University of Pittsburgh reported the results on 503 patients with idiopathic trigeminal neuralgia treated with Gamma Knife radiosurgery. A total of 644 radiosurgery procedures were performed. Of these 503 patients, 89 were additional radiosurgery procedures. A single 4-mm isocenter was used in 99% of the patients and two 4-mm isocenters were used in 1% of the patients. The position of a single isocenter was 3–8 mm anterior from the junction of the trigeminal nerve and pons. When two isocenters were used, these were placed to create an oval dose distribution in which a longer nerve segment extending more anteriorly was irradiated. The most common dose of radiosurgery was 80 Gy (88.1% of patients) with a range of 60–90 Gy. Forty-two did not have any follow-up data and were excluded from the analysis. All patients had long-standing pain refractory to medical management to a variety of medications. Twenty-nine percent of patients required additional surgical procedures for better pain control. Additional procedures included repeat radiosurgery, glycerol rhizotomy, microvascular decompression, and balloon microcompression. Pain was measured using the BNI (Barrow Neurological Institute, see Table 17.2) pain intensity score.

Eighty-nine percent of patients responded (BNI score I–IIIb) to radiosurgery after a median latency period of 1 month. Eleven percent of patients had poor pain relief (BNI score IV or V). Forty percent of patients achieved a complete initial pain relief (BNI score I). Factors associated with initial complete pain relief (BNI score I), significant pain relief (BNI scores I–IIIa), and adequate pain relief (BNI scores I–IIIb) were trigeminal neuralgia without additional symptoms (Type 1 trigeminal neuralgia defined as more than 50% episodic pain).

The probability of maintaining significant pain relief was achieved in 73% of patients at 1 year, 65% at 2 years, 41% at 5 years, and 26% at 10 years. The probability of maintaining adequate pain relief was 80% at 1 year, 71% at 2 years, 46% at 5 years, and 30% at 10 years. Pain recurred in 193 patients. The median time to recurrence was 48 months. No patient experienced an early complication from

Table 17.2 Barrow Neurological Institute pain score [3]

Class I	No pain, no medication
Class II	Occasional pain, no medication
Class IIIa	No pain, medication
Class IIIb	Pain, medication controlled
Class IV	Pain, not well controlled
Class V	No pain relief

radiosurgery. Ten percent developed increased facial sensory dysfunction which occurred during the first 2 years after radiosurgery. The 1-, 3-, and 5-year rates for maintenance of sensation in patients who noted sensory dysfunction were 96, 82, and 78%, respectively.

University of Arkansas Series [4]

The University of Arkansas reported the results of 44 patients with typical trigeminal neuralgia treated with Gamma Knife radiosurgery. This group was compared to 36 patients treated for the same condition but with microvascular decompression. This was not a randomized study. For patients who were young and healthy, microvascular decompression was recommended and proceeded to radiosurgery if patient refused microvascular decompression. For those patients who were older, had significant comorbidities, or refused microvascular decompression, radiosurgery was performed. Radiosurgery dose prescription was 80 Gy for 42 patients and 90 Gy in 2 patients. A single 4-mm isocenter was used for all patients. The isocenter was placed 2–4 mm anterior to the junction of the trigeminal nerve and the pons. Of the total number of patients, only 15 of 80 patients had atypical features. Both patient cohorts were comparable in terms of sex, laterality of involved nerve, and race. However, the cohorts differed in terms of age, duration of symptoms, and incidence of medical comorbidities. Patients self-rated their postoperative pain relief on a 10-point visual analog scale (0 being completely pain-free and 10 being no change from preoperative pain level and frequency of pain).

All patients that had microvascular decompression were initially pain-free. By the time of last follow-up, 80.6% of the microvascular decompression group of patients remained pain-free. There were seven recurrences in the microvascular decompression group. These developed between 3 and 36 months after the procedure. Initial, 2-, and 5-year actuarial rates of pain-free outcome were 100, 88, and 80% for microvascular decompression. In the radiosurgery group, 77.3% of patients were pain-free at a median of 4 weeks after radiosurgery. By the last follow-up, 46.6% of patients remained pain-free without medication. There were 14 recurrences between 3 and 4.42 years after an initial pain-free outcome. The initial, 2-, and 5-year rates of pain-free outcome were 78, 50, and 33%, respectively. There was no death or major morbidity in the microvascular decompression cohort. There were no cases of facial weakness, permanent severe facial numbness, or anesthesia dolorosa. Two patients suffered permanent mild paresthesias or numbness. In the radiosurgery cohort, there was no death, major morbidity, trigeminal motor weakness, or anesthesia dolorosa. Three patients experienced permanent new mild paresthesias or numbness. One patient developed severe permanent sensory numbness.

Ruber International Hospital Series [5]

The Ruber International Hospital series reported the results on 117 patients with trigeminal neuralgia treated with Gamma Knife radiosurgery. Minimum follow-up was 2 years. Radiosurgery was the first procedure for 103 patients and a second procedure for 14 patients. Sixty-one percent of patients received 90 Gy, 31% of patients received 80 Gy, and 8% of patients received 85 Gy. A single 4-mm collimator isocenter, located in the anterior portion of the cisternal segment of the trigeminal nerve, was used for all patients. The BNI pain score was used for pain classification (see Table 17.2). Mean follow-up was 66 months (range, 24–170 months). At the end of the study, clinical response to radiosurgery was classified as BNI Class I in 52% of patients, Class II in 6% of patients, Class IIIa–IIIb in 13% of patients, and Class IV in 29% of patients. Mean time to pain relief was 3.4 months (range, 0–27 months). There was no statistically significant relationship with patient's sex or age, pain laterality or distribution, previous facial numbness, or elapsed time from onset of pain to radiosurgery. Recurrence was defined as a change from response Class I or II to a lower class. BNI Class I rate was 85% at 3 years, 81% at 5 years, and 76% at 7 years. Complete response rates (BNI Class I and II) were 91% at 3 years, 86% at 5 years, and 82% at 7 years. Significant association was seen between good response and patients without any previous radiosurgery and with good initial response to medication and between facial altered sensation and patients previously treated by surgery.

Toxicity was limited to facial altered sensation in the territory of the treated nerve. De novo or worsened facial numbness was seen in 38 patients. Facial altered sensation occurred in a mean time of 14 months with 85% manifesting in the first 2 years.

The Combined Cleveland Clinic and Mid-Michigan Medical Center Hospital Series [6]

The combined Cleveland Clinic and Mid-Michigan Medical Center series reported the results on 870 patients with trigeminal neuralgia treated with Gamma Knife radiosurgery. For treatment a single 4-mm isocenter was placed at the dorsal root entry zone of the trigeminal nerve. The prescribed dose varied from 70 to 95 Gy. For patients treated before the year 2000, the prescribe dose was recalculated (from 75 to 82 Gy) using a collimator-corrected output factor. Outcome measures were

Table 17.3 Barrow Neurological Institute numbness score [3]

Class I	No numbness
Class II	Mild numbness, not bothersome
Class III	Numbness, somewhat bothersome
Class IV	Numbness, very bothersome

limited to pain response and facial numbness. The BNI pain score (see Table 17.2) was used to characterized pain response in one institution, and in the other institution, pain response was evaluated using an excellent (pain-free and off medication), good (rare pain or pain-free on medication not causing side effects), fair (persistent pain but less severe than before treatment), and poor (no significant response to therapy) scoring system. For scoring facial numbness, both institutions used the BNI facial numbness scale (see Table 17.3). For analysis, patients were divided into three dose groups: ≤82 Gy (40% of patients), 83–86 Gy (10% of patients), and ≥90 Gy (50% of patients). Ninety-five percent of patients had typical trigeminal neuralgia, and 9% of patients had a diagnosis of multiple sclerosis. In total, 69 patients did not have a pain response recorded at follow-up and were omitted from the study.

The 4-year rate of excellent to good pain relief across all patients was 86.7%. The 4-year rate of excellent or good pain response as a function of dose was 79%, 81.6%, and 92% in patients treated to ≤82 Gy, 83–86 Gy, and ≥90 Gy, respectively. This was statistically significant. Patients treated to doses ≥90 Gy had statistically significant longer times to pain failure as compared to patients treated to doses ≤82 Gy. The dose prescribed, age at time of radiosurgery, and a history of prior procedure were predictors of pain failure after radiosurgery. Patients treated to lower doses (≤82 Gy) were at a statistically significant higher risk of having pain recurrence compared with patients treated to ≥90 Gy. Additionally, patients who had a prior surgical procedure were at higher risk for pain failure after radiosurgery. At last follow-up, 62% of patients reported excellent and 19% of patients reported good pain control.

The 5-year rate of freedom from BNI Class III or Class IV facial numbness was 58.4%. The 4-year rates of freedom from BNI Class III/IV numbness were similar among patients treated to 83–86 Gy (50.7%) and ≥90 Gy (59.7%) and were significantly lower than the 4-year rate for patients treated to ≤82 Gy (74.9%). One percent of patients were diagnosed with anesthesia dolorosa, all of whom were treated to doses ≤86 Gy.

Isocenter Placement

There is variation in the literature regarding placement of the isocenter for trigeminal neuralgia. No clear consensus could be found in the literature regarding whether an anterior [7–9], middle [10], or posterior [11–13] placement is preferred. The pain-free rates appear to be similar regardless isocenter placement. However, there is one report comparing anterior vs. posterior placement of the isocenter. This showed that posterior placement of the isocenter provides better short-term pain control [14].

Dose Prescription

The standard dose of radiosurgery for trigeminal neuralgia with Gamma Knife is in the range of 80–90 Gy. This dose is prescribed to the 100% isodose line [15–17].

Repeat Gamma Knife Radiosurgery for Recurrent Trigeminal Neuralgia

University of Pittsburgh Series [18]

The University of Pittsburgh reported on 119 patients, with a median follow-up of 48 months, diagnosed with recurrent trigeminal neuralgia that received repeat Gamma Knife radiosurgery. For treatment, a single 4-mm isocenter was used. The target was placed anterior to the first procedure's target so that the two radiosurgical volumes overlapped by 50%. The median target dose was 70 Gy. The median cumulative target dose was 145 Gy. BNI pain score of I to IIIb was considered as successful treatment, whereas a score of IV or V was considered a treatment failure. Initial pain response considered successful treatment was seen in 103 of 119 patients (86%). Median time to initial response was 1.5 months. At last evaluation pain response considered successful was seen in 57 of 108 patients (53%). Three percent and 18% of patients developed new or increased facial sensory dysfunction that was temporary or permanent, respectively.

Wake Forest University Series [19]

Wake Forest University reported on 37 patients, with a mean follow-up of 3.8 years, who had undergone repeat Gamma Knife for trigeminal neuralgia. A 4-mm collimator was used in all patients. The location of the isocenter was generally moved distally from the initial procedure's isocenter. If the initial procedure's isocenter was placed distally, then the repeat procedure's isocenter was placed closer to the brainstem to minimize overlap. The initial mean target dose was 87.3 Gy. The mean repeat treatment dose was 84.4 Gy. Pain relief was categorized as excellent (complete pain relief without medications), good (complete pain relief or minimal residual pain still requiring medication), fair (persistent pain with >50% pain relief with or without medication), or poor (persistent pain with <50% pain relief regardless of medication status). Overall 17 patients (46%) had excellent pain relief, 9 (24%) had good pain relief, 5 (14%) had fair pain relief, and 6 (16%) had poor pain relief. The mean interval to complete pain relief was 10.5 weeks. Of the 37 patients, 21 had some degree of trigeminal nerve dysfunction after repeat Gamma Knife. Of the 26 patients who had had no numbness before the second Gamma Knife procedure, 10 (38%) had developed numbness after the second Gamma Knife procedure. Of the 11 patients with pre-existing numbness before repeat Gamma Knife, 3 (27%) experienced worsening of this numbness after the second procedure. Fourteen of 21 patients (67%) who had experienced some degree of numbness had an excellent outcome. In addition, 21 (100%) of 21 patients experiencing numbness had >50% pain relief, and 9 (60%) of 15 patients experiencing no numbness had >50% pain relief. None of 6 patients with poor outcomes had sensory disturbances after GKRS. The incidence of numbness was 78% in patients who received >108.5 Gy to the surface of the pons and 39% in patient who received <108.5 Gy. Cumulative doses equal or higher than 84.3 Gy to the dorsal root entry zone carried a toxicity rate of 72% vs. 44% if the cumulative dose was less than 84.3 Gy.

In a subsequent report [20], the institution reported on 152 patients with recurrent trigeminal neuralgia after Gamma Knife radiosurgery. Eighty-four percent of patients achieved at least BNI score of IIIb, with 46% achieving BNI score of I. The 1-, 3-, and 5-year rates of BNI I pain relief were 63%, 50%, and 37%, respectively. The 1-, 3-, and 5-year rates of BNI IIIb or better pain relief were 74%, 59%, and 46%, respectively. Two patients developed anesthesia dolorosa. The main predictive factors for pain relief were facial numbness after and a positive pain response to the first Gamma Knife procedure.

Gamma Knife Radiosurgery in Multiple Sclerosis-Related Trigeminal Neuralgia

The University of Pittsburgh [21] reported on 37 patients with multiple sclerosis-related trigeminal neuralgia with a median follow-up time of 56.7 months. A single 4-mm isocenter targeting 2–8 mm anterior to the junction of the trigeminal nerve and pons was used. Median prescribed dose was 80 Gy. The median time to achieve complete pain relief (BNI score I) and reasonable pain control (BNI score I–IIIb) were 10 days and 7 days, respectively. Eventual complete pain relief and reasonable pain relief were noted in 62.1% and 97.3% of patients. One patient had no improvement. Reasonable pain control was maintained in 82.6%, 73.9%, and 54% of patients after 1, 3, and 5 years. Recurrent pain occurred in 37.8% of patients. Two patients described new unilateral facial sensory dysfunction after radiosurgery.

The Marseille [22] group reported on 43 patients with multiple sclerosis-associated trigeminal neuralgia that were treated with Gamma Knife radiosurgery. Median follow-up was 53.8 months. A single 4-mm collimator was used and positioned in the cisternal portion of the trigeminal nerve at a median distance of 8 mm anterior to the entrance of the trigeminal nerve into the brainstem. Median prescribed dose was 85 Gy. Pain was scored using three different scales: BNI (see

Table 17.4 Burchiel classification of facial pain [23]

Class I	Pain free, no medication
Class II	Pain free, on medication
Class IIIa	Pain improved, no medication
Class IIIb	Pain improved, on medication
Class IV	Pain not improved

Table 17.5 Regis classification of facial pain [24]

Class I	No trigeminal pain, no medication
Class II	No pain, with medication
Class III	Pain frequency reduction >90%
Class IV	Pain frequency, reduction 50–90%
Class V	No pain reduction
Class VI	Pain worsening

Table 17.2), Burchiel (see Table 17.4), and Regis (see Table 17.5). For hypoesthesia evaluation, the BNI facial hypoesthesia classification was used. Thirty-nine patients (90.7%) had initial pain cessation in a median time of 30 days. Their actuarial probability of remaining pain free without medication at 6 months and 1, 3, 5, and 10 years was 87.2, 71.8, 43.1, 38.3, and 20.5%, respectively, and remained stable until 12 years. The hypoesthesia actuarial rate at 6 months, 1 year, and 2 years was 11.5, 11.5, and 16% and remained stable until 12 years.

Gamma Knife Radiosurgery for Medically Refractory Atypical Trigeminal Neuralgia

The University of Maryland and Boston University [25] reported their results in the use of Gamma Knife radiosurgery in 35 patients with atypical trigeminal neuralgia. A single 4-mm isocenter was placed adjacent to the region where the trigeminal nerve exits the brainstem. The median prescription dose was 75 Gy. Pain outcome was classified using the BNI pain score. Before treatment all patients classified their pain as severe (BNI IV or V). With a median follow-up of 29 months, 72% reported excellent/good outcomes (BNI I, 22%; BNI II, 6%; BNI III, 44%). The mean time to pain relief was 5.8 weeks. The mean duration of pain relief was 62.4 weeks. Eighty-eight percent of patients reported a decrease in the use of pain medication. The 1-year, 2-year, and 3-year actuarial rates of freedom from pain were 53%, 39%, and 39%, respectively. During the follow-up period, 39% of patients who initially experienced pain relief reported a recurrence of their pain. There were no major complications. Persistent facial numbness (BNI III–IV) was reported in 19% of patients.

Which Patients Should Receive Gamma Knife Radiosurgery for Trigeminal Neuralgia?

Gamma Knife radiosurgery for medically refractory or multiple sclerosis-related trigeminal neuralgia is considered first-line treatment along with microvascular decompression and rhizotomy. However, before selecting candidates for Gamma Knife, the treating radiosurgeon takes into consideration several patient factors such as existing comorbidities, prior treatments, pain severity, and patient's choice. In general, for patients refusing non-radiosurgical treatments but are candidates for microvascular decompression, Gamma Knife is an option with the understanding that microvascular decompression has twice the rate of durable pain relief of Gamma Knife radiosurgery. That is, microvascular decompression is superior to Gamma Knife radiosurgery in achieving long-lasting pain relief [26–28]. In addition, following microvascular decompression, most patients have immediate pain relief, whereas for Gamma Knife, there is a latent period of approximately 1 month [29, 3]. These considerations are important in cases where the pain is so severe that the patient's activities of daily living are affected.

Frameless Radiosurgery for Trigeminal Neuralgia

Over the past 10 years, there has been several manuscripts published regarding frameless radiosurgery for trigeminal neuralgia [30–35]. These studies have reported results in a small number of patients as compared to the frame-based radiosurgery literature presented above. In addition, the follow-up of these studies is relatively short with median or average follow-up ranging between 15 and 37 months. One study [36] investigated the accuracy of frameless stereotactic intracranial radiosurgery utilizing the BrainLab mask and Exac Trac table. Results showed an accuracy of the positioning system of approximately 0.3 mm in each direction. The intrafraction motion was 0.35 ± 0.21 mm with a maximum of 1.15 mm. The clinical studies showed that frameless SRS is safe and effective in the management of trigeminal neuralgia.

References

1. Leksell L. Stereotaxic radiosurgery in trigeminal neuralgia. Acta Chir Scand. 1971;137(4):311–4.
2. Kondziolka D, Zorro O, Lobato-Polo J, Kano H, Flannery T, Flickinger J, Lunsford L. Gamma Knife stereotactic radiosurgery for idiopathic trigeminal neuralgia. J Neurosurg. 2010;112(4):758–65.

3. Rogers CL, Shetter AG, Fiedler JA, et al. Gamma Knife radiosurgery for trigeminal neuralgia: the initial experience of the Barrow Neurological Institute. Int J Radiat Oncol Biol Phys. 2000;47:1013–9.
4. Linskey M, Ratanatharathorn V, Penagaricano J. A prospective cohort study of microvascular decompression and Gamma Knife surgery in patients with trigeminal neuralgia. J Neurosurg. 2008;109(Suppl 2):190–72.
5. Martinez Moreno N, Gutierrez-Sarraga J, Rey-Portoles G, Jimenez-Huete A, Martinez Alvarez R. Long-term outcomes in the treatment of classical trigeminal neuralgia by Gamma Knife radiosurgery: a retrospective study in patients with minimum 2-year follow-up. Neurosurgery. 2016;79(6):879–88.
6. Kotecha R, Kotecha R, Modugula S, Murphy E, Jones M, Kotecha R, Reddy C, Suh J, Barnett G, Neyman G, Machado A, Nagel S, Chao S. Trigeminal neuralgia treated with stereotactic radiosurgery: the effect of dose escalation on pain control and treatment outcomes. Int J Radiat Oncol Biol Phys. 2016;96(1):142–8.
7. Lorenzoni JG, Massager N, David P, Devriendt D, Desmedt F, Brotchi J, Levivier M. Neurovascular compression anatomy and pain outcome in patients with classical trigeminal neuralgia treated by radiosurgery. Neurosurgery. 2008;62(2):368–75.
8. Massager N, Lorenzoni JG, Devriendt D, Desmedt F, Brotchi J, Levivier M. Gamma Knife surgery for idiopathic trigeminal neuralgia performed using a far-anterior cisternal target and a high dose of radiation. J Neurosurg. 2004;100(4):597–605.
9. Regis J, Arkha Y, Yomo S, Murata N, Roussel P, Donnet A, Peragut JC. Radiosurgery in trigeminal neuralgia: long-term results and the influence of operative nuances. Neurochirurgie. 2009;55(2):213–22.
10. Kondziolka D, Lunsford LD, Flickinger JC. Stereotactic radiosurgery for the treatment of trigeminal neuralgia. Clin J Pain. 2002;18(1):42–7.
11. Han J, Dg K, Chung HT, Paek SH, Kim YH, Cy K, Kim JW, Kim YH, Jeong SS. Long-term outcome of Gamma Knife radiosurgery for treatment of typical trigeminal neuralgia. Int J Radiat Oncol Biol Phys. 2009;75(3):822–7.
12. Huang CF, Tu HT, Liu WS, Chiou SY, Lin LY. Gamma Knife surgery used as primary and repeated treatment for idiopathic trigeminal neuralgia. J Neurosurg. 2008;109(Suppl):179–84.
13. Longhi M, Rizzo P, Nicolato A, Foroni R, Reggio M, Gerosa M. Gamma Knife radiosurgery for trigeminal neuralgia: results and potentially predictive parameters-part I: idiopathic trigeminal neuralgia. Neurosurgery. 2007;61(6):1254–60.
14. Matsuda S, Serizawa T, Nagano O, Ono J. Comparison of the results of 2 targeting methods in Gamma Knife surgery for trigeminal neuralgia. J Neurosurg. 2008;109(Suppl):185–9.
15. Kondziolka D, Lunsford LD, Flickinger JC, Young RF, Vermeulen S, Duma CM, Jacques DB, Rand RW, Regis J, Peragut JC, Manera L, Epsatein MH, Lindquist C. Stereotactic radiosurgery for trigeminal neuralgia: a multiinstitutional study using the gamma unit. J Neurosurg. 1996;84(6):940–5.
16. Cheuk AV, Chin LS, Petitt JH, Herman JM, Fang HB, Regine WF. Gamma Knife surgery for trigeminal neuralgia: outcome, imaging, and brain stem correlates. Int J Radiat Ocol Biol Phys. 2004;60(2):537–41.
17. Maesawa S, Salame C, Flickinger JC, Pirris S, Kondziolka D, Lunsford LD. Clinical outcomes after stereotactic radiosurgery for idiopathic trigeminal neuralgia. J Neurosurg. 2001;94(1):14–20.
18. Park K, Kondziolka D, Berkowitz O, Kano H, Novotny J, Niranjan A, Flickinger J, Lunsford L. Repeat Gamma Knife radiosurgery for trigeminal neuralgia. Neurosurgery. 2012;70:295–305.
19. Aubuchon AC, Chan MD, Lovat JF, Balamucki CJ, Ellis TL, Tatter SB, McMullen KP, Munley MT, Deguzman AF, Ekstrand KE, Bourland JD, Shaw EG. Repeat Gamma Knife radiosurgery for trigeminal neuralgia. Int J Radiat Oncol Biol Phys. 2011;81(4):1059–65.
20. Helis CA, Lucas JT, Bourland JD, Chan MD, Tatter SB, Laxton AW. Repeat radiosurgery for trigeminal neuralgia. Neurosurgery. 2015;77:755–61.

21. Zorro O, Lobato-Polo J, Kano H, Flickinger J, Lunsford L, Kondziolka D. Gamma Knife radiosurgery for multiple sclerosis-related trigeminal neuralgia. Neurology. 2009;73:1149–54.
22. Tuleasca C, Carron R, Resseguier N, Donnet A, Roussel P, Gaudart J, Levivier M, Regis J. Multiple-sclerosis related trigeminal neuralgia: a prospective series of 43 patients treated with Gamma Knife surgery with more than one year of follow-up. Streotact Funct Neurosurg. 2014;92:203–10.
23. Eller JL, Raslan AM, Burchiel KJ. Trigeminal neuralgia: definition and classification. Neurosurg Focus. 2005;18:E3.
24. Regis J, et al. Prospective controlled trial of gamma knife surgery for essential trigeminal neuralgia. J Neurosurg. 2006;104:913–24.
25. Dhople A, Kwok Y, Chin I, Shepard D, Slawson R, Amin P, Regine W. Efficacy and quality of life outcomes in patients with atypical trigeminal neuralgia treated with Gamma Knife radiosurgery. Int Radiat Oncology Biol Phys. 2007;69(2):397–403.
26. Brisman R. Microvascular decompression vs. Gamma Knife for typical trigeminal neuralgia: preliminary findings. Stereotact Funct Neurosurg. 2007;85:94–8.
27. Linskey ME, Ratanatharathorn V, Penagarciano J. A prospective cohort study of microvascular decompression and Gamma Knife surgery in patients with trigeminal neuralgia. J Neurosurg. 2008;109(Suppl):160–72.
28. Pollock BE, Schoeberl KA. Prospective comparison of posterior fossa exploration and stereotactic radiosurgery dorsal root entry zone target as a primary surgery for patients with idiopathic trigeminal neuralgia. Neurosurgery. 2010;67:633–9.
29. Barker FGII, Jannetta PJ, Bissonette DJ, et al. The long-term outcome of microvascular decompression for trigeminal neuralgia. N Engl J Med. 1996;334:1077–83.
30. Patil CG, Veeravagu A, Bower RS, Li G, Chang SD, Lim M, Adler JR Jr. CyberKnife radiosurgical rhizotomy for the treatment of atypical trigeminal nerve pain. Neurosurg Focus. 2007;23(6):E9.
31. Fariselli L, Marras C, De Santis M, Marchetti M, Milanesi I, Broggi G. CyberKnife radiosurgery as a first treatment for idiopathic trigeminal neuralgia. Neurosurgery. 2009;64(Suppl):A96–101.
32. Chen JC, Rahimian J, Rahimian R, Arellano A, Miller MJ, Girvigian MR. Frameless image-guided radiosurgery for initial treatment of typical trigeminal neuralgia. World Neurosurg. 2010;74(4–5):538–43.
33. Conti A, Pontoriero A, Latì G, Esposito F, Siniscalchi EN, Crimi S, Vinci S, Brogna A, De Ponte F, Germanò A, Pergolizzi S, Tomasello F. Frameless stereotactic radiosurgery for treatment of multiple sclerosis-related trigeminal neuralgia. World Neurosurg. 2017;103:702–12.
34. Shields LBE, Shanks TS, Shearer AJ, Shelton LA, Shelton BJ, Howe J, Coons JM, Plato B, Spalding AC. Frameless image-guided radiosurgery for trigeminal neuralgia. Surg Neurol Int. 2017;26:87.
35. Kerolus MG, Sen N, Mayekar S, Templeton A, Turian J, Diaz A, Munoz L, Byrne RW, Sani S. Truebeam radiosurgery for the treatment of trigeminal neuralgia: preliminary results at a single institution. Cureus. 2017;9(6):e1362.
36. Verbakel WF, Lagerwaard FJ, Verduin AJ, Heukelom S, Slotman BJ, Cuijpers JP. The accuracy of frameless stereotactic intracranial radiosurgery. Radiother Oncol. 2010;97(3):390–4.

Chapter 18
Percutaneous Procedures for Trigeminal Neuralgia

Michael D. Staudt, Maricruz Rivera, and Jonathan P. Miller

Introduction

Treatment of trigeminal neuralgia (TN) by percutaneous rhizotomy has long been considered a safe and effective alternative to medical or open surgical management. Although medical management with anticonvulsants remains the first-line treatment for TN, symptoms are sometimes refractory, and side effects are often intolerable. Microvascular decompression (MVD) can provide excellent, long-term pain relief in patients with neurovascular compression, although it may not be an option in elderly patients or those with extensive comorbidities. As such, percutaneous lesioning procedures, including radiofrequency rhizotomy (RR), glycerol rhizotomy (GR), and percutaneous balloon compression (PBC), are an attractive and effective alternative with relatively low surgical risk.

In 1911, Härtel described the treatment of TN using percutaneous injection of ethanol through the foramen ovale, identified via simple anatomic landmarks [1]. However, technical limitations in the ability to produce lesions of precisely controlled intensity limited the use of percutaneous techniques for the next several decades. Operative management commonly consisted of open surgical decompression based on the belief that TN was related to compressive scar tissue within the trigeminal ganglion or nerve fibers [2, 3]. Subsequently, it became clear that trauma to the trigeminal nerve causing facial numbness correlated well with pain relief [4–6]. For some time, middle fossa craniotomy was used to approach the trigeminal

M. D. Staudt · J. P. Miller (✉)
Department of Neurological Surgery, University Hospitals Cleveland Medical Center, Case Western Reserve University, Cleveland, OH, USA
e-mail: Michael.staudt@londonhospitals.ca; jonathan.miller@uhhospitals.org

M. Rivera
Case Western Reserve University, School of Medicine, Cleveland, OH, USA
e-mail: mxr354@case.edu

J. Y. Suen, E. Petersen (eds.), *Diagnosis and Management of Head and Face Pain*, https://doi.org/10.1007/978-3-319-90999-8_18

ganglion to produce a lesion. The development of techniques allowing precise lesion creation led to a resurgence in the use of the less invasive percutaneous approach.

The modern use of percutaneous techniques continues to adhere to the basic principles and landmarks initially described by Härtel. Each of these procedures causes direct injury to the trigeminal ganglion and nerves. Radiofrequency rhizolysis (RR), described by Wall and Sweet [7], refers to thermocoagulation of the trigeminal ganglion and nerve fibers. RR underwent a number of refinements to maximize clinical efficacy while reducing the risk of inducing painful dysesthesias, including temperature monitoring, short-acting anesthetics to allow patient feedback, and the development of fine electrodes for highly selective lesion creation [8, 9]. The discovery of glycerol rhizotomy (GR) was serendipitous: injection of radiopaque tantalum powder suspended in glycerol to localize the trigeminal ganglion for radiosurgical targeting was found to lead to pain relief [10], and the modern usage of this technique has changed little since its discovery [11–13]. Percutaneous balloon compression (PBC) was developed as a percutaneous modification of the middle fossa approach based on the observation that facial pain responded better to compression of the nerve [6, 14]. Subsequent preclinical studies demonstrated that PBC preferentially damages large myelinated pain fibers while sparing small unmyelinated fibers [13, 15], corresponding to the sensory trigger of TN [16].

Percutaneous lesioning techniques treat the symptoms of TN by injuring the trigeminal nerve, producing hypesthesia within the affected distribution. Pain recurrence rates are relatively high as the nerve recovers over time, although repeat procedures are effective [17, 18]. The minimally invasive nature and relative ease of use has encouraged widespread adoption and can confer excellent clinical efficacy in appropriately chosen patients. The aim of this chapter is to describe patient selection and surgical technique of percutaneous procedures, with a review of clinical efficacy and outcomes.

Patient Selection

Careful consideration of clinical characteristics of facial pain is essential in order to choose the appropriate intervention. TN is a heterogeneous pain disorder with a variety of clinical manifestations and potential etiologies [19]. The most important consideration when considering surgical approach is the preponderance of intermittent lancinating pain (Type 1 TN) as opposed to constant pain (Type 2 TN); other features of TN include identifiable triggers, memorable onset of pain, pain-free intervals, and good response to antiepileptics, particularly carbamazepine [20]. TN may also be caused by nerve injury, trauma, or multiple sclerosis [19]. The first-line treatment involves the use of antiepileptic medications. An MRI is commonly obtained during the diagnostic work-up to rule out other etiologies and identify vascular compression at the root entry zone [21, 22]. If neurovascular compression is identified, microvascular decompression (MVD) leads to more durable pain relief without sensory loss, although it is considerably more invasive [23].

The choice of a percutaneous procedure is appropriate for patients who have failed medical management or developed intolerable side effects and who are not considered candidates for MVD due to elevated surgical risk or personal preference. Percutaneous treatments can also be effective in patients with recurrent TN symptoms despite previous MVD. Patients with symptoms suggestive of trigeminal neuropathic pain or deafferentation are not considered candidates for percutaneous techniques, since lesioning procedures may exacerbate symptoms by causing additional damage to the nerve.

Symptomatic TN develops in 1–2% of patients with multiple sclerosis and responds to percutaneous rhizotomy [24, 25], although outcome is suboptimal compared with patients with idiopathic TN, with a higher recurrence rate and worse side effect profile [24, 26, 27]. RR has somewhat better outcome compared with GR and PBC in this population [28, 29]. Retrospective studies of percutaneous treatment of TN secondary to multiple sclerosis or herpes are significantly limited due to small sample sizes [24, 26–30]. Patients with symptomatic TN also acquire less benefit from MVD compared with idiopathic TN [31, 32].

The three percutaneous techniques differ in the ability to target individual trigeminal nerve distributions. In general, RR is the most selective, as the ability to perform awake mapping using stimulation allows for selective localization of the lesion to the painful area. RR for the treatment of V1 distribution pain is rarely performed because of the elevated risk of corneal anesthesia. GR can be used to treat pain in only V3, in both V3 and V2, or in all three distributions by injecting a precise volume of glycerol; special techniques can allow for treatment of isolated V1 distribution pain. PBC is less selective but rarely produces corneal anesthesia due to preferential compression of large diameter fibers [15].

Perioperative Preparation

Anatomic Considerations

An understanding of the anatomic relationship of the foramen ovale to its surrounding structures is essential to ensure clinical efficacy and safety. Access to the foramen ovale is based on the anatomic landmarks of Härtel [1]: the entry point is 2–3 cm lateral and 1 cm inferior to the oral commissure, and the trajectory is chosen to approach the mid-pupillary line at 3 cm anterior to the external auditory canal (Fig. 18.1).

Meckel's cave is accessed through the foramen ovale, which is located in the greater wing of the sphenoid bone (Fig. 18.2). Meckel's cave is a cerebrospinal fluid-filled cistern containing the trigeminal (Gasserian) ganglion, which comprises the three divisions of the trigeminal nerve: V1 or ophthalmic, V2 or maxillary, and V3 or mandibular. Cannulation of Meckel's cave may result in spontaneous egress of cerebrospinal fluid, which may be correlated with clinical efficacy [33]; however, the lack of cerebrospinal fluid does not necessarily indicate an extracisternal location nor does spontaneous flow indicate accurate placement. If necessary, injection of contrast medium can be used to confirm position.

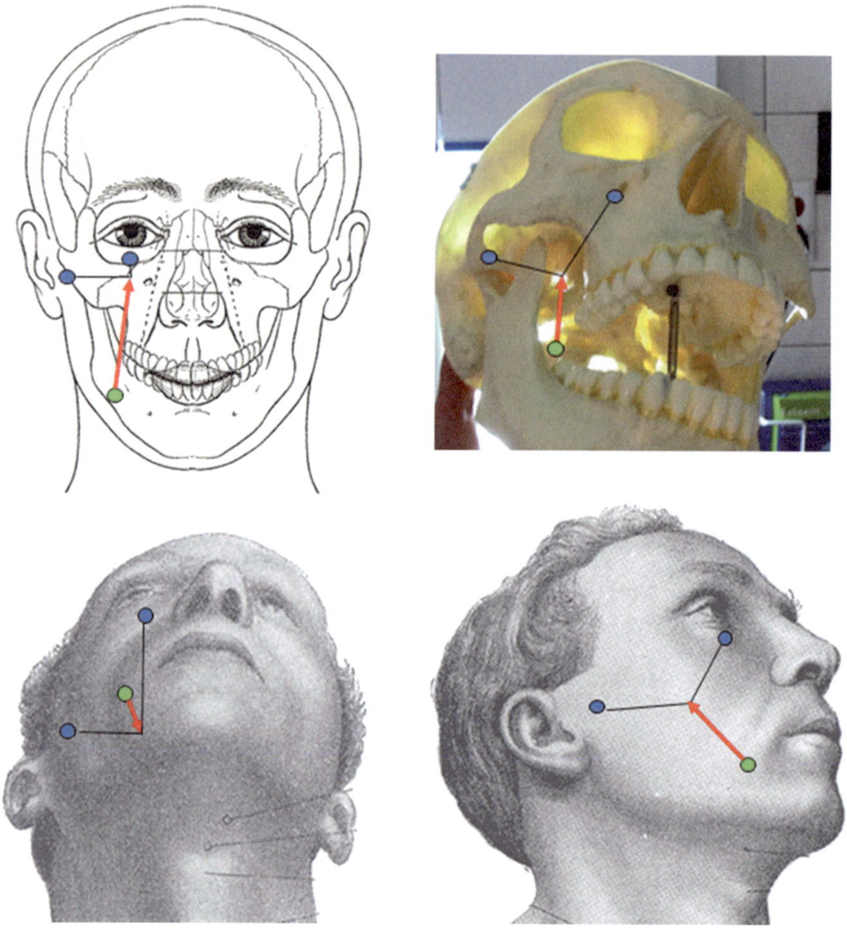

Fig. 18.1 Anatomic landmarks for foramen ovale cannulation. Entry point (green circle) is identified 2 cm lateral and 1 cm inferior to the corner of the mouth. Target is identified by the intersection of the mid-pupillary line and a point 2 cm in front of the tragus (blue circles). It is important not to drape off these landmarks during preparation (Adapted from Ref. 53, Figs. 1199, 1194, and 1195)

Other nearby foramen in the vicinity of the foramen ovale should not be cannulated in order to avoid injury to neurovascular structures (Fig. 18.2). The carotid canal lies posterolaterally and the foramen lacerum posteromedially, so an inappropriately posterior needle trajectory may injure the C2 or C3 segment of the carotid artery, respectively. Pulsatile blood flow through the needle or a rapidly enlarging buccal hematoma may be indicative of internal carotid artery penetration. If this occurs, the needle is immediately withdrawn, and pressure is applied to the posterior pharyngeal space and the patient admitted for observation. Further vascular imaging may be required, as well outpatient follow-up to monitor potential complications such as the development of a carotid-cavernous fistula [34]. However, if there are no complications, the procedure may be safely performed a few days later.

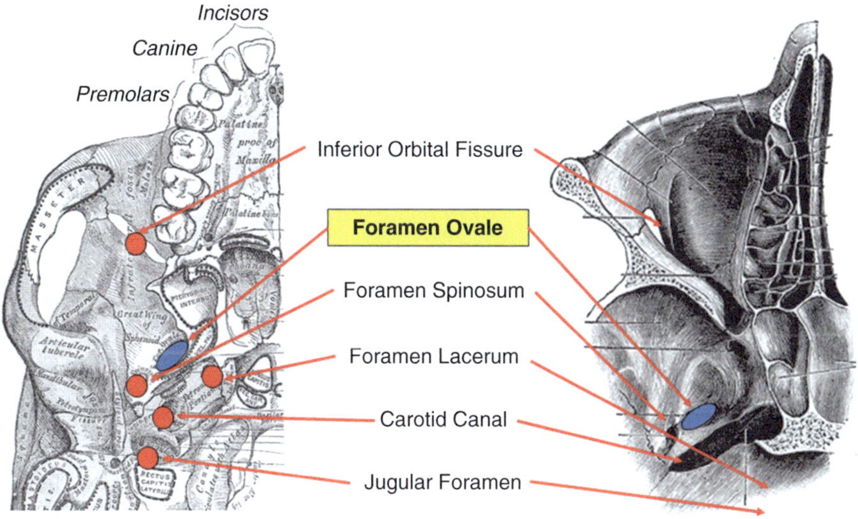

Fig. 18.2 Overview of relevant skull base anatomy for foramen ovale cannulation. Foramen ovale is highlighted and indicated by blue oval. Nearby foramen which may be potentially cannulated if trajectory is off-target is indicated by right circles (Adapted from Ref. 53, Figs. 187 and 191)

General Operative Principles

Percutaneous techniques may be performed in the operating room or angiography suite. A radiolucent operative table is useful to allow visualization by fluoroscopy. The patient is positioned supine with the neck placed in a neutral position, supported by towels, a foam, or gel donut, or placed in horseshoe headrest. It is helpful to mark the three anatomic landmarks to aid in visualization.

The perioral area is then cleaned with sterile preparation. During application of surgical drapes, it is essential to maintain adequate exposure of the anatomic landmarks in order to confirm the correct trajectory. For RR, the patient is anesthetized during needle placement and lesioning but awake for mapping, whereas GR and PBC may be performed under general anesthesia. This should be discussed with the anesthesiologist beforehand to optimize patient comfort and clinical response. The surgeon may choose to insert a piece of gauze or oral airway into the patient's mouth to prevent involuntary biting during needle localization.

The entry point is infiltrated with local anesthetic, and a small stab incision is made with a #11 or #15 blade. The surgeon's index finger is placed in the mouth along the buccal mucosa on the lateral pterygoid wing, taking care not to place the finger between the teeth, and a cannulated needle is inserted and guided toward the foramen ovale just inside the mucosa along the correct trajectory. If the needle penetrates the mucosa and enters the mouth, the procedure is aborted. On lateral fluoroscopy, the target is at the intersection of the clivus and planum sphenoidale (Fig. 18.3a). It is also possible to visualize the foramen using a submental vertex view with the patient's head fully extended (Fig. 18.3b). The cannula is guided by placing the surgeon's index finger within the patient's mouth.

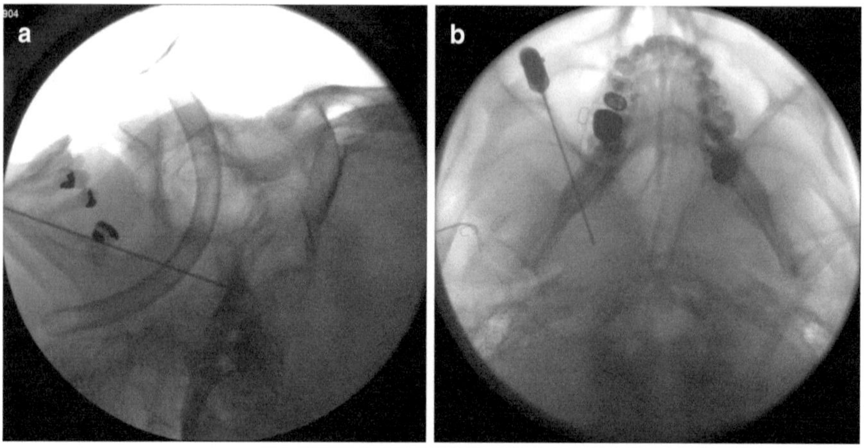

Fig. 18.3 Radiographic localization of foramen ovale. Lateral (**a**) and submental vertex (**b**) XR views demonstrate appropriate needle placement at the skull base. Overlapping of the clivus and planum sphenoidale is evident in the lateral view (**a**)

Entry into the foramen ovale is often accompanied by contraction of the ipsilateral masseter muscle and wincing of the patient's face. Penetration of the foramen can elicit a vasovagal response resulting in significant bradycardia and blood pressure fluctuations [35]; anticholinergics (typically atropine) may be administered before starting the procedure to blunt these effects. An intracisternal location may also be verified by the spontaneous egress of cerebrospinal fluid, although this is not always seen. Fluoroscopy should always be used once the foramen has been cannulated to ensure the needle placement remains below the clival line.

Percutaneous Techniques

Radiofrequency Rhizotomy

As the patient will be awake during part of the procedure, it is necessary to use a short-acting anesthetic such as methohexital or propofol. After cannulation of the foramen ovale, a specially designed electrode is introduced and placed in the location of the pain distribution as assessed on fluoroscopy. The patient is awakened, and stimulation (50 Hz, 1 ms) is delivered until tingling is described. If the needle is in the correct location, the threshold for paresthesia is usually much less than 1 V. If necessary, the needle is repositioned until the area of the patient's symptoms is covered without involving V1.

The patient is then sedated again for thermal lesioning. Temperatures 60–70 °C are generally used for the first lesion, with additional lesions performed at greater temperatures as necessary to produce mild hypesthesia. The lesion duration is typically 60 s but can range from 30 to 120 s. During this time, cutaneous erythema in the affected distribution may be visible, consistent with vasodilation of the region supplied by the stimulated fibers. Once a lesion has been made, the patient is awakened for sensory testing to light touch and pinprick in all three trigeminal distributions. A successful lesion produces slight numbness or a throbbing sensation within the desired distribution, which corresponds with lasting clinical efficacy. If there is minimal analgesia or the patient maintains symmetrical sensory discrimination, then the lesion may be repeated at higher temperatures.

Once a successful lesion has been created, the electrode and cannula are withdrawn. The entry site may be covered with a small dressing or liquid adhesive; a suture is not commonly required due to the small size of the entry incision. The patient is returned to the postanesthetic recovery room for observation.

Glycerol Rhizotomy

It is not necessary to have the patient awake during GR, and some surgeon's may prefer deeper anesthesia for patient comfort. A 20-gauge spinal needle is advanced to the foramen ovale as previously described, and the patient is brought to a sitting or semi-sitting position. Iodinated contrast (typically iohexol) is then injected into the trigeminal cistern to estimate the volume of glycerol, which tends to range from 0.25 to 0.4 mL. Following contrast injection, the stylet is replaced and radiographs are taken to confirm appropriate filling of the cistern. The contrast is then drained passively via removal of the stylet in preparation for glycerol injection. If the contrast does not drain completely, the patient can be positioned supine or in slight Trendelenburg to allow drainage into the posterior fossa.

The glycerol injection is also performed with the patient in a sitting or semi-sitting position. The injection can be modified based on the patient's pain distribution: the full volume of glycerol can be injected for pain within multiple distributions, one-third of the estimated volume can be injected to isolate the mandibular distribution, and glycerol can be injected prior to complete contrast drainage to isolate the ophthalmic distribution (the glycerol rises above the contrast medium). As with RR, cutaneous erythema in the affected distribution may be visualized.

After the procedure, the patient is returned to the postanesthetic recovery room for observation and is maintained in a sitting or semi-sitting position for 2 h with instructions not to extend the neck in order to prevent glycerol leakage into the posterior fossa.

Balloon Compression

As with GR, PBC may be performed under deep or general anesthesia. A 14-gauge needle is positioned at the entry of the foramen as previously described, either to enter the foramen [36] or dock the needle and insert the guiding stylet [16]. The position is confirmed with fluoroscopy, followed by removal of the stylet and insertion of a 4-French diameter balloon with a radiopaque inner wire to aid in visualization.

Positioning of the balloon dictates the distribution that will be affected. The balloon should be placed in a medial and superior direction for the ophthalmic distribution, in a central position for the maxillary distribution or for pain in multiple distributions, and in a lateral and inferior direction for the mandibular distribution. Submental vertex positioning of the intraoperative fluoroscopy may aid in achieving an appropriate medial-lateral trajectory. Air is then withdrawn from the balloon catheter, followed by connection to the insufflation syringe which measures intraluminal pressure. The balloon is then inflated from between 1000 and 1200 mmHg for at least 60 s, although up to 6 min may be necessary for maximal efficacy [37]. Inflation occurs via injection of radiopaque iohexol until a classical "pear shape" is visible on fluoroscopy. If the pressure or balloon shape is inadequate, a larger balloon may be used. Bradycardia is more commonly observed during PBC than other techniques.

Patient Outcomes

Radiofrequency Rhizotomy

Percutaneous treatment of TN can provide significant relief for patients who fail medical management. Patient selection, acceptable risk tolerance, and type of pain are important factors to consider when determining which is the best procedure. Large, single-institution studies demonstrate RR to have high rates of acute pain relief, with 92–97.6% of patients reporting complete pain resolution [28, 38–44]. A retrospective analysis of 1200 patients reported an acute pain relief rate of 93% and recurrence rate of 20% with a mean follow-up time of 9 years (range, 1–21 years) [38]. The recurrence rate included patients with mild pain not requiring medication to severe pain requiring additional surgical intervention. The rate of recurrence is inversely proportional to the degree of sensory loss, so the objective of RR is to generate a lesion resulting in dense hypesthesia in V2 and V3 divisions and mild hypalgesia in V1 division to preserve the corneal reflex. Patients with anesthesia or dense hypesthesia following RR had a median pain-free survival greater than 15 years, with a recurrence rate of 20% and 25%, respectively. Patients with mild hypalgesia had a median pain-free survival less than 3 years, with a recurrence rate of 60%.

RR is associated with a higher rate of acute pain relief and lower rate of recurrence compared with the other percutaneous procedures, but the frequency and severity of complications is somewhat higher. Corneal sensory impairment occurs at a rate of 1–20.3% and is not exclusive to lesions involving the V1 division [39]. Corneal sensory impairment can be transient or lead to other complications such as keratitis enucleation which is rarely necessary [39]. Masseter weakness occurs after 3–65% of procedures; a retrospective analysis of 1000 procedures demonstrated an overall incidence of 10.5% [39]. Painful dysesthesia occurs in 6.5% of cases (range,

1–8%), which rarely leads to anesthesia dolorosa (0.6–12%) [39]. Other less common side effects include diplopia, cranial nerve palsy, and meningitis.

Glycerol Rhizotomy

Of all three percutaneous treatment options for TN, GR has the largest variability in rates of both initial pain relief and recurrence. Initial pain relief occurs after 53.1–98% of procedures [28, 29, 45, 46], with intact preoperative facial sensation as a positive prognostic indicator [47]. In a retrospective study of 32 patients undergoing GR, 56% developed recurrence within 5 years, requiring additional procedures to achieve pain relief [28], and another study documented a 5-year recurrence rate of 69% [29]. Experiencing some degree of postoperative sensory loss is associated with long-term pain relief [47]. Patients with recurrence were treated with GR or with RR, achieving the same initial pain relief rates.

The development of complications following GR is similar to RR. The most common side effect is the development of dysesthesia, with rates ranging from 0.7% to 23% [28, 29, 45]. Due to the difficulty of isolating specific branches during this procedure, development of dysesthesia can occur in previously unaffected trigeminal divisions [46]. Corneal sensory impairment is also a common side effect, with rates as high as 16% [47]. Reactivation of herpes occurs in approximately 8% of patients after GR [29], which is also seen following PBC. Prophylactic acyclovir treatment prior to GR can decrease the risk of reactivation. Incidence of anesthesia dolorosa and masseter muscle weakness is generally low, with rates less than 5% [29, 47]. Treatment of TN due to multiple sclerosis with GR may be associated with excellent outcome [29].

Balloon Compression

Immediately following surgery, PBC yields high rates of acute pain relief (range, 83–100%) [37, 48–50] with a recurrence rate ranging from 19% to 29% at 5 years [49, 50]. Comparing patient outcomes between studies is hindered by the lack of an established protocol, since differences in balloon shape, compression pressure, and compression time may generate divergent results. Abdennebi et al. [37] evaluated 901 patients and concluded a "pear-shaped" balloon and compression time of 6 min were ideal. Skirving et al. [50] report compression times of greater than 5 min, while Lobato et al. [48] report compression for only 1 min.

The most common complications of balloon compression are transient masseter muscle weakness and dysesthesia, which occur at a frequency of 6.2–12% and 1.5–19%, respectively [49, 50]. Reactivation of herpes labialis as a result of PBC occurs in a minority of patients and resolves with acyclovir treatment [36, 37]. Transient oculomotor nerve palsy occurs in less than 2% of patients [37]. Unlike RR, PBC spares small fibers resulting in minimal risk of developing anesthesia dolorosa and corneal sensory impairment rates (range, 0–0.6% and 0–2.3%, respectively), making PBC a better option for patients with V1 division TN.

Alternatives

The durability and complication profile of MVD is superior to percutaneous lesioning techniques and is commonly used in patients with neurovascular compression without surgical contraindication [44, 51]. Radiosurgery is much less invasive, although onset of effect is delayed and there is lower likelihood of cessation of medication [52].

Conclusions

Percutaneous procedures including RR, GR, and PBC play an important role in the treatment of medically refractory TN. Relief of acute pain is excellent in appropriately selected patients, particularly patients with idiopathic triggerable Type 1 TN, and complications are rare. Recurrence is common, but repeated procedures can be effective.

References

1. Härtel F. Die Leitungsans thesie und injektions behandlung des Ganglion Gasseri und der Trigem inusstmme langenbecks. Arch Klin Chir. 1911;100:193.
2. Taarnhoj P. Decompression of the trigeminal root and the posterior part of the ganglion as treatment in trigeminal neuralgia; preliminary communication. J Neurosurg. 1952;9:288–90. https://doi.org/10.3171/jns.1952.9.3.0288.
3. Svien HJ, Love JG. Results of decompression operation for trigeminal neuralgia four years plus after operation. J Neurosurg. 1959;16:653–5. https://doi.org/10.3171/jns.1959.16.6.0653.
4. Woodhall B, Odom GL. Stilbamidine isethionate therapy of tic douloureux. J Neurosurg. 1955;12:495–500. https://doi.org/10.3171/jns.1955.12.5.0495.
5. Brown JA, Preul MC. Percutaneous trigeminal ganglion compression for trigeminal neuralgia. Experience in 22 patients and review of the literature. J Neurosurg. 1989;70:900–4. https://doi.org/10.3171/jns.1989.70.6.0900.
6. Shelden CH, Pudenz RH, Freshwater DB, Crue BL. Compression rather than decompression for trigeminal neuralgia. J Neurosurg. 1955;12:123–6. https://doi.org/10.3171/jns.1955.12.2.0123.
7. Sweet WG. Proceedings: analgesia dolorosa after differential retrogasserian thermal or mechanical rhizotomy: tactics employed to decrease its influence. J Neurol Neurosurg Psychiatry. 1975;38:407.
8. Nugent GR. Radiofrequency treatment of trigeminal neuralgia using a cordotomy-type electrode. A method. Neurosurg Clin N Am. 1997;8:41–52.

9. Taha JM, Tew JM Jr. Treatment of trigeminal neuralgia by percutaneous radiofrequency rhizotomy. Neurosurg Clin N Am. 1997;8:31–9.
10. Leksell L. Trigeminal neuralgia. Some neurophysiologic aspects and a new method of therapy. Lakartidningen. 1971;68:5145–8.
11. Hakanson S. Trigeminal neuralgia treated by the injection of glycerol into the trigeminal cistern. Neurosurgery. 1981;9:638–46.
12. Lunsford LD, Bennett MH. Percutaneous retrogasserian glycerol rhizotomy for tic douloureux: Part 1. Technique and results in 112 patients. Neurosurgery. 1984;14:424–30.
13. Bennett MH, Lunsford LD. Percutaneous retrogasserian glycerol rhizotomy for tic douloureux: Part 2. Results nd implications of trigeminal evoked potential studies. Neurosurgery. 1984;14:431–5.
14. Mullan S, Lichtor T. Percutaneous microcompression of the trigeminal ganglion for trigeminal neuralgia. J Neurosurg. 1983;59:1007–12. https://doi.org/10.3171/jns.1983.59.6.1007.
15. Brown JA, Hoeflinger B, Long PB, Gunning WT, Rhoades R, Bennett-Clarke CA, Chiaia NL, Weaver MT. Axon and ganglion cell injury in rabbits after percutaneous trigeminal balloon compression. Neurosurgery. 1996;38:993–1003; discussion 1003–4.
16. Brown JA. Percutaneous balloon compression for trigeminal neuralgia. Clin Neurosurg. 2009;56:73–8.
17. Laghmari M, El Ouahabi A, Arkha Y, Derraz S, El Khamlichi A. Are the destructive neurosurgical techniques as effective as microvascular decompression in the management of trigeminal neuralgia? Surg Neurol. 2007;68:505–12. https://doi.org/10.1016/j.surneu.2006.11.066.
18. Lopez BC, Hamlyn PJ, Zakrzewska JM. Systematic review of ablative neurosurgical techniques for the treatment of trigeminal neuralgia. Neurosurgery. 2004;54:973–982; discussion 982–3.
19. Burchiel KJ. A new classification for facial pain. Neurosurgery. 2003;53:1164–1166; discussion 1166–7.
20. Eller JL, Raslan AM, Burchiel KJ. Trigeminal neuralgia: definition and classification. Neurosurg Focus. 2005;18:E3.
21. Haines SJ, Jannetta PJ, Zorub DS. Microvascular relations of the trigeminal nerve. An anatomical study with clinical correlation. J Neurosurg. 1980;52:381–6. https://doi.org/10.3171/jns.1980.52.3.0381.
22. Jannetta PJ. Arterial compression of the trigeminal nerve at the pons in patients with trigeminal neuralgia. J Neurosurg. 1967;26(Suppl):159–62. https://doi.org/10.3171/jns.1967.26.1part2.0159.
23. Barker FG 2nd, Jannetta PJ, Bissonette DJ, Larkins MV, Jho HD. The long-term outcome of microvascular decompression for trigeminal neuralgia. N Engl J Med. 1996;334:1077–83. https://doi.org/10.1056/NEJM199604253341701.
24. Mallory GW, Atkinson JL, Stien KJ, Keegan BM, Pollock BE. Outcomes after percutaneous surgery for patients with multiple sclerosis-related trigeminal neuralgia. Neurosurgery. 2012;71:581–586; discussion 586. https://doi.org/10.1227/NEU.0b013e31825e795b.
25. Cheng JS, Sanchez-Mejia RO, Limbo M, Ward MM, Barbaro NM. Management of medically refractory trigeminal neuralgia in patients with multiple sclerosis. Neurosurg Focus. 2005;18:e13.
26. Martin S, Teo M, Suttner N. The effectiveness of percutaneous balloon compression in the treatment of trigeminal neuralgia in patients with multiple sclerosis. J Neurosurg. 2015;123:1507–11. https://doi.org/10.3171/2014.11.JNS14736.
27. Mathieu D, Effendi K, Blanchard J, Seguin M. Comparative study of Gamma Knife surgery and percutaneous retrogasserian glycerol rhizotomy for trigeminal neuralgia in patients with multiple sclerosis. J Neurosurg. 2012;117(Suppl):175–80. https://doi.org/10.3171/2012.6.GKS12987.
28. Fraioli B, Esposito V, Guidetti B, Cruccu G, Manfredi M. Treatment of trigeminal neuralgia by thermocoagulation, glycerolization, and percutaneous compression of the gasserian ganglion and/or retrogasserian rootlets: long-term results and therapeutic protocol. Neurosurgery. 1989;24:239–45.

29. Bender MT, Pradilla G, Batra S, See AP, James C, Pardo CA, Carson BS, Lim M. Glycerol rhizotomy and radiofrequency thermocoagulation for trigeminal neuralgia in multiple sclerosis. J Neurosurg. 2013;118:329–36. https://doi.org/10.3171/2012.9.JNS1226.
30. Wang J, Zhou Y, Zhang ZF, Li CQ, Zheng WJ, Liu J. Comparison of one-level minimally invasive and open transforaminal lumbar interbody fusion in degenerative and isthmic spondylolisthesis grades 1 and 2. Eur Spine J. 2010;19:1780–4. https://doi.org/10.1007/s00586-010-1404-z.
31. Gass A, kitchen N, MacManus DG, Moseley LF, Hennerici MG, Miller DH. Trigeminal neuralgia in patients with multiple sclerosis: lesion localization with magnetic resonance imaging. Neurology. 1997;49:1142–4.
32. Ariai MS, Mallory GW, Pollock BE. Outcomes after microvascular decompression for patients with trigeminal neuralgia and suspected multiple sclerosis. World Neurosurg. 2014;81:599–603. https://doi.org/10.1016/j.wneu.2013.09.027.
33. Jagia M, Bithal PK, Dash HH, Prabhakar H, Chaturvedi A, Chouhan RS. Effect of cerebrospinal fluid return on success rate of percutaneous retrogasserian glycerol rhizotomy. Reg Anesth Pain Med. 2004;29:592–5.
34. Rish BL. Cerebrovascular accident after percutaneous rf thermocoagulation of the trigeminal ganglion. Case report. J Neurosurg. 1976;44:376–7. https://doi.org/10.3171/jns.1976.44.3.0376.
35. Brown JA, Preul MC. Trigeminal depressor response during percutaneous microcompression of the trigeminal ganglion for trigeminal neuralgia. Neurosurgery. 1988;23:745–8.
36. Cheng JS, Lim DA, Chang EF, Barbaro NM. A review of percutaneous treatments for trigeminal neuralgia. Neurosurgery. 2014;10(Suppl 1):25–33.; discussion 33. https://doi.org/10.1227/NEU.0000000000001687.
37. Abdennebi B, Guenane L. Technical considerations and outcome assessment in retrogasserian balloon compression for treatment of trigeminal neuralgia. Series of 901 patients. Surg Neurol Int. 2014;5:118. https://doi.org/10.4103/2152-7806.137838.
38. Tew JMJ, Morgan CJ, Grande AW. Percutaneous stereotactic rhizotomy in the treatment of intractable facial pain. In: Quinones-Hinojosa A, editor. Schmidek and sweet operative neurosurgical techniques. New York: Elsevier; 2012. p. 1409–18.
39. Broggi G, Franzini A, Lasio G, Giorgi C, Servello D. Long-term results of percutaneous retrogasserian thermorhizotomy for "essential" trigeminal neuralgia: considerations in 1000 consecutive patients. Neurosurgery. 1990;26:783–786; discussion 786–7.
40. Kanpolat Y, Savas A, Bekar A, Berk C. Percutaneous controlled radiofrequency trigeminal rhizotomy for the treatment of idiopathic trigeminal neuralgia: 25-year experience with 1600 patients. Neurosurgery. 2001;48:524–32.
41. Scrivani SJ, Keith DA, Mathews ES, Kaban LB. Percutaneous stereotactic differential radiofrequency thermal rhizotomy for the treatment of trigeminal neuralgia. J Oral Maxillofac Surg. 1999;57:104–11.
42. Smith HP, McWhorter JM, Challa VR. Radiofrequency neurolysis in a clinical model: neuropathological correlation. J Neurosurg. 1981;55:246–53.
43. Taha JM, Tew JMJ, Buncher CR. A prospective 15-year follow up of 154 consecutive patients with trigeminal neuralgia treated by percutaneous stereotactic radiofrequency thermal rhizotomy. J Neurosurg. 1995;83:989–93.
44. Tronnier VM, Rasche D, Hamer J, Kienle A, Kunze S. Treatment of idiopathic trigeminal neuralgia: comparison of long-term outcome after radiofrequency rhizotomy and microvascular decompression. Neurosurgery. 2001;48:1261–8.
45. Asplund P, Blomstedt P, Bergenheim AT. Percutaneous balloon compression vs percutaneous retrogasserian glycerol rhizotomy for the primary treatment of trigeminal neuralgia. Neurosurgery. 2016;78:421–8.; discussion 428. https://doi.org/10.1227/NEU.0000000000001059.
46. Erdem E, Alkan A. Peripheral glycerol injections in the treatment of idiopathic trigeminal neuralgia: retrospective analysis of 157 cases. J Oral Maxillofac Surg. 2001;59:1176–80. https://doi.org/10.1053/joms.2001.26721.

47. Steiger HJ. Prognostic factors in the treatment of trigeminal neuralgia. Acta Neurochir. 1991;113:11–7.
48. Lobato RD, Rivas JJ, Sarabia R, Lamas E. Percutaneous microcompression of the gasserian ganglion for trigeminal neuralgia. J Neurosurg. 1990;72:546–53.
49. Chen JF, Tu PH, Lee ST. Long-term follow-up of patients treated with percutaneous balloon compression for trigeminal neuralgia in Taiwan. World Neurosurg. 2011;76:586–91. https://doi.org/10.1016/j.wneu.2011.05.021.
50. Skirving DJ, Dan NG. A 20-year review of percutaneous balloon compression of the trigeminal ganglion. J Neurosurg. 2001;94:913–7.
51. Lovely TJ, Jannetta PJ. Microvascular decompression for trigeminal neuralgia. Surgical technique and long-term results. Neurosurg Clin N Am. 1997;8:11–29.
52. Kondziolka D, Zorro O, Lobato-Polo J, Kano H, Flannery TJ, Flickinger JC, Lunsford LD. Gamma Knife stereotactic radiosurgery for idiopathic trigeminal neuralgia. J Neurosurg. 2010;112:758–65. https://doi.org/10.3171/2009.7.JNS09694.
53. Gray H, Lewis WH. Anatomy of the human body. Philadelphia: Lea and Febiger; 1918.

Chapter 19
Microvascular Decompression of the Trigeminal Nerve for Trigeminal Neuralgia

Taylor Anne Wilson and John Diaz Day

Introduction

Facial pain is a relatively common complaint with many different etiologies and anatomical origins. Trigeminal neuralgia (TN), also known as *tic douloureux*, is one of the most common causes of facial pain [1]. Classically, TN is characterized by excruciating, episodic, lancinating pain in the distribution of one or more branches of cranial nerve V (CNV) that is triggered by a sensory stimulus. The pathophysiology of TN is not completely understood nor agreed upon; however, the prevailing hypothesis is that neurovascular compression of the trigeminal nerve by an artery or vein damages the nerve, resulting in neuronal dysfunction and development of neuropathic pain. Compression may result in damage to the myelin sheath which results in ephaptic transmission of impulses that are perceived as pain. Injured neurons often respond abnormally with heightened sensitivity, increased excitability, spontaneous signaling activity, or aberrant neuronal connectivity. Other neurovascular compression syndromes include hemifacial spasm and glossopharyngeal neuralgia, which involve, respectively, the facial nerve, cranial nerve VII (CNVII), and the glossopharyngeal nerve, cranial nerve IX (CNIX).

These cephalic neuralgias are often complex, chronic conditions that have proven difficult to treat. Many medical and surgical modalities have been investigated to

T. A. Wilson · J. D. Day (✉)
Department of Neurosurgery, University of Arkansas for Medical Sciences, Little Rock, AR, USA
e-mail: twilson@uams.edu; jdday@uams.edu

J. Y. Suen, E. Petersen (eds.), *Diagnosis and Management of Head and Face Pain*, https://doi.org/10.1007/978-3-319-90999-8_19

improve treatment of patients with TN and other compressive cephalic neuralgias. Most of these modalities are aimed at providing symptomatic relief. Microvascular decompression (MVD), however, is a neurosurgical procedure designed to target the underlying pathophysiology to treat the disease pathology, providing symptomatic relief. MVD is one of the most effective treatments for TN and other vascular compression syndromes, with high rates of long-term pain relief and/or cure.

Trigeminal Neuralgia: Clinical Presentation and Epidemiology

TN is classically characterized by episodes of electric shock-like, severe, lancinating pain in the distribution of one of more branches of the trigeminal nerve. Episodes usually only last several seconds and rarely last >2 min, and there are periods without pain or symptoms between episodes. Pain and symptoms are almost always unilateral and without associated neurologic deficits. Episodes are typically triggered by normally non-noxious sensory stimuli, such as eating, brushing teeth, or chewing, in the distribution of the effected trigeminal branch.

TN is reported to have an annual incidence of approximately 4 per 100,000 population. The majority of patients who develop TN are over 50 years old with a mean age of 63 at diagnosis [2–6]. TN is more common in females than males with a 1.8:1 ratio [4, 5]. TN almost always occurs unilaterally with only 1% of TN occurring bilaterally, and these patients with bilateral TN almost always have pain and symptoms more consistent with atypical TN. Of the 99% of patients with unilateral TN, 60% have pain and symptoms on the right and 39% have pain and symptoms on the left. TN may affect any one branch or branches of the trigeminal nerve. Most commonly, as seen in 42% of patients, V2 and V3 are both involved. Involvement of V2 alone is seen in 20% of patients, V3 alone in 17% of patients, and both V1 and V2 in 14% of patients, and much less commonly, all three divisions are seen in 5% of patients and V1 alone in 2% of patients [3, 6, 7].

TN, however, does not always fit this classic description; thus, TN has been divided into two clinical types—typical TN and atypical TN, also referred to as TN type 1 (TN1) and TN type 2 (TN2), respectively. Typical TN refers to those patients with the classic TN symptoms described above. Atypical TN refers to facial pain also in the distribution of one or more branches of the trigeminal nerve, but the quality of pain is different, characterized by more constant aching, burning pain. Interestingly, some patients with atypical TN initially presented with a typical TN picture, but over time, their symptoms evolve to include additional symptoms more characteristic of atypical TN. In the author's experience, this picture tends to occur in patients treated medically, with the change occurring as a consequence of the medication. The underlying cause of the pain is unchanged. TN may be viewed as a spectrum of disease states versus distinct clinical types; however, the clinical type of TN has important implications for diagnosis, treatment, and prognosis [8, 9].

Pathophysiology

In more than 90% of patients, TN is due to neurovascular compression of the trigeminal nerve by an artery or vein. The superior cerebellar artery (SCA) is most commonly the offending vessel. Less commonly, branches of the anterior inferior cerebellar (AICA), an ectatic basilar artery, or veins may compress the trigeminal nerve and produce TN. Other, much less common, causes of TN include compression from a posterior fossa tumor or demyelination from multiple sclerosis. Pain secondary to non-compressive causes is overwhelmingly atypical in nature [10, 11].

TN is a type of neuropathic pain syndrome. Other neuropathic pain syndromes include the other cephalic neuralgias, hemifacial spasm and glossopharyngeal neuralgia, diabetic neuropathy, and postherpetic neuralgia [12]. Neuropathic pain is characterized by abnormal, often complex, unpleasant sensation caused by neuronal damage or dysfunction [2, 13]. In TN, the pathophysiology is not completely understood; however, the prevailing hypothesis is that compression of the trigeminal nerve at its dorsal root entry zone damages the nerve [14–19]. Damage to these first-order neurons in the trigeminal pathway then leads to neuronal dysfunction, demyelination, and development of neuropathic pain. The dorsal root entry zone is where the transition exists between central myelin synthesized by the oligodendrocytes and the peripheral myelin synthesized by the Schwann cells [20–22]. Thus, the dorsal root entry zone is particularly vulnerable, and compression at that site may lead to micro-injury of nerve fibers with neuronal dysfunction and subsequent segmental demyelination. Injured neurons respond abnormally to normal signals in their normal environment with heightened sensitivity, increased excitability, spontaneous signaling activity, or aberrant neuronal connectivity [23, 24]. Additionally, the partially demyelinated large A fibers are able to form aberrant synapses with nearby smaller, poorly myelinated A-delta fibers and unmyelinated C (nociceptive) fibers, leading to ephaptic transmission and abnormal neuronal signaling. These pathophysiological changes trigger downstream changes in secondary pain pathways that ultimately manifest clinically with the pain and symptoms of TN [25]. Hemifacial spasm and glossopharyngeal neuralgia are also hypothesized to occur via similar pathophysiological changes [11, 14, 20, 23].

Interestingly, most patients with TN2 initially began with symptoms more consistent with TN1, but over time, as the disease progressed, they gradually began developing more atypical symptoms. One study found that the mean time from onset of typical TN symptoms to more atypical TN symptoms is over several years [1]. This suggests that typical and atypical TN may represent two ends of a spectrum with TN existing as a continuum of disease rather than having distinct clinical entities [8]. As a cautionary note, many patients with TN1 will experience a change in the character of their pain as a consequence of taking anticonvulsant medications that are typically prescribed, i.e., carbamazepine. Therefore, in taking the patient's history, it is important to inquire what the symptoms were like before initiating medical therapy. This will mitigate against the possibility of misdiagnosis as TN2 based upon only having the pain history after medical treatment, which has changed from the initial quality of symptoms.

Historical Perspective

More than 900 years ago, Avicenna described a clinical syndrome consistent with what is now known as TN [26]. In 1756, Nicholas Andre officially named this condition *tic douloureux* reflecting his notion that the disease entity was a form of convulsive disorder involving the nervous system [18, 26, 27]. In the 1820s, Charles Bell determined the trigeminal nerve, and its sensory function was anatomically and physiologically distinct from the facial nerve and its motor function. This anatomical distinction allowed him to localize the pain and symptoms of *tic douloureux* to the trigeminal nerve, and it was subsequently renamed *trigeminal neuralgia* [18, 26, 27]. With an anatomical basis for TN, surgical approaches were developed to access and section affected fibers of the trigeminal ganglion to block the transmission of pain; however, these approaches were associated with high rates of morbidity [18, 27, 28].

In the late 1920s/early 1930s, Walter Dandy first described the basis for the modern day MVD and developed the hypothesis that the pathophysiology of MVD is related to vascular compression of the trigeminal nerve [29]. In 1929, Dandy published his suboccipital, cerebellar approach, which he used to access and partially section the trigeminal ganglion [30]. While performing this procedure, Dandy observed arterial loops often obstructing his view of the trigeminal ganglion, and these vessels also appeared to exert mass effect on the root entry zone of the trigeminal nerve. Subsequently, Dandy hypothesized that the pathophysiology of TN is related to vascular compression of the trigeminal nerve [26, 27, 29, 30]. Dandy never formally tested this theory, and over time, his approach was largely forgotten [18].

Dandy's observations and hypothesis regarding the pathophysiology of trigeminal neuralgia is the basis for modern day MVD. In the late 1950s/early 1960s, Jannetta began to popularize MVD for the treatment of TN by studying and elaborating on the pathophysiology behind Dandy's theory that neurovascular compression of the trigeminal nerve at the dorsal root entry zone leads to the clinical manifestation of TN. Before the MVD procedure gained popularity as a treatment modality for TN, the widely held hypothesis was that manipulation, or trauma, to the nerve itself was the cause of symptomatic relief in TN [14, 18]. In the late 1970s/1980s, as Jannetta built his series of patients treated by MVD, the hypothesis that alleviating the compression by separating the offending vessel and the nerve became more widely accepted by the neurosurgical community [18].

In 1996, Jannetta solidified his popularization of MVD when he published the landmark study that established MVD as safe with a high rate of long-term success in relieving pain and symptoms of TN. In this study, there were 1185 patients with TN who underwent MVD between 1972 and 1991. In this study, MVD consisted of a suboccipital craniotomy with microsurgical separation of compressing arteries and veins from the nerve, maintaining the separation with a cotton or Teflon felt. The primary endpoint of this study was relief of pain. An excellent outcome was defined as complete relief of pain with >98% of pain relieved without need for medication. A good outcome was defined by partial relief of pain with >75% reduction in pain, and a poor outcome, considered a failure of treatment, was defined by recurrence of >25% preoperative pain or need for additional intervention. Jannetta had an excellent outcome in 82% of patients immediately postop and in 75% and 64% of patients at 1-year and 10-year follow-up, respectively. Most recurrences occurred at 2 years after surgery with recurrence rates less than 2% at 5 years and less than 1% at 10 years. Several risk factors for recurrence were identified. Lack of immediate postoperative relief, symptoms for >8 years prior to surgery, female sex, and venous compression were identified as negative prognostic indicators. This study demonstrated a low rate of morbidity with MVD, but when there was a complication, CSF leak, hearing loss, and facial numbness were the most common [31].

Treatment Options

There have been many different treatment modalities, both medically and surgically, aimed at treating TN. Medical management is generally the initial treatment strategy for TN. Many different pharmacological agents have been and are used for treating TN. Pharmacological agents with antiepileptic properties have been the most effective in relieving pain [32]. Thus, carbamazepine and oxcarbazepine are first line for treatment of TN. Carbamazepine has been reported to relieve pain in 69% of patients with newly treated TN. Other medications commonly used in patients with TN include baclofen, gabapentin, phenytoin, clonazepam, lamotrigine, and amitriptyline. These medications can be highly efficacious in relieving pain; however, pain relief from these medications often decreases over time, necessitating higher doses to maintain the same effect. Unfortunately, these medications are not without side effects that may limit their use [22, 33, 34]. Thus, medications may fail by no longer providing pain relief, in which patients are considered to have medication-refractory TN, or the side effect profile becomes such that it precludes continued use as treatment [13, 15, 18, 32, 35].

When medical therapies fail for whichever reasons, more invasive, surgical procedures are considered. Surgical options include chemoneurolysis, radiofrequency ablation, percutaneous balloon ablation, stereotactic radiosurgery (e.g., Gamma Knife®), and MVD [27, 36–39]. MVD, which involves a lateral suboccipital craniotomy followed by microsurgical technique to dissect and separate the offending blood vessel or vessels away for the nerve, is considered the most efficacious treatment for medication-refractory TN based upon available data [15, 18, 33, 40]. The technique as performed by the senior author is described below. In the author's practice, all surgical methods are employed, and patients' individual characteristics are taken into account when recommending one treatment over another. In general, physiologically younger patients with imaging evidence of vascular compression are offered MVD as the treatment of choice. Elderly patients with multiple comorbidities are considered better candidates for an ablative option, either radiofrequency rhizolysis or Gamma Knife® radiosurgery. Radiofrequency rhizolysis is preferred for these patients with TN1 owing to the ability to target the involved division specifically. It is also the preferred treatment for patients with TN2, especially secondary to multiple sclerosis. Gamma Knife® radiosurgery is preferred in elderly patients with multiple comorbidities that are poor surgical candidates in the author's practice.

Microvascular Decompression

MVD is generally considered the most efficacious treatment for medication-refractory TN in neurosurgical practice [31, 33, 41–44]. This procedure involves a small lateral suboccipital craniotomy followed by microsurgical technique to dissect and separate the offending blood vessel or vessels away from the nerve. Teflon felt pledgets are placed between the vessel and nerve to prevent compression from recurring. MVD has a high success rate in relieving pain in patients with TN. Depending on certain patient characteristics and TN symptoms, the overall rate of successful pain relief is approximately 90%. Of these patients with successful pain relief, 75–80% have complete or near-complete resolution of their pain after surgery and no longer need medication, and the other 10% have some pain relief from surgery but continue to require medication to completely or near completely control pain. Unfortunately, TN can recur despite successful pain relief initially with MVD [31, 45]. In the author's practice, recurrence tends to be secondary to arachnoid scarring that appears at surgery to be exerting torque or a pull on the nerve. Release of this scar tissue typically resolves the pain.

Recurrence rates following MVD have been reported anywhere from 1.5 to 3.5% annually [42, 46]. Recurrence rates are higher in females than males. Patients whose trigeminal nerve is compressed by a vein also have much higher recurrence rates than those compressed by an artery [46–48]. Venous compression of the trigeminal nerve has also been shown to be associated with lower rates of pain relief immediately postoperatively compared with arterial compression.

Although this procedure is generally well tolerated and efficacious in relieving pain in patients with TN, no procedure is without risks. More common complications of MVD include facial sensory loss (25%), trochlear nerve palsy (4.3%), hearing loss (3%), aseptic meningitis (2%), facial nerve palsy (1.6%), deafness (1%), and bacterial meningitis (0.9%). CSF leak and cerebellar injury may also occur. Mortality has been reported at 0.2–2.0% for MVD [47, 49]. Cranial nerve palsies (facial sensory loss, trochlear palsy, facial palsy) tend to be transient, with most improving shortly after surgery [48, 50]. Aseptic meningitis is generally hemogenic in nature and responds well to dexamethasone, usually lasting 3–7 days [51].

Surgical Technique

There are many variations in surgical technique for microvascular decompression. The following description represents the preferences of the senior author.

Patient Selection

Selection of candidates for MVD involves taking an accurate history and obtaining advanced imaging studies that may reliably demonstrate the compressive pathology. All patients with facial pain should have high-resolution MRI imaging of the brain, including thin cuts through the region of the pons with FIESTA (fast imaging employing steady-state acquisition, a.k.a. True FISP, T2-FFE) sequences (Fig. 19.1). These images have a high chance of demonstrating the compressive vessel. Otherwise MRI is necessary to rule out the presence of tumor or aneurysm causing compression. Patients with TN1 that demonstrate evidence of vascular contact with the nerve at the brain stem on MRI and a lack of comorbidities that would contraindicate general anesthesia should be considered for MVD. Patients with TN2 that have evidence of compressive pathology may be considered as well; however, it must be stressed to these patients prior to surgery that the outcomes are not always optimal in such cases.

Patient Position and Preparation

After the induction of general anesthesia, patients are placed in the lateral decubitus position with the head fixed in a Mayfield skull clamp. The chin is tucked and the head rotated slightly so that the nose is in neutral position, with the crown of the head slightly tilted downward. The upper arm is rested on a padded arm rest and is angled obliquely away from the body with the shoulder pulled gently. This helps to open the angle between the lateral subocciput and the shoulder, mitigating the possibility of the shoulder blocking the surgeon's access to the area. The patient is well padded and secured to the table.

The author prefers to perform this operation in a "keyhole" fashion; therefore, exact positioning of the incision and craniotomy are critical to obtain adequate exposure. A "lazy S" type of incision is planned, with its center over a point approximately 1 cm posterior to the body of the mastoid and 1 cm below the superior nuchal line. The superior nuchal line is traced by connecting the root of the zygomatic process with the inion. This line marks the level of the distal transverse sinus, delineating the level of the posterior fossa (Fig. 19.2). Total incision length is approximately 4 cm. After sterile preparation and draping, the incision is made and the soft tissues elevated and retracted with multiple blunt scalp hooks. The

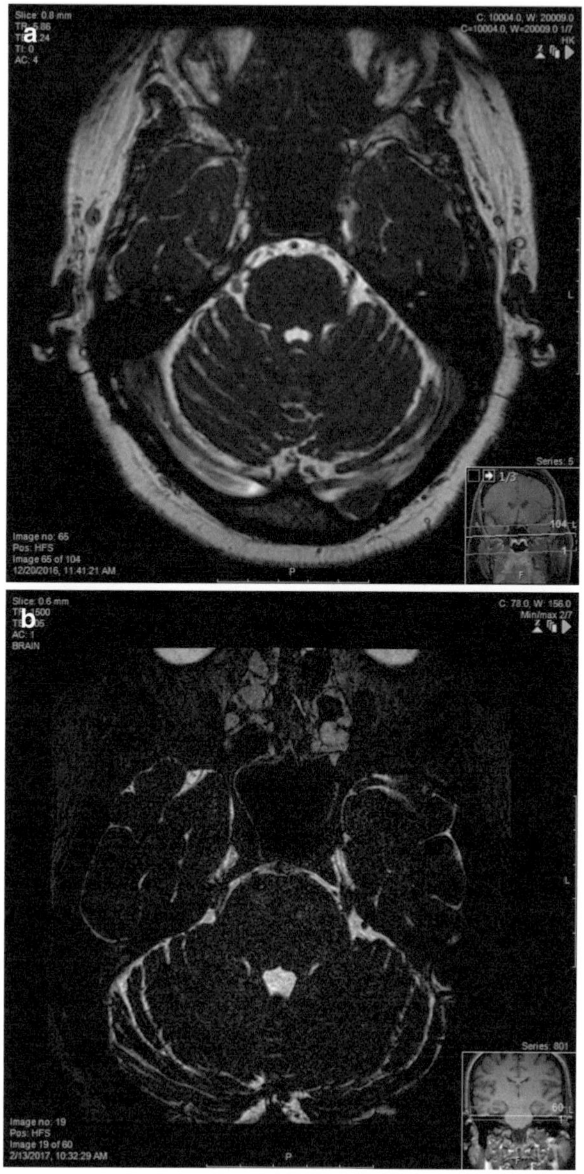

Fig. 19.1 Axial high-resolution T2 MRI views of TN1 patients with typical findings of vascular contact causing symptoms (arrows)

craniotomy is then made, measuring approximately 15 mm in diameter. Critical is to position the craniotomy such that the posterior margin of the upper curve of the sigmoid sinus is at the anterior margin. The dura is then opened in a curved fashion with a "Y" extension posterior and superior. This positions the opening at the petrotentorial angle. It is most helpful to allow CSF to drain while gently elevating the cerebellum away from the petrotentorial angle. Patience to allow sufficient CSF to drain results in relaxation of the cerebellum and provides operative space.

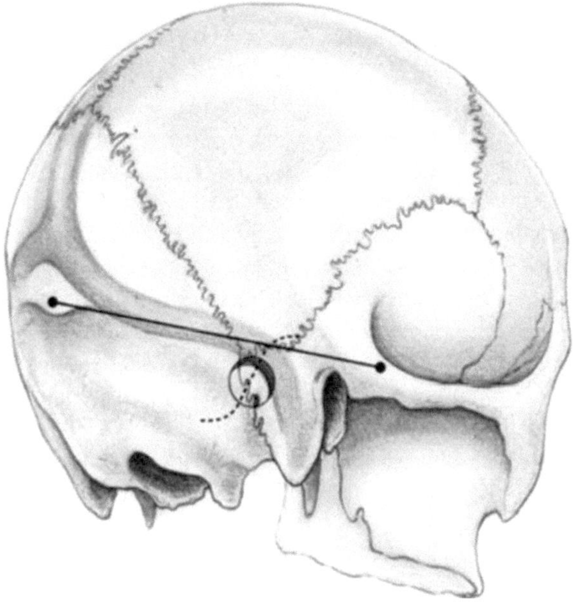

Fig. 19.2 Optimal placement of the keyhole craniotomy is judged based upon external landmarks to expose the posterior superior curve of the sigmoid sinus at the anterior edge. This places the surgeon at the petrotentorial angle with an optimal view, avoiding the need for retraction (From Day JD, Kellogg J, Tschabitscher M, Fukushima T: Surface and Superficial Surgical Anatomy of the Posterolateral Skull Base: Significance for Surgical Planning and Approach. **Neurosurgery** 38:1079–1084, 1996)

Intradural Dissection

The key landmark in approaching the prepontine cistern and trigeminal nerve root entry zone is to locate the petrotentorial angle and follow this medial. The petrosal vein complex is invariably encountered lateral to the operative region and is enveloped in arachnoid. The arachnoid membrane is sharply dissected away from the petrosal vein complex which will result in relaxation of the cerebellum away from the dural surface. Drainage of cerebrospinal fluid increases the operative space and obviates the need for fixed retraction. Arachnoid is then further opened above and below the petrosal vein complex to fully expose the nerve root entry zone. Dural dissection inferior to the petrosal vein complex should avoid arachnoid around just superior to the cochlear nerve and internal auditory meatus. Dissection of this region of arachnoid risks damaging the subarcuate artery, resulting in hearing loss.

It is important to preserve the petrosal vein complex when possible to avoid an unexpected complication owing to poor venous drainage of the cerebellum and middle cerebellar peduncle. The petrosal vein can usually be sacrificed with impunity; however, it is never certain, and there are no preoperative tests that will reliably predict the reliance of the structures on this outflow route. Therefore, it is best to preserve this venous complex whenever possible. If it is not possible to navigate surgically around this vein complex and it must be sacrificed, closure of the confluence of the vein as near as possible to its junction with the superior petrosal sinus is the best strategy. The key is to maintain a confluence that is open such that there is the possibility of redirected venous outflow through one or more tributaries.

The nerve is then inspected for vascular contact. The most frequent artery to contact the nerve is the superior cerebellar artery, compressing the vessel on its superior aspect. Much less frequent is the anterior inferior cerebellar artery or an ectatic basilar artery. The arachnoidal attachments of the artery are divided with sharp microsurgical dissection and the vessel moved gently away from the nerve. Small pledgets of Teflon felt are then placed to prevent the artery from making further contact with the nerve (Fig. 19.3). It is best to place the pledgets in such a way that they are unlikely to move, in effect "shingling" them in place. The senior author describes this as "building a fence" between the vessel and the nerve. Recurrence secondary to slippage of a pledget is unlikely when done in this manner.

Venous compression constitutes a different situation in terms of whether the vessel is excluded from contact either by pledget placement or sacrifice of the vein. The most common vein to be pathologic is the trigeminal vein, which accompanies the nerve in its course across the prepontine space to its entrance into Meckel's cave. This vein tends to be quite large in these situations, and a judgment is required regarding whether it is reasonably safe to sacrifice the vessel. In general, as with the petrosal vein complex, it is best to preserve major venous structures to avoid complications from venous insufficiency. However, if the patient has a robust petrosal vein complex, it is generally safe to sacrifice a trigeminal vein causing compression. If the petrosal vein is absent or underdeveloped, a large trigeminal vein is more likely to be important to the venous drainage of the brain stem and anterior cerebellum and should be preserved. Freeing the vein and placing pledgets to obviate contact with the nerve is then the necessary maneuver.

In some cases of venous compression, the area of contact with the nerve has been observed to be more distal along the nerve, at the cisternal segment and not at the entry zone. What can be very difficult in this situation is adequate visualization of the affected segment of the nerve. The view may be obstructed by the suprameatal eminence, located superior to the internal auditory meatus. In such situations visualization will be improved by reduction of the suprameatal eminence by drilling or utilizing a bone tip with an ultrasonic aspirator. An alternative strategy in this situation is to utilize an endoscope, typically a 30° instrument, to obtain an adequate working view.

Another anatomical situation that may present particular challenges is compression of the nerve by an ectatic basilar artery. Maintaining Teflon pledgets in position between the nerve and a large artery with higher amplitude pulsations owing to its size is less secure. Therefore, taking steps to reduce the potential effects of movement that could dislodge the pledgets becomes necessary. The senior author has found it best in these situations to augment the decompression by placing a cotton loop around the artery, avoiding stretch or compression of perforating branches, and securing the loop to the petrous dura with suture (Fig. 19.4). This "sling" around the vessel is fashioned such that the course of the artery is altered enough to decrease the force of contact on the nerve. Pledgets are then placed between the artery and nerve to complete the decompression.

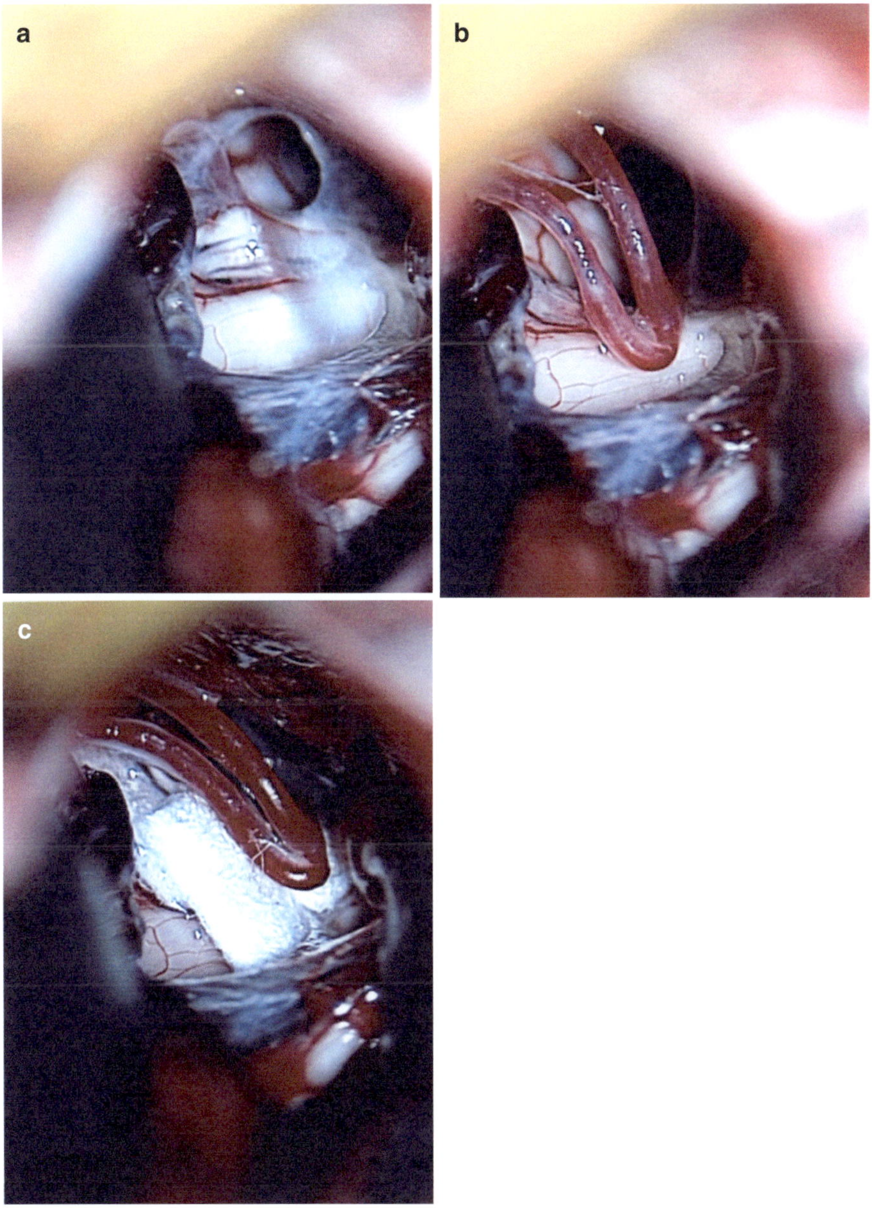

Fig. 19.3 Operative microscope views of a typical situation of superior cerebellar artery compression of the trigeminal nerve. (**a**) Prior to arterial dissection. (**b**) The artery is freed from contact with the nerve. (**c**) Multiple Teflon felt pledgets are placed to prevent further arterial contact with the nerve

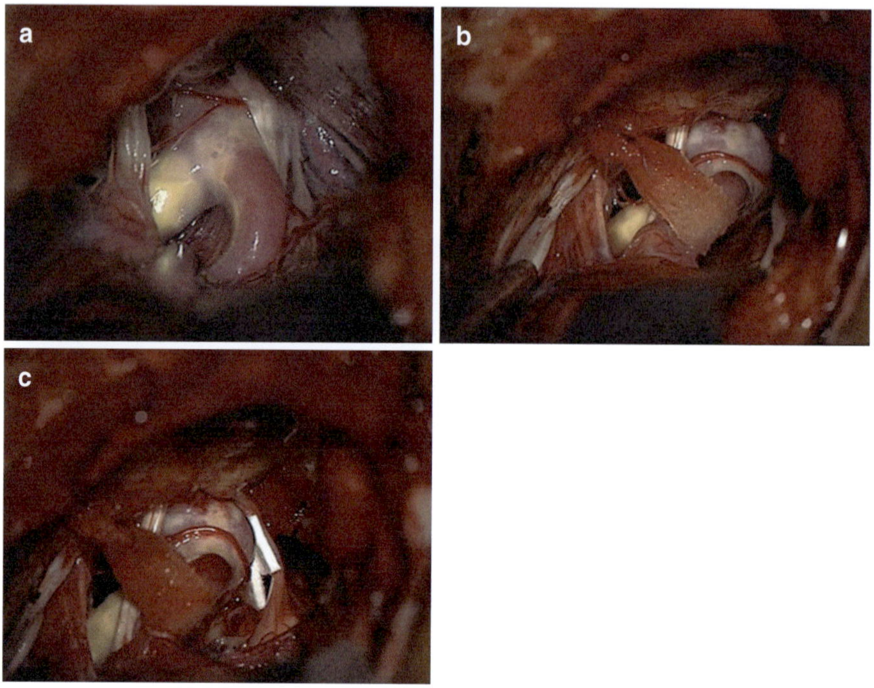

Fig. 19.4 Operative views of an ectatic basilar artery compressing the trigeminal nerve in an elderly patient with recalcitrant neuralgia. (**a**) The basilar artery compresses the left trigeminal nerve with the vertebrobasilar junction visible just below. (**b**) The artery is deviated inferior and lateral without kinking by placing a sling around the left vertebral artery. (**c**) After redirecting the vessel Teflon is placed to pad the vessel completing the decompression

Reconstruction and Closure

After concluding the intradural work, the field is flooded with irrigant. It is advisable to recheck the pledget positions after vigorous irrigation to make certain nothing will easily dislodge. After this final check, the dura is closed. Reconstruction of the bone defect is important to mitigate against the risk of postoperative headache. With keyhole openings as described above, bone defect reconstruction with hydroxyapatite cement is effective, especially if any openings into mastoid air cells occurred with bone removal. Closure of these openings are necessary to prevent leakage of cerebrospinal fluid postoperatively via the mastoid to the middle ear space and through to the Eustachian tube. The muscle layers and scalp are then sutured and a simple dressing applied.

Discussion: Outcomes with MVD for TN

Considering surgical treatments for TN, MVD is one of the most efficacious treatments for patients with medication-refractory TN. However, results are not consistent when treating patients with atypical TN with MVD [3, 52–54]. Several studies have compared outcomes for MVD between these two types of TN and found that patients with typical TN have much better outcomes in terms of immediate and long-term pain relief compared with those with atypical TN [3]. Outcomes are categorized as excellent, complete pain relief without addition of medication; good, mild or intermittent pain relief controlled with addition of medication; or poor, minimal or no pain relief even with addition of medications. Immediately postop, 80–90% of patients with typical TN have been reported to have an excellent outcome with complete pain relief, but only 45–50% with atypical TN had complete pain relief [9]. Regarding the other patients with atypical TN, partial pain relief is reported in 30% and poor pain relief or recurrence is reported in 20% [1, 54–56].

Regarding long-term follow-up of 5 years, it has been found that 73% of patients with typical TN continued to have an excellent outcome with sustained complete pain relief, whereas only 35% with atypical TN continued to have complete pain relief [9]. Depending on the source, recurrence rates are also much higher in patient with atypical TN, reported as high as 40–50%, compared with 10% in patients with typical trigeminal neuralgia. Thus, patients with typical TN are more likely to have both immediate pain relief and sustained, long-term pain relief following MVD [52, 54, 57, 58].

Predictors of outcome regarding immediate and long-term pain relief vary depending on the study [9, 57]. The presence of lancinating pain is the strongest predictor of successful outcome, and this should be strongly taken into consideration when deciding treatment modality in patients with TN [56, 57]. There is variability among studies regarding other positive or negative predictors of pain relief. One study found that memorable onset and the presence of clear trigger factors were associated with better outcomes in both typical and atypical TN [9]. This same study found that preoperative sensory loss, however, is associated with worse outcomes in patients with atypical TN, but not typical TN [9, 52, 57]. There is mixed evidence regarding postoperative facial numbness with some studies finding either no association with long-term pain relief or associated with worse outcomes and postoperative burning and aching pain [55, 59–61].

Aside from MVD, other procedures involve lesioning the nerve to block abnormal neuronal signal conduction that is interpreted as pain. MVD, on the other hand, addresses the underlying pathophysiology. MVD is now generally regarded as the most effective treatment for TN as it is associated with the lowest rates of recurrence and sensory loss. With good patient selection and attention to meticulous microsurgical technique, outcomes with MVD should remain the patient's best chance of an optimal outcome.

References

1. Hai J, Li S-T, Pan Q-G. Treatment of atypical trigeminal neuralgia with microvascular decompression. Neurol India. 2006;54:53–6; discussion 57. Available: http://www.ncbi.nlm.nih.gov/pubmed/16679644
2. Kumar S, Rastogi S, Mahendra P, Bansal M, Chandra L. Pain in trigeminal neuralgia: neurophysiology and measurement: a comprehensive review. J Med Life. 2013;6:383–8. Available: http://www.pubmedcentral.nih.gov/articlerender.fcgi?artid=3973876&tool=pmcentrez&rendertype=abstract
3. Li S-T, Wang X, Pan Q, Hai J, Liu N, Shen F, et al. Studies on the operative outcomes and mechanisms of microvascular decompression in treating typical and atypical trigeminal neuralgia. Clin J Pain. 2005;21:311–6. Available: http://www.ncbi.nlm.nih.gov/pubmed/15951648
4. Obermann M. Treatment options in trigeminal neuralgia. Ther Adv Neurol Disord. 2010;3:107–15.
5. Obermann M, Katsarava Z. Update on trigeminal neuralgia. Expert Rev Neurother. 2009;9:323–9. Available: http://www.ncbi.nlm.nih.gov/pubmed/19271941
6. Taha JM, Tew JM. Comparison of surgical treatments for trigeminal neuralgia: reevaluation of radiofrequency rhizotomy. Neurosurgery. 1996;38:865–71.
7. Perkin GD, Brandt T. Trigeminal and glossopharyngeal neuralgia. In: Brandt T, Caplan LR, Dichgans J, Christoph Diener H, Kennard C, editors. Neurological disorders: course and treatment. 2nd ed. San Diego: Academic Press; 2003. p. 67–75.
8. Burchiel KJ, Slavin KV. On the natural history of trigeminal neuralgia. Neurosurgery. 2000;46:152–4.
9. Tyler-Kabara EC, Kassam AB, Horowitz MH, Urgo L, Hadjipanayis C, Levy EI, et al. Predictors of outcome in surgically managed patients with typical and atypical trigeminal neuralgia: comparison of results following microvascular decompression. J Neurosurg. 2002;96:527–31.
10. Jannetta PJ, Abbasy M, Maroon JC, Ramos FM, Albin MS. Etiology and definitive microsurgical treatment of hemifacial spasm. Operative techniques and results in 47 patients. J Neurosurg. 1977;47:321–8.
11. Jannetta PJ. Vascular compression is the cause of trigeminal neuralgia. APS J. 1993;2:217–27.
12. Truini A, Galeotti F, Cruccu G. New insight into trigeminal neuralgia. J Headache Pain. 2005;6:237–9. Available: http://www.pubmedcentral.nih.gov/articlerender.fcgi?artid=3452002&tool=pmcentrez&rendertype=abstract
13. Zakrzewska JM, Linskey ME: Trigeminal neuralgia. BMJ. 2014;348:g474 Available: http://books.google.com/books?id=vAbU8rfb-OoC&pgis=1%5Cnhttp://www.ncbi.nlm.nih.gov/pubmed/24534115%5Cnhttp://www.ncbi.nlm.nih.gov/pubmed/25299564
14. Adams CB. Microvascular compression: an alternative view and hypothesis. J Neurosurg. 1989;70:1–12. Available: http://www.ncbi.nlm.nih.gov/pubmed/2642544
15. Al-Quliti KW. Update on neuropathic pain treatment for trigeminal neuralgia. The pharmacological and surgical options. Neurosciences (Riyadh). 2015;20:107–14. Available: http://www.ncbi.nlm.nih.gov/pubmed/25864062%5Cnhttp://www.pubmedcentral.nih.gov/articlerender.fcgi?artid=PMC4727618
16. Barrett AP, Schifter M. Trigeminal neuralgia. Aust Dent J. 1993;38:198–203.
17. Chen GQ, Wang XS, Wang L, Zheng JP. Arterial compression of nerve is the primary cause of trigeminal neuralgia. Neurol Sci. 2014;35:61–6.
18. Cole CD, Liu JK, Apfelbaum RI. Historical perspectives on the diagnosis and treatment of trigeminal neuralgia. Neurosurg Focus. 2005;18:1–15.
19. Scrivani SJ, Mathews ES, Maciewicz RJ. Trigeminal neuralgia. Oral Surg Oral Med Oral Pathol Oral Radiol Endod. 2005;100:527–38. Available: http://www.ncbi.nlm.nih.gov/pubmed/16243236
20. Love S, Coakham HB. Trigeminal neuralgia: pathology and pathogenesis. Brain. 2001;124:2347–2360. Available: papers3://publication/uuid/88F8C9A6-6290-4688-BDF2-05E37B5D6354

21. Maarbjerg S, Di Stefano G, Bendtsen L, Cruccu G. Trigeminal neuralgia – diagnosis and treatment. Cephalalgia. 2017;37:33310241668728. Available: http://journals.sagepub.com/doi/10.1177/0333102416687280
22. Van Kleef M, Van Genderen WE, Narouze S, Nurmikko TJ, Van Zundert J, Geurts JW, et al. 1. Trigeminal neuralgia. Pain Pract. 2009;9:252–9.
23. Devor M, Amir R, Rappaport ZH. Pathophysiology of trigeminal neuralgia: the ignition hypothesis. Clin J Pain. 2002;18:4–13.
24. Sabalys G, Juodzbalys G, Wang H-L. Aetiology and pathogenesis of trigeminal neuralgia: a comprehensive review. J Oral Maxillofac Res. 2013;3:e2. Available: http://www.pubmedcentral.nih.gov/articlerender.fcgi?artid=3886096&tool=pmcentrez&rendertype=abstract
25. Fromm GH, Terrence CF, Maroon JC. Trigeminal neuralgia. Current concepts regarding etiology and pathogenesis. Arch Neurol. 1984;41:1204–7. Available: http://www.ncbi.nlm.nih.gov/pubmed/6487105
26. DANDY WE. An operation for the cure of tic douloureux. Arch Surg. 1929;18:687. Available: http://archsurg.jamanetwork.com/article.aspx?articleid=538939
27. Patel SK, Liu JK. Overview and history of trigeminal neuralgia. Neurosurg Clin N Am. 2016;27:265–76.
28. Eboli P, Stone JL, Aydin S, Slavin KV. Historical characterization of trigeminal neuralgia. Neurosurgery. 2009;64:1183–6.
29. Dandy WE. Glossopharyngeal neuralgia (tic douloureux): its diagnosis and treatment. Arch Surg. 1927;15:198–214. https://doi.org/10.1001/archsurg.1927.01130200046002.
30. Dandy WE. The treatment of trigeminal neuralgia by the cerebellar route. Ann Surg. 1932;96:787–95.
31. Barker FG, Jannetta PJ, Bissonette DJ, Larkins MV, Jho HD. The long-term outcome of microvascular decompression for trigeminal neuralgia. N Engl J Med. 1996;334:1077–83. Available: http://www.ncbi.nlm.nih.gov/pubmed/8598865
32. Zakrzewska JM, Coakham HB. Microvascular decompression for trigeminal neuralgia: update. Curr Opin Neurol. 2012;25:296–301.
33. Cruccu G, Gronseth G, Alksne J, Argoff C, Brainin M, Burchiel K, et al. AAN-EFNS guidelines on trigeminal neuralgia management. Eur J Neurol. 2008;15:1013–28.
34. Zakrzewska JM, Linskey ME. Neurosurgical interventions for the treatment of trigeminal neuralgia (Protocol). Cochrane Database Syst Rev. 2008;(3):CD007312. Cochrane Review ID 102. https://doi.org/10.1002/14651858.CD007312.
35. Belber CJ, Rak RA. Balloon compression rhizolysis in the surgical management of trigeminal neuralgia. Neurosurgery. 1987;20:908–13.
36. Liu JK, Apfelbaum RI. Treatment of trigeminal neuralgia. Neurosurg Clin N Am. 2004;15:319–34.
37. Loeser JD. Tic douloureux. Pain Res Manag. 2001;6:156–65.
38. Ong KS, Keng SB. Evaluation of surgical procedures for trigeminal neuralgia. Anesth Prog. 2003;50:181–8.
39. Pagni CA, Fariselli L, Zeme S. Trigeminal neuralgia. Non-invasive techniques versus microvascular decompression. It is really available any further improvement? Acta Neurochir Suppl. 2008:27–33.
40. Burchiel KJ, Steege TD, Howe JF, Loeser JD. Comparison of percutaneous radiofrequency gangliolysis and microvascular decompression for the surgical management of tic douloureux. Neurosurgery. 1981;9:111–9.
41. Elias WJ, Burchiel KJ. Microvascular decompression. Clin J Pain. 2002;18:35–41. Available: http://www.ncbi.nlm.nih.gov/entrez/query.fcgi?cmd=Retrieve&db=PubMed&dopt=Citation&list_uids=11803301
42. Elias WJ, Burchiel KJ. Microvascular decompression. Clin J Pain. 2002;18:35–41. Available: http://www.ncbi.nlm.nih.gov/pubmed/11803301
43. Kabatas S, Karasu A, Civelek E, Sabanci AP, Hepgul KT, Teng YD. Microvascular decompression as a surgical management for trigeminal neuralgia: Long-term follow-up and review of the literature. Neurosurg Rev. 2009;32:87–93.

44. Sade B, Lee JH. Microvascular decompression for trigeminal neuralgia. Neurosurg Clin N Am. 2014;25:743–9.
45. Chakravarthi PS, Ghanta R, Kattimani V. Microvascular decompression treatment for trigeminal neuralgia. J Craniofac Surg. 2011;22:894–8. Available: http://www.ncbi.nlm.nih.gov/pubmed/21558885
46. Burchiel KJ, Clarke H, Haglund M, Loeser JD. Long-term efficacy of microvascular decompression in trigeminal neuralgia. J Neurosurg. 1988;69:35–8. Available: http://www.ncbi.nlm.nih.gov/pubmed/2454303
47. Kolluri S, Heros RC. Microvascular decompression for trigeminal neuralgia. A five-year follow-up study. Surg Neurol. 1984;22:235–40. Available: http://www.ncbi.nlm.nih.gov/pubmed/6463831
48. Smith JH, Cutrer FM. Numbness matters: a clinical review of trigeminal neuropathy. Cephalalgia. 2011;31:1131–44. Available: http://www.ncbi.nlm.nih.gov/pubmed/21628435
49. McLaughlin MR, Jannetta PJ, Clyde BL, Subach BR, Comey CH, Resnick DK. Microvascular decompression of cranial nerves: lessons learned after 4400 operations. J Neurosurg. 1999;90:1–8.
50. Shah AA. Microvascular decompression for trigeminal neuralgia. J Pak Med Assoc. 1993;43:134–5.
51. Cohen-Gadol AA. Microvascular decompression surgery for trigeminal neuralgia and hemifacial spasm: nuances of the technique based on experiences with 100 patients and review of the literature. Clin Neurol Neurosurg. 2011;113:844–53.
52. Elias WJ, Burchiel KJ. Trigeminal neuralgia and other craniofacial pain syndromes: an overview. Semin Neurosurg. 2004;15:59–69.
53. Eller JL, Raslan AM, Burchiel KJ. Trigeminal neuralgia: definition and classification. Neurosurg Focus. 2005;18:E3.
54. W han H, Zhang K, guo ZJ. Atypical trigeminal neuralgia: a consequence of central sensitization. Med Hypotheses. 2010;75:65–6.
55. Hong W, Zheng X, Wu Z, Li X, Wang X, Li Y, et al. Clinical features and surgical treatment of trigeminal neuralgia caused solely by venous compression. Acta Neurochir. 2011;153:1037–42.
56. Zhang H, Lei D, You C, Mao BY, Wu B, Fang Y. The long-term outcome predictors of pure microvascular decompression for primary trigeminal neuralgia. World Neurosurg. 2013;79:756–62.
57. Miller JP, Magill ST, Acar F, Burchiel KJ. Predictors of long-term success after microvascular decompression for trigeminal neuralgia. J Neurosurg. 2009;110:620–6. Available: http://www.ncbi.nlm.nih.gov/pubmed/19231931
58. Lichtor T, Mullan JF. A 10-year follow-up review of percutaneous microcompression of the trigeminal ganglion. J Neurosurg. 1990;72:49–54. Available: http://www.ncbi.nlm.nih.gov/pubmed/2294184
59. Barker FG, Jannetta PJ, Bissonette DJ, Shields PT, Larkins MV Jho HD. Microvascular decompression for hemifacial spasm. J Neurosurg. 1995;82:201–10. Available: http://content.wkhealth.com/linkback/openurl?sid=WKPTLP:landingpage&an=00006123-900000000-97910%5Cnhttp://www.ncbi.nlm.nih.gov/pubmed/7815147
60. Barker FG, Jannetta PJ, Bissonette DJ, Jho HD. Trigeminal numbness and tic relief after microvascular decompression for typical trigeminal neuralgia. Neurosurgery. 1997;40:39–45.
61. Matsushima T, Huynh-Le P, Miyazono M. Trigeminal neuralgia caused by venous compression. Neurosurgery. 2004;55:334–8.

Chapter 20
Advanced Neurosurgical Interventions

Sharona Ben-Haim, Ahmed M. Raslan, and Andre Machado

Introduction

There are many etiologies causing the various phenotypic patterns of facial pain, some of which are more likely to be refractory to both medical management and often to first and sometimes second lines of more common surgical interventions. These surgical interventions usually target the peripheral component of the trigeminal nerve from its most distal aspect in the subcutaneous nerve endings of the face, to the location of its cell bodies in the dorsal root ganglion located within Meckel's cave, to its entry into the brainstem. When these approaches fail to provide relief, or when destructive interventions exacerbate pain, advanced neurosurgical interventions in central nervous system targets should be considered.

Pain and temperature fibers of the face are circuitous in their course from peripheral nerves to their widespread representation in the cerebral cortex. Upon entering the lateral aspect of the pons, these fibers take a sharp turn caudally in the spinal trigeminal tract before synapsing in the spinal trigeminal nucleus. The inferior aspect of this nucleus is named the nucleus caudalis, and nociceptive afferent fibers are thought to synapse with second-order neurons in this region. This nucleus

S. Ben-Haim (✉)
Department of Neurosurgery, University of California San Diego, La Jolla, CA, USA
e-mail: sbenhaim@ucsd.edu

A. M. Raslan
Department of Neurological Surgery, OHSU, Portland, OR, USA
e-mail: raslana@ohsu.edu

A. Machado
The Cleveland Clinic, Center for Neurological Restoration, Cleveland, OH, USA
e-mail: machada@ccf.org

J. Y. Suen, E. Petersen (eds.), *Diagnosis and Management of Head and Face Pain*, https://doi.org/10.1007/978-3-319-90999-8_20

extends caudally to the spinal trigeminal tract, which together is often called the trigeminocervical complex (TCC), thought to project down to the level of the C2 spinal segment [1, 2]. Second-order neurons cross midline and synapse mainly on the medial ventral posterior (or ventral caudal) nucleus of the thalamus (VPM), as well as other thalamic targets. From here, third-order neurons travel up to various regions of the cerebral cortex including primary and secondary somatosensory cortex, anterior cingulate gyrus, posterior parietal cortex, and insula, among others. Other salient brainstem pathways have been described which involve both ascending and descending control of these fibers, most notably areas including the periaqueductal gray (PAG) and ventral medulla [1, 3]. These complex networks of cortical and subcortical regions that in concert process pain information and experience are referred to as the "pain matrix."

Advanced neurosurgical interventions of the CNS pathways of head and facial pain have attempted to target most of these anatomic locations often with lesioning procedures subsequently followed by neuromodulatory techniques. In this chapter, we will discuss interventions in the spinal cord/brainstem regions as well as both lesioning and neuromodulation of cerebral targets.

Advanced Neurosurgical Interventions: The Spine and Brainstem

Nucleus Caudalis Dorsal Root Entry Zone (DREZ) Lesioning

The descending trigeminal tract and spinal trigeminal nucleus comprise fibers from several cranial nerves. The nucleus can be parsed into three subdivisions from rostral to caudal including the nucleus oralis, the nucleus interpolaris, and the nucleus caudalis, located at the level of the spinomedullary junction to the C2 segment, which carries pain and temperature fibers from the trigeminal nerve [4]. The nucleus caudalis has thus been the target of intervention in the treatment of facial pain, particularly at the root entry zone where pain and temperature fibers enter the dorsal horn gray matter of the spinal cord. The spinocerebellar pathway and the pyramidal tract are within close proximity to the nucleus caudalis and thus pose a significant risk to this procedure. Akin to the spinal dorsal root entry zone surgery, nucleus caudalis DREZ is intended to destroy second-order neurons involved in chronic pain syndromes that lead to their hyperactivity, as is thought to be the case in certain clinical syndromes including anesthesia dolorosa.

This technique commonly employs a unilateral approach, although a bilateral approach has recently been described [5]. A midline incision is made from the inion to the spinous process of C3, and C1 hemilaminectomy is performed along with a suboccipital craniectomy. Using microsurgical technique and employing a special curved probe designed to mitigate the risk of postoperative ipsilateral ataxia [6], a single line of lesions is made at 1-mm intervals directly above the C2 dorsal rootlets and extended to approximately 5 mm above the obex on a line between the cervical dorsal roots and the rootlets of the spinal accessory nerve [7]. Lesions are made using RF probes for 15 s each at a temperature of 70 C. Neurophysiologic monitoring to safeguard against extension of lesioning into the neighboring corticospinal tract is critical.

In one recent series, 11 nucleus caudalis DREZ procedures were reported for varied pathologies of head and face pain including pain resulting from tumors, atypical facial pain, and trigeminal neuralgia, among others. After the procedure 72.5% of patients reported initial pain relief, and 1 year after surgery, 62% of patients still considered their pain relief satisfactory [4]. Bullard and Nashold reported 25 nucleus caudalis DREZ operations for severe facial pain, with good to excellent pain relief in 96% of patients at the time of discharge and sustained relief in 67% of patients at 1 year [8]. In a more recent retrospective study involving nucleus caudalis DREZ in 16 patients with head and face pain, 68.9% reported being at least very satisfied with their pain relief after lesioning, and an average of 58.1% had pain relief that lasted more than 1 year. In this series, two patients reported transient postoperative ataxia, and two patients reported a permanent new neuropathy/radiculopathy. Eighty percent of patients in this study believed it improved their quality of life [7].

Nucleus Caudalis Tractotomy-Nucleotomy

The elucidation of the brainstem components of the spinal trigeminal tract, which send descending postganglionic projections to the nucleus caudalis, similarly led to interventions targeted toward the treatment of intractable facial pain starting in the late 1930s. This technique was further refined by applying stereotactic and minimally invasive percutaneous techniques that target the tract at the cervicomedullary junction [4, 9]. Although not commonly used, this remains a viable treatment option for patients suffering from a variety of head and face pain syndromes including malignancy-related facial pain, neuropathic pain, and various cranial nerve neuralgias. The trigeminal tractotomy-nucleotomy is a miniature nucleus caudalis DREZ that produces a complete lesion of the trigeminal tract but only a single or dual lesion into the nucleus; therefore, it is more appropriate for conditions such as cancer pain of the face or neuropathic facial pain such as facial pain after dental procedures. The procedure is done in the prone position using RF electrodes that are also used for cordotomy and recently has been done using general anesthesia with the aid of intraoperative CT scans. Two tandem lesions are created at 75 C for 60 s [10, 11].

In one series, ten patients underwent a percutaneous trigeminal tractotomy-nucleotomy with initial pain relief reported as 98%, with 80% relief observed at 6-month follow-up [10]. While some authors believe that the procedure may not have enough coverage of the nucleus caudalis to achieve maximal efficacy [6], some recommend this procedure to be considered prior to more invasive techniques including nucleus caudalis DREZ, particularly in the treatment of cancer-related head and neck pain [12].

High Cervical Spinal Cord Neuromodulation

Neuromodulation of the dorsal aspect of the spinal cord is well described in the treatment of intractable pain of the body, and more recently spinal cord stimulation of the high cervical region has been showed to be efficacious in the treatment of both headache and facial pain syndromes [13]. These interventions target the spinal trigeminal nucleus and nucleus caudalis region, with an aim to modulate similar pathways as nucleus caudalis dorsal root entry zone procedures.

There has been a relative dearth of reported cases in the literature, with some conflicting results. An initial case report by Barolat et al. revealed successful treatment of trigeminal neuralgia by two leads in the cervical spinal cord between C1 and C2 [14]. Another study of 41 patients with implanted dual two-contact paddle electrodes (four contacts per system) in the cervical spinal cord for both upper limb as well as face pain concluded that facial pain did not respond well to this treatment modality [15]. In another study of 35 patients, cervicomedullary junction SCS with quadripolar paddle leads was used for the treatment of intractable head and face pain and reports that 71.4% of patients had a successful trial with subsequent implantation of stimulating electrodes between the occiput and C2. Of these patients, 75% retained their implants and reported continued pain relief, with 50% reporting decreased use of oral pain medications [16]. There is suggestion that adequate pain relief in high cervical SCS may be highly dependent upon location of the electrodes with adequate coverage of the nucleus caudalis region and attention to its anatomic variability [17]. Successful use of this approach may necessitate modifications of the technique for adequate placement at the cervicomedullary junction and may require small occipital craniectomy in addition to a C1 laminotomy to achieve ideal coverage [16, 18].

Stereotactic Mesencephalotomy

Stereotactic mesencephalotomy aims to lesion the spinothalamic, trigeminothalamic, and/or spinoreticular tracts at the midbrain level to treat medically refractory, nociceptive, contralateral pain and is most widely utilized in the setting of cancer-related head and neck pain. It was initially reported in 1952 by Spiegel and Wycis for the treatment of intractable facial pain [19] but despite its efficacy has been rarely utilized in the twenty-first century [20]. Anatomical target points indicate that effective lesions are 5 mm behind the posterior commissure and 5–10 mm lateral to and 5 mm below the intercommissural plane [21] targeting the spinothalamic/trigeminothalamic tract and avoiding the medial lemniscus. The major potential side effects from this procedure are severe dysesthesias following damage to the medial lemniscus as well as disorders of ocular motility [20].

Advanced Neurosurgical Interventions: Cerebrum

Lesions

The creation of lesions in the brain for the treatment of chronic pain comprised some of the earliest targeted functional neurosurgical interventions and continues to be further refined with the aid of stereotactic methods and the utilization of new technology. Currently, this treatment modality is often superseded by neuromodulatory techniques; however, it nonetheless remains highly effective and may in fact be superior in certain circumstances including, most notably, in the setting of cancer pain.

Lesioning of the thalamus for the treatment of pain has been utilized for several decades, and target regions for intractable pain involving the head and face include both lateral and medial thalamic regions such as the ventroposteromedial (VPM), mediodorsal, centromedian, intralaminar, and parafascicular nuclei, thought to play a critical role in both the sensory-discriminative and the affective-motivational components of pain.

Over the past several decades, however, open ablative techniques often involving radiofrequency lesions have been largely replaced by incisionless techniques including Gamma Knife radiosurgery [22] and most recently MR-guided high-intensity focused ultrasound [23] with similar overall success rates. A recent meta-analysis review of Gamma Knife thalamotomy for the treatment of pain found that 23–44% of patients undergoing Gamma Knife (treated with a maximum cumulative dose ranging from 140 to 250 Gy) for both malignant and nonmalignant sources of pain achieved "significant" long-term pain relief [22]. Methodologies and exact targets are not consistent between series nor are indications for treatment, making comparison studies difficult to interpret.

The anterior cingulate cortex (ACC) is thought to play a role in the affective component of pain and has been the target of lesioning procedures for the treatment of chronic, medically refractory pain for decades. Although some variations have been reported, the target is typically described as being located 7 mm from midline, 20 mm posterior to the anterior tip of the fontal horns of the lateral ventricle, and 1 mm above the roof of the ventricles, bilaterally [24]. In a recent meta-analysis, a total of 224 patients who underwent anterior cingulotomy were reviewed including 36 patients with head and neck cancer, 6 patients with face pain, 2 patients with "atypical" face pain, 2 patients with postherpetic neuralgia, and 1 patient with thalamic face pain. It was found that greater than 60% of patients across all studies were reported to have significant pain relief postoperatively, which was sustained at least 1 year after surgery [25]. There was no significant difference in patients who underwent the procedure for a neoplastic source of pain compared to a nonneoplastic source. A significant correlation was found between pain relief outcome and the position of the lesion, with better outcomes found as the lesion target approached the tip of the frontal horns, possibly due to proximity to rostral emotional subdivision of the ACC [25].

Deep Brain Stimulation

Deep brain stimulation for the amelioration of chronic pain has been performed since the early 1950s and became a widely used treatment modality in the 1970s and mid-1980s. The technique fell out of favor in the late 1990s after two multicenter trials were conducted with neither satisfying its endpoint criteria. DBS is currently FDA approved for the management of Parkinson's disease and essential tremor, with a humanitarian device exemption for the treatment of dystonia and obsessive-compulsive disorder, and is currently performed for pain in the USA on an investigational basis or occasionally as off-label use of the hardware. It has been utilized, in the past, for a variety of chronic neuropathic and nociceptive pain syndromes including trigeminal neuropathy, postherpetic neuralgia, deafferentation facial pain, "atypical" facial pain, as well as other head and neck pathologies. Criticisms from previous literature have involved variability in patient selection as well as inconsistencies in neurosurgical technique [26], and more recent studies have benefited from new imaging modalities, procedural and hardware improvements, as well as advancements in patient and target selection.

Currently there is no consensus as to the best target to treat chronic pain, with the sensory thalamus (ventral posterior lateral and medial) being the most common [27]. Modulation of descending control pathways by targeting the periaqueductal and periventricular gray matter has also been utilized with success, with some contending that it is more effective specifically in the treatment of nociceptive pain [28]. Other targets such as the posterior hypothalamus have been tried successfully for the treatment of chronic trigeminal autonomic cephalalgia however were unsuccessful in the treatment of "atypical" facial pain [29].

In a series of 85 patients undergoing deep brain stimulation of the contralateral ventral posterior nucleus of the thalamus and/or periventricular gray area for pain, approximately 66% gained benefit and efficacy at long-term follow-up. In this cohort, 15 patients presented specifically for head and face pain pathologies, 11 of which were implanted and had sufficient follow-up data. In this subset, 54.5% of patients experienced pain relief at a mean of 23 months of follow-up [30].

More recently, targets have sought to modulate the affective sphere of pain circuitry based on the concept that the overall pain experience is determined by the integration of sensory-discriminative information combined with the affective-motivational and evaluative-cognitive processing of pain [31]. Electrodes have been placed in the anterior cingulate cortex [32] as well as the ventral striatum/anterior limb of internal capsule (VS/ALIC) [33] with success in relieving some of the affective components of pain while frequently not changing the nociceptive experience of pain. In one series, Boccard and colleagues describe their experience with 16 patients who underwent deep brain stimulation placement of the dorsal anterior cingulate cortex for chronic neuropathic pain, in which 11 patients had long-term follow-up data at a mean of 13.2 months [34]. In this cohort, there was an insignificant reduction in improvement of pain as measured on the visual analog scale (VAS); however, there was statistically significant improvement in the physical functioning and bodily pain domains of the SF-36 as well as on the EuroQol (EQ-3D), which evaluates dimensions including anxiety, pain, usual activities, self-care, and mobility.

Motor Cortex Stimulation

Electrical modulation of the motor cortex was initially employed after animal models revealed that stimulation in this region was sufficient to induce complete, long-term inhibition of thalamic burst hyperactivity in a thalamic pain model [35]. In this procedure, a combination of intraoperative image guidance as well as electrophysiology can be used to locate the motor cortex, and a small craniotomy or burr hole is made. Paddle electrodes are then most often placed epidurally and aligned either parallel or perpendicular to the central sulcus, although operative technique varies considerably between centers.

A review of the use of motor cortex stimulation for pain found that among the 210 patients identified, a good response (>40–50% pain relief) was found in approximately 55% of patients and in approximately 45% of patients with postoperative follow-up >1 year. Results were slightly better in patients with facial pain etiologies compared to poststroke pain syndrome. A good response was achieved in 68% of the 44 patients with trigeminal neuropathic pain [36]. Several other case series have similarly documented good results of using MCS for the treatment of trigeminal neuropathic pain, with one review noting that 75–100% of patients achieve "good to excellent" pain relief [28]. A recent randomized controlled trial using a high- and low-frequency stimulation crossover model for a variety of neuropathic pain syndromes enrolled 12 patients, 6 of whom withdrew from the study due to transient adverse events. In the remaining six patients, there was no significant change in pain relief with low or high stimulation [37]. There is still significant debate over the efficacy of this treatment modality, and larger randomized studies are underway with greater attention to patient selection and utilization of a more standardized set of techniques.

Future Directions

When necessary, interventions of the central nervous system can be effective at targeting severe neuropathic facial pain refractory to other medical and first-line surgical treatment modalities. As we achieve further sophistication in understanding the varied anatomic pathways and cortical representations of head and facial pain, potential targets and methodologies will be refined. This, in combination with improvements in the technological aspects of both increasingly less invasive lesioning and neuromodulatory procedures, will serve to add to our armamentarium of continually more efficacious interventions.

References

1. Goadsby PJ, Bartsch T, Dodick DW. Occipital nerve stimulation for headache: mechanisms and efficacy. Headache. 2008;48:313–8.
2. Goadsby PJ, Zagami AS. Stimulation of the superior sagittal sinus increases metabolic activity and blood flow in certain regions of the brainstem and upper cervical spinal cord of the cat. Brain. 1991;114(Pt 2):1001–11.
3. Hoskin KL, Bulmer DC, Lasalandra M, et al. Fos expression in the midbrain periaqueductal grey after trigeminovascular stimulation. J Anat. 2001;198:29–35.
4. Kanpolat Y, Tuna H, Bozkurt M, et al. Spinal and nucleus caudalis dorsal root entry zone operations for chronic pain. Neurosurgery. 2008;62:235–42; discussion 42–4.
5. Kanpolat Y, Al-Beyati E, Yakupoglu H. Staged bilateral nucleus caudalis DREZ lesioning for persistent idiopathic facial pain: exceptional case report. Turk Neurosurg. 2017;27:316–20.
6. Nashold BS Jr, el-Naggar AO, Ovelmen-Levitt J, et al. A new design of radiofrequency lesion electrodes for use in the caudalis nucleus DREZ operation. Technical note. J Neurosurg. 1994;80:1116–20.
7. Chivukula S, Tempel ZJ, Chen CJ, et al. Spinal and nucleus caudalis dorsal root entry zone lesioning for chronic pain: efficacy and outcomes. World Neurosurg. 2015;84:494–504.
8. Bullard DE, Nashold BS Jr. The caudalis DREZ for facial pain. Stereotact Funct Neurosurg. 1997;68:168–74.
9. Kanpolat Y, Deda H, Akyar S, et al. CT-guided trigeminal tractotomy. Acta Neurochir (Wien). 1989;100:112–4.
10. Raslan AM. Percutaneous computed tomography-guided radiofrequency ablation of upper spinal cord pain pathways for cancer-related pain. Neurosurgery. 2008;62:226–33; discussion 33–4.
11. Thompson EM, Burchiel KJ, Raslan AM. Percutaneous trigeminal tractotomy-nucleotomy with use of intraoperative computed tomography and general anesthesia: report of 2 cases. Neurosurg Focus. 2013;35(3):E5.
12. Kanpolat Y, Caglar S, Akyar S, et al. CT-guided pain procedures for intractable pain in malignancy. Acta Neurochir Suppl. 1995;64:88–91.
13. Deer TR, Mekhail N, Petersen E, et al. The appropriate use of neurostimulation: stimulation of the intracranial and extracranial space and head for chronic pain. Neuromodulation Appropriateness Consensus Committee. Neuromodulation. 2014;17:551–70; discussion 70.
14. Barolat G, Knobler RL, Lublin FD. Trigeminal neuralgia in a patient with multiple sclerosis treated with high cervical spinal cord stimulation. Case report. Appl Neurophysiol. 1988;51:333–7.
15. Simpson BA, Bassett G, Davies K, et al. Cervical spinal cord stimulation for pain: a report on 41 patients. Neuromodulation. 2003;6:20–6.
16. Tomycz ND, Deibert CP, Moossy JJ. Cervicomedullary junction spinal cord stimulation for head and facial pain. Headache. 2011;51:418–25.
17. Sandwell SE, El-Naggar AO, Nettleton GS, et al. Trigeminal nucleus caudalis anatomy: guidance for radiofrequency dorsal root entry zone lesioning. Stereotact Funct Neurosurg. 2010;88:269–76.
18. Chivukula S, Tempel ZJ, Weiner GM, et al. Cervical and cervicomedullary spinal cord stimulation for chronic pain: efficacy and outcomes. Clin Neurol Neurosurg. 2014;127:33–41.
19. Spiegel EA, Wycis HT. Mesencephalotomy in intractable facial pain. Trans Am Neurol Assoc. 1952;56:186–9.
20. Ivanishvili Z, Pujara S, Honey CM, et al. Stereotactic mesencephalotomy for palliative care pain control: a case report, literature review and plea to rediscover this operation. Br J Neurosurg. 2016;30:444–7.
21. Kim DR, Lee SW, Son BC. Stereotactic mesencephalotomy for cancer—related facial pain. J Korean Neurosurg Soc. 2014;56:71–4.

22. Roberts DG, Pouratian N. Stereotactic radiosurgery for the treatment of chronic intractable pain: a systematic review. Oper Neurosurg (Hagerstown). 2017;13(5):543–51.
23. Jeanmonod D, Werner B, Morel A, et al. Transcranial magnetic resonance imaging-guided focused ultrasound: noninvasive central lateral thalamotomy for chronic neuropathic pain. Neurosurg Focus. 2012;32:E1.
24. Spangler WJ, Cosgrove GR, Ballantine HT Jr, et al. Magnetic resonance image-guided stereotactic cingulotomy for intractable psychiatric disease. Neurosurgery. 1996;38:1071–6; discussion 6–8.
25. Sharim J, Pouratian N. Anterior cingulotomy for the treatment of chronic intractable pain: a systematic review. Pain Physician. 2016;19:537–50.
26. Bittar RG, Kar-Purkayastha I, Owen SL, et al. Deep brain stimulation for pain relief: a meta-analysis. J Clin Neurosci. 2005;12:515–9.
27. Abreu V, Vaz R, Rebelo V, et al. Thalamic deep brain stimulation for neuropathic pain: efficacy at three years' follow-up. Neuromodulation. 2017;20:504–13.
28. Levy R, Deer TR, Henderson J. Intracranial neurostimulation for pain control: a review. Pain Physician. 2010;13:157–65.
29. Broggi G, Franzini A, Leone M, et al. Update on neurosurgical treatment of chronic trigeminal autonomic cephalalgias and atypical facial pain with deep brain stimulation of posterior hypothalamus: results and comments. Neurol Sci. 2007;28(Suppl 2):S138–45.
30. Boccard SG, Pereira EA, Moir L, et al. Long-term outcomes of deep brain stimulation for neuropathic pain. Neurosurgery. 2013;72:221–30; discussion 31.
31. Melzack R. From the gate to the neuromatrix. Pain. 1999;Suppl 6:S121–6.
32. Russo JF, Sheth SA. Deep brain stimulation of the dorsal anterior cingulate cortex for the treatment of chronic neuropathic pain. Neurosurg Focus. 2015;38:E11.
33. Lempka SF, Malone DA Jr, Hu B, et al. Randomized clinical trial of deep brain stimulation for poststroke pain. Ann Neurol. 2017;81:653–63.
34. Boccard SG, Fitzgerald JJ, Pereira EA, et al. Targeting the affective component of chronic pain: a case series of deep brain stimulation of the anterior cingulate cortex. Neurosurgery. 2014;74:628–35; discussion 35–7.
35. Tsubokawa T, Katayama Y, Yamamoto T, et al. Treatment of thalamic pain by chronic motor cortex stimulation. Pacing Clin Electrophysiol. 1991;14:131–4.
36. Fontaine D, Hamani C, Lozano A. Efficacy and safety of motor cortex stimulation for chronic neuropathic pain: critical review of the literature. J Neurosurg. 2009;110:251–6.
37. Radic JA, Beauprie I, Chiasson P, et al. Motor cortex stimulation for neuropathic pain: a randomized cross-over trial. Can J Neurol Sci. 2015;42:401–9.

Chapter 21
Surgical Management of Migraines

Eric J. Wright and William G. Austen Jr.

Introduction

Migraines are a common neurological disorder that are characterized by episodically debilitating headaches that affect millions of patients. Associated symptoms of migraines include nausea and emesis, various sensory hypersensitivities and auras, and photophobia. With a prevalence of 18% in women and 6% in men, the socioeconomic burden of healthcare costs and lost work productivity of the estimated 35 million patients that suffer is greater than $13 billion dollars per year [1]. Patients' physical and psychological well-being are also greatly affected.

Several different classification systems exist describing migraines. The frequency and chronicity can be used to classify migraines as episodic or chronic in nature. Chronic migraines are defined as having migraine symptoms for a minimum of 15 days per month occurring more than three consecutive months. Chronic migraine patients have three times the annual medical cost than episodic migraine patients [2].

OnabotulinumtoxinA is the only FDA-approved treatment for prevention of chronic migraines [3]. However, the majority of pharmacologic treatments are focused on the abortive therapy after a migraine episode begins, with the most common class of medications being the serotonin receptor agonists, triptans.

E. J. Wright
Division of Plastic and Reconstructive Surgery, Department of Surgery, University of Arkansas for Medical Sciences, Little Rock, AR, USA
e-mail: plasticsurgery@drericwright.com

W. G. Austen Jr. (✉)
Division of Plastic and Reconstructive Surgery, Harvard Medical School, Massachusetts General Hospital, Boston, MA, USA
e-mail: wausten@mgh.harvard.edu

J. Y. Suen, E. Petersen (eds.), *Diagnosis and Management of Head and Face Pain*, https://doi.org/10.1007/978-3-319-90999-8_21

Nonpharmacological treatments revolve around the avoidance of migraine "triggers." This varies from patient to patient but commonly includes light, temperature variances, tobacco, alcohol, and certain foods. Despite the long list of medications currently utilized, no medication is 100% effective. Each medication has contraindications, side effects, and overall lack of efficacy.

The etiology of migraines has yet to completely be described. Numerous theories have been reported including vascular, neurogenic, neurovascular, extra-sensitive nerve fiber, medication overuse, and peripheral. The current surgeries support the peripheral trigger point theory of migraine etiology. It is believed that due to compression, migraine or migraine-type pain is experienced.

The goal of any treatment of migraines is to reduce the intensity, severity, and duration so that the individual can function within society. This is most commonly achieved by medical therapies as described. However, there remains a distinct population of patients who do not receive adequate benefit from current treatment strategies. Other groups of patients suffer from the treatment-related side effects or have poor medical compliance leading to continued symptoms. Together, these groups of patients can be considered "refractory" to the medical treatment of migraines. It is this refractory group of migraine patients that has pushed for the continued evolution of migraine treatments beyond medication.

History

Beginning in the 1930s and 1940s, attempts to surgically cure migraines were introduced [4]. These early case reports involved transectioning segments of the trigeminal nerve fibers with resolution of the patients' migraines. This field continued to expand, addressing various nerves around the calvarium that were believed to be causing the migraine symptoms. In 1969, the greater occipital neurectomy was described with good results [5]. The majority of early studies were to address peripheral neuralgias around the head and neck.

In 2000, the first study was published showing a reduction in migraine headaches in patients that had undergone cosmetic forehead rejuvenation, a surgery where the corrugator supercilii was resected to prevent glabellar skin wrinkling [6]. This was followed in 2002 by a prospective trial of surgical peripheral nerve decompression for the treatment of migraines [7]. Patients that were preoperatively diagnosed by the neurologist with having migraines based upon the International Headache Society classification system were injected with Botox to screen for surgical candidates. If improvement was noted, then surgery was offered to the patient. Improvement, defined as a reduction in frequent or intensity, was found in 95% of surgically treated patients. Numerous additional studies have been published with findings of successful outcomes following surgery [8–12]. A placebo study including a "sham" surgery control found the patients undergoing the actual surgery had a statistically significant improvement at 1 year [8].

Anatomical Basis

Due to the increasing number of studies showing improvement in migraine patients' symptoms following surgery, anatomical studies have been conducted in an attempt to explain how the surgeries can be beneficial. Four areas are believed to contribute to the majority of peripheral nerve compression, known as trigger areas.

The frontal trigger area involves the supraorbital and supratrochlear nerves. These nerves can have compression from muscle, fascia, blood vessels, or bone [13–15]. Anatomical studies have shown the initial area of compression to the supraorbital nerve can occur after exiting from the superior orbital fissure along the intraconal path due to a periosteal sleeve. The nerve exits the orbit through either a foramen or notch. This nonexpanding segment can be another area of compression. Close involvement with the supraorbital artery and constant irritation by the contraction of the corrugator muscle fibers as the nerve continues to the subcutaneous location are also common areas of compression.

The temporal trigger area involves the compression of the zygomaticotemporal nerve. This nerve is completely sensory in nature and is a branch of the trigeminal nerve, maxillary division (V2). As the nerve emerges from the zygomatic bone to enter the temporal fossa, areas of compression can occur as it ascends through the deep temporal fascia and temporalis muscle. Three paths have been described for the transition of the nerve, long or short intramuscular paths or a completely extra muscular path [16, 17].

Six anatomical compression points have been described for the greater occipital nerve, the medial branch of the C2 dorsal root. As the nerve is followed from deep to superficial, it traverses several different muscles. Initially, the nerve exits from deep to the obliquus capitis inferior muscle and enters the semispinalis muscle. It travels through this muscle exiting to enter the trapezius muscle. It then exits through the tendinous portion as it travels adjacent to the occipital artery before entering the subcutaneous tissue, providing sensation to the posterior scalp. At each of the transitions, areas of compression have been described based upon anatomical studies [18].

The fourth area described as a migraine trigger is the septum, which involves irrigation or compression of the ethmoidal nerves. Another branch of the maxillary division of the trigeminal nerve is the anterior and posterior ethmoidal nerves. Deviated septums or hypertrophied turbinates have been implicated in leading to nerve irritation and subsequent pain located behind the eye.

Diagnosis and Preoperative Planning

Though patients suffering from migraines are desperate to have improvement, the goal of the initial evaluation is to determine which subset of migraine patients would actually benefit from surgery. Ideal patients are chronic migraine sufferers who have had relief from neither nonpharmacologic nor pharmacologic therapies. Patients

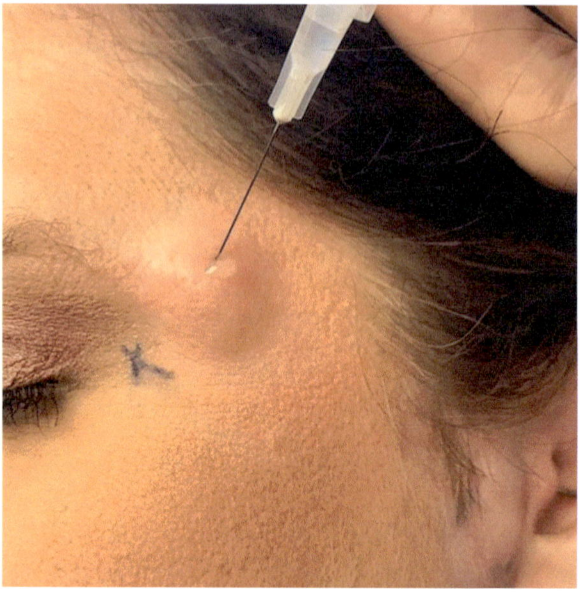

Fig. 21.1 Local anesthetic nerve injection in office

should have established neurology care that has thoroughly evaluated the patient and has diagnosed the migraine. For patients that have yet to find any relief, studies have supported the role of surgery in the treatment of specific neuralgias. Though neurologists have different diagnosis criteria, the surgery can address either diagnosis.

A thorough migraine history is obtained. Candidates for surgery are patients that have failed or have not achieved adequate control of the migraines (chronic refractory migraines). Any history of previous onabotulinumtoxinA or local anesthetic injections performed for nerve blocks is reviewed as well as the postinjection outcomes. Patients with tender trigger points, at areas of known nerve compression as discussed above, favor peripheral migraine etiology. The single most important history is the location of the pain at the time of onset. This is the site that can have a small amount of local anesthetic injected in clinic to help with diagnosis (Fig. 21.1). Patients that have improvement with local anesthetic injection are believed to be excellent candidates for surgical intervention. Physical exam includes location of the tender areas. It is not uncommon on physical exam, when locating the trigger area, that an arterial signal can be found with the use of a Doppler. For patients that present with a history suggestive of a nasal trigger etiology, thorough intranasal exam is performed to evaluate for a deviated septum or turbinate hypertrophy. CT scans are also beneficial for a thorough workup.

Surgery

With the comprehensive anatomical studies demonstrating the various sites of potential compression, the surgeries have been refined to address each area. It is unlikely that a specific compression point can be identified and in an isolated fashion

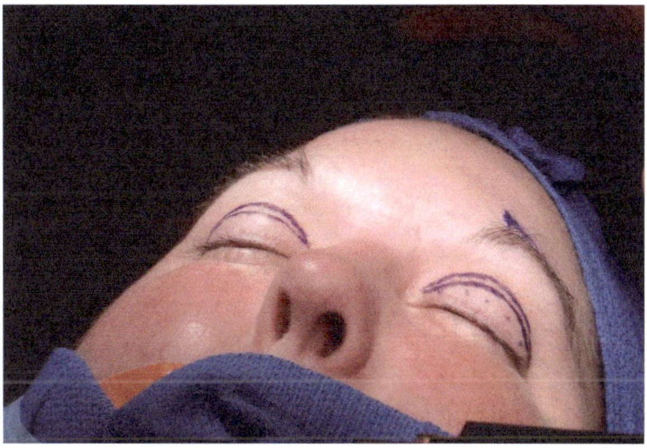

Fig. 21.2 Transpalpebral approach for frontal migraine release

released without releasing adjacent compression areas. It is the authors' recommendations to fully release the entire nerve from all defined compression areas. Since the anatomical exposure has already been obtained, additional decompression steps do not overly add to the complexity of the surgery. But more importantly, this will ensure adequate release and prevent any repetitive surgeries that may be considered if patients continue to have symptoms in the postoperative period [19].

For the frontal trigger area, the surgical approach can be either through an open transpalpebral incision or an endoscopic approach (Fig. 21.2). The benefits of an open approach are direct visualization of the supraorbital foramen or notch as well as the intraorbital path of the supraorbital nerve. The open approach utilizes an upper eyelid incision in the superior tarsal crease, similar to a blepharoplasty incision. The skin and orbicularis oculi muscle are elevated from the septum up to the superior orbital rim. At this location, dissection medially will identify the supraorbital and supratrochlear nerves (Fig. 21.3). The nerves are released from the orbital notch or foramen. An osteotome may be required to decompress the bony foramen when present (Figs. 21.4 and 21.5). As the nerves travel superiorly, there can be a close anatomical relation to the supraorbital artery and vein. The vessels are isolated and removed when found in close proximity to the nerves. Care must be taken to ensure complete ligation to prevent retraction into the globe where bleeding is more difficult to control. As the nerve continues, the glabellar muscles will be visualized. The depressor supercilii and corrugator supercilii muscles are removed along the path of the nerves. At this point, the nerves should have a nonrestrictive path exiting the globe to the subcutaneous tissue where the nerve continuously branches. In order to prevent subsequent scarring, a component of the medial compartment fat is released to act as a graft. Endoscopic decompression is an alternative method with access incisions being placed in the hair-bearing frontal scalp area.

The zygomaticotemporal nerve can also be accessed through either the open or endoscopic approach. With the open approach, dissection is extended from the lateral aspect of the upper eyelid incision (Fig. 21.6). Dissection proceeds laterally along the superficial surface of the deep temporal fascia. Once the nerve is identified, a long

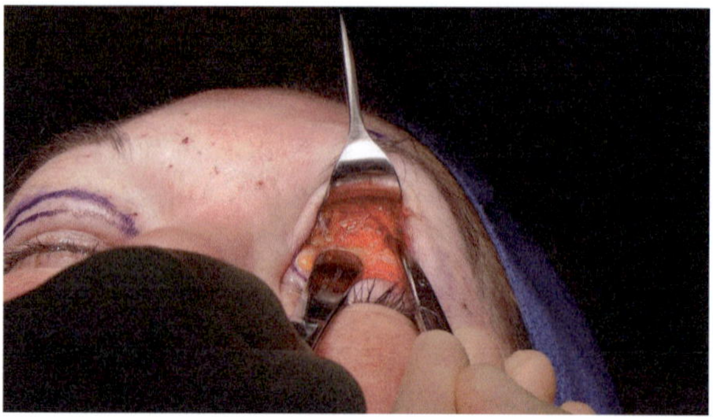

Fig. 21.3 Identification of the supratrochlear and supraorbital nerves

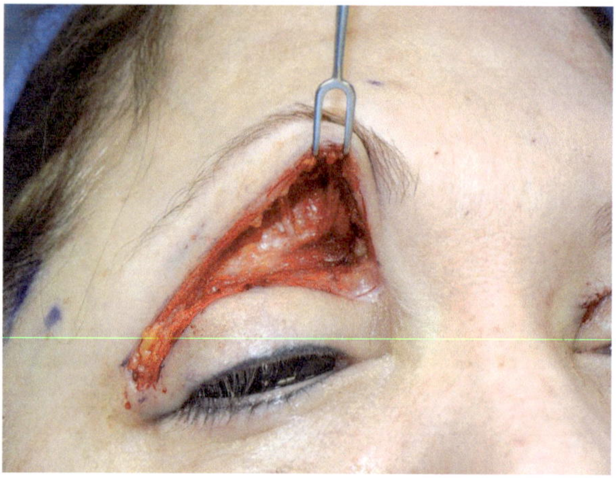

Fig. 21.4 Supraorbital nerve exiting through a bony foramen

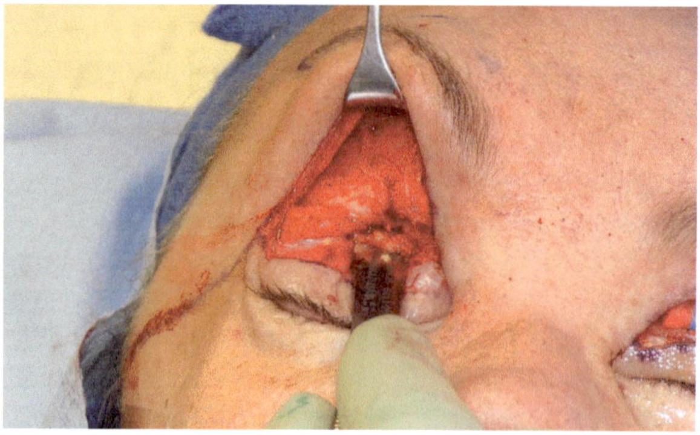

Fig. 21.5 Osteotomy of the bony foramen to release the supraorbital nerve

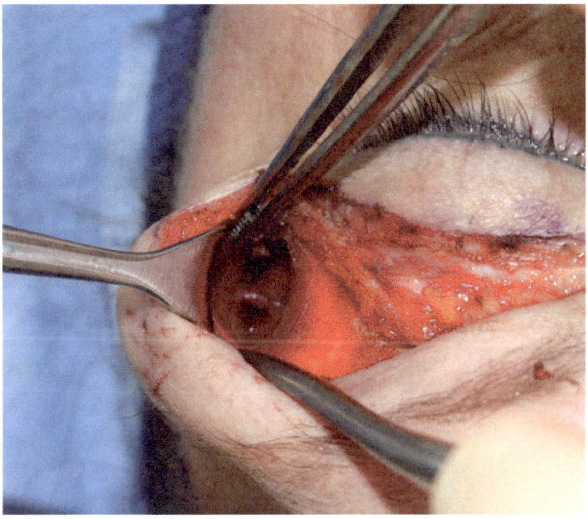

Fig. 21.6 Approach for the zygomaticotemporal nerve through the transpalpebral incision

hemostat is used to avulse the nerve. If an isolated zygomaticotemporal neuralgia is expected, a direct incision over the lateral orbital brow can be made. This provides for excellent access to the nerve (Figs. 21.7 and 21.8). Once the nerve is identified, it can be transected at the bony foramen. With the endoscopic approach from the hairline, the key point is identifying the deep temporal fascia. Once in the correct plane, the nerve is identified and avulsed in a similar fashion.

Patients will have postoperative edema and ecchymosis for 1–2 weeks. Paresthesia of the forehead will occur due to the manipulation of the nerves during the decompression. Contour irregularities related to the muscle resection in the glabellar area can be seen in some cases as well as asymmetric movement if any residual muscle remains. For endoscopic procedures, alopecia can occur in the incision site. With the open procedure, a compression wrap is applied and worn for 24 h postoperatively. With endoscopic procedures, a drain may be added due to the extra dissection area.

The occipital area is accessed with the patient in the prone position. It is beneficial to have the head slightly flexed as the upper shoulder area can block access in certain patients. This can be obtained with flexion of the bed or with the use of a shoulder roll. A small 2-inch area of hair is shaved extending from the occipital protuberance inferiorly. It is beneficial to mark this area with the patient awake and in the upright position to ensure the midline is appropriately marked. The midline incision gives easy access to performing bilateral greater occipital nerve releases. After incising through the midline fascia, the trapezius fascia is opened in the area corresponding to location of the nerve (3 cm inferior to the occipital protuberance, 1.5 cm lateral from the midline). The nerve is identified and followed both superficial and deep, removing a small cuff of muscle when encountered. As the nerve is traced superficially, it is common to find a close approximation of the nerve and the occipital artery (Fig. 21.9). The artery is ligated and removed.

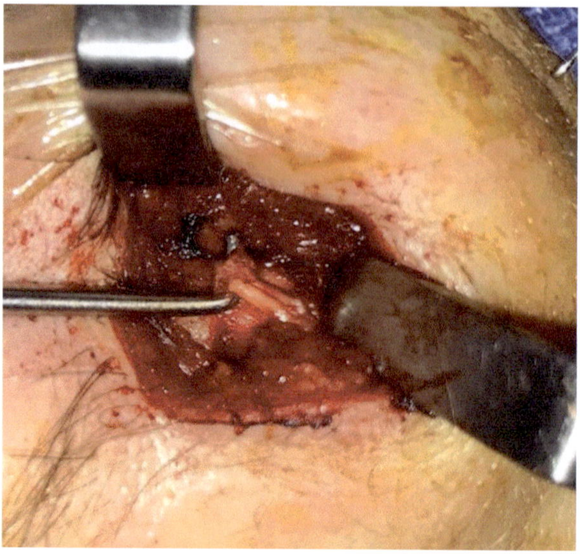

Fig. 21.7 Direct approach to the zygomaticotemporal nerve

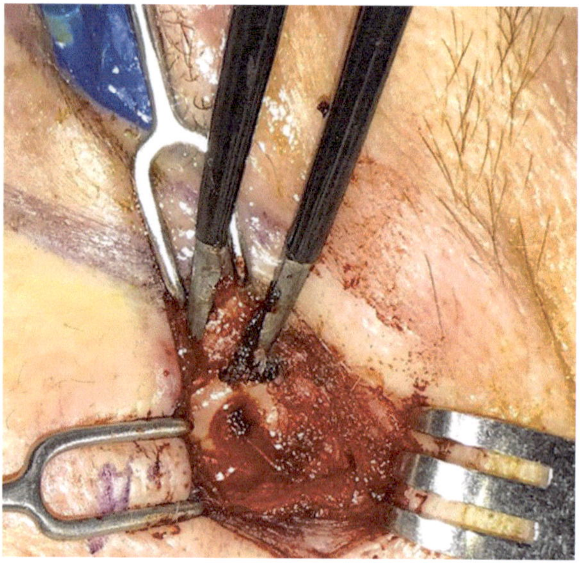

Fig. 21.8 Complete transection of the zygomaticotemporal nerve

For the nasal trigger procedure, standard septoplasty techniques are performed to remove any irritation or compression that is occurring. Though not all patients will have a functional respiratory obstruction before the surgery, correction of the deviation and alleviation of any compressing areas that are touching the septum will lead to improvements in the migraine symptoms.

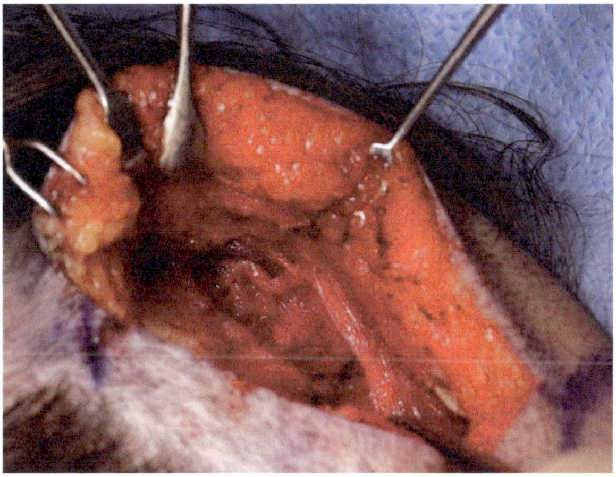

Fig. 21.9 Occipital nerve release. Occipital artery and nerve shown in close approximation

The auriculotemporal nerve and lesser occipital nerve are two other common nerves that can be surgically addressed. These nerves are localized to the exact location of irritation based upon the results of preoperative nerve blocks. Operatively, the nerve is identified by direct incision and resected. This concept can be applied to numerous sensory nerves around the head and neck that are found to be contributing to pain. With thorough anatomical knowledge, these procedures can be performed safely with low risk.

All of the above surgical procedures carry risks. Risks include bleeding, infection, injury, or damage to surrounding anatomical structures and the risk of general anesthesia. All patients will experience numbness following the procedure that last for several months. If the nerve is only decompressed, the numbness is expected to resolve. If the nerve is transected or avulsed, then the numbness is permanent. These risks must be weighed against the expected benefits based upon a thorough history and physical.

Conclusion

Migraine treatment will continue to revolve around pharmacologic interventions. However, there is a subset of patients that are considered "refractive" to current pharmacologic therapy that have peripheral nerve compression triggers that can be ameliorated by decompression surgery. Practitioners providing comprehensive migraine care should explore this possibility of surgery for patients with chronic or refractory migraine symptoms.

References

1. Hu XH, Markson LE, Lipton RB, Stewart WF, Berger ML. Burden of migraine in the United States: disability and economic costs. Arch Intern Med. 1999;159(8):813–8.
2. Messali A, Sanderson JC, Blumenfeld AM, Goadsby PJ, Buse DC, Varon SF, et al. Direct and indirect costs of chronic and episodic migraine in the United States: a web-based survey. Headache. 2016;56(2):306–22.
3. Sun-Edelstein C, Rapoport AM. Update on the pharmacological treatment of chronic migraine. Curr Pain Headache Rep. 2016;20(1):6–015.
4. Haynes WO. Surgical treatment of intractable unilateral cephalalgia. J Am Med Assoc. 1948;136(8):538–41.
5. Murphy JP. Occipital neurectomy in the treatment of headache. Results in 30 cases. Md State Med J. 1969;18(6):62–6.
6. Guyuron B, Varghai A, Michelow BJ, Thomas T, Davis J. Corrugator supercilii muscle resection and migraine headaches. Plast Reconstr Surg. 2000;106(2):429–34; discussion 435.
7. Guyuron B, Tucker T, Davis J. Surgical treatment of migraine headaches. Plast Reconstr Surg. 2002;109(7):2183–9.
8. Guyuron B, Reed D, Kriegler JS, Davis J, Pashmini N, Amini S. A placebo-controlled surgical trial of the treatment of migraine headaches. Plast Reconstr Surg. 2009;124(2):461–8.
9. Poggi JT, Grizzell BE, Helmer SD. Confirmation of surgical decompression to relieve migraine headaches. Plast Reconstr Surg. 2008;122(1):115–22; discussion 123.
10. Dirnberger F, Becker K. Surgical treatment of migraine headaches by corrugator muscle resection. Plast Reconstr Surg. 2004;114(3):652–7; discussion 658.
11. Guyuron B, Kriegler JS, Davis J, Amini SB. Comprehensive surgical treatment of migraine headaches. Plast Reconstr Surg. 2005;115(1):1–9.
12. Gfrerer L, Lans J, Faulkner HR, Nota S, Bot AGJ, Austen WG Jr., Ability to Cope with Pain Puts MigraineSurgery Patients in Perspective. Plastic and Reconstructive Surgery 141 (1):169–74.
13. Janis JE, Ghavami A, Lemmon JA, Leedy JE, Guyuron B. Anatomy of the corrugator supercilii muscle: part I. Corrugator topography. Plast Reconstr Surg. 2007;120(6):1647–53.
14. Fallucco M, Janis JE, Hagan RR. The anatomical morphology of the supraorbital notch: clinical relevance to the surgical treatment of migraine headaches. Plast Reconstr Surg. 2012;130(6):1227–33.
15. Hagan RR, Fallucco MA, Janis JE. Supraorbital rim syndrome: definition, surgical treatment, and outcomes for frontal headache. Plast Reconstr Surg Glob Open. 2016;4(7):e795.
16. Totonchi A, Pashmini N, Guyuron B. The zygomaticotemporal branch of the trigeminal nerve: an anatomical study. Plast Reconstr Surg. 2005;115(1):273–7.
17. Janis JE, Hatef DA, Thakar H, Reece EM, McCluskey PD, Schaub TA, et al. The zygomaticotemporal branch of the trigeminal nerve: part II. Anatomical variations. Plast Reconstr Surg. 2010;126(2):435–42.
18. Janis JE, Hatef DA, Ducic I, Reece EM, Hamawy AH, Becker S, et al. The anatomy of the greater occipital nerve: part II. Compression point topography. Plast Reconstr Surg. 2010;126(5):1563–72.
19. Gfrerer L, Maman DY, Tessler O, Austen WG, Nonendoscopic Deactivation of Nerve Triggers in Migraine Headache Patients. Plastic and Reconstructive Surgery 134 (4):771–8.

Chapter 22
Vestibular Migraine

Matthew D. Cox, Julien Arden Norton, and John L. Dornhoffer

Introduction

Vestibular migraine (VM) describes the condition of episodic vertigo occurring in patients with a history of migraine or other clinical manifestations of migraine. Other terms that have been used nearly interchangeably with vestibular migraine include migrainous vertigo, migraine-associated vertigo, migraine-related vestibulopathy, benign recurrent vertigo, and benign paroxysmal vertigo of childhood.

Vestibular migraine is a distinct clinical entity from migraine with brainstem aura (MBA), which was previously known as basilar migraine. The diagnosis of MBA requires the presence of at least one neurologic symptom of brainstem or bilateral cortical origin as part of the aura [1].

The importance of vestibular migraine may be simply illustrated by its high prevalence and the fact that it represents one of the most common causes (if not the most common) [2] of episodic vertigo. In a series of 200 consecutive patients referred for evaluation of dizziness, 38% were diagnosed with vestibular migraine [3]. Vestibular migraine is thought to account for around 10% of patients examined in vertigo clinics [4].

A large population study (4869 German patients) observed a lifetime incidence of 0.98% for VM, spontaneous episodic vertigo was reported by 67% of VM patients, and positional vertigo was reported in 24%. Age-adjusted, health-related quality of life scores were consistently lower for individuals with VM, as compared

M. D. Cox (✉) · J. L. Dornhoffer
Division of Otology/Neurotology, Department of Otolaryngology/Head and Neck Surgery, University of Arkansas for Medical Sciences, Little Rock, AR, USA
e-mail: mdcox@uams.edu; dornhofferjohnl@uams.edu

J. A. Norton
Department of Otolaryngology/Head and Neck Surgery, University of Arkansas for Medical Sciences, Little Rock, AR, USA
e-mail: mathewdcoxmd@gmail.com

J. Y. Suen, E. Petersen (eds.), *Diagnosis and Management of Head and Face Pain*, https://doi.org/10.1007/978-3-319-90999-8_22

to controls without vertigo. This study also found that only 20% of affected patients had been diagnosed with vestibular migraine by a physician [5].

Ménière's disease, vestibular migraine, and benign paroxysmal positional vertigo (BPPV) represent the most common causes of episodic vertigo. While BPPV is usually readily distinguished from the others by a short duration of symptoms and characteristic physical examination findings (i.e., positive Dix-Hallpike maneuver), differentiation of BPPV from VM may be complicated in some patients, as positional vertigo is observed in 24% of patients with VM [5]. Positional nystagmus was observed in 29% of vestibular migraine patients in one series. While this was definite central-type positional nystagmus in 18%, the remaining 11% of patients had positional nystagmus with peripheral features [6].

In other cases, it may similarly be challenging to differentiate between Ménière's disease and vestibular migraine due to significant overlap of clinical features between these two [7–9]. A relationship between Ménière's disease and VM has been proposed as early as Prosper Ménière's initial description of MD.

Migraine

Migraine is classified as migraine with or without aura. Vertigo and/or other vestibular symptoms may be associated with migraine, but these symptoms are not classified as aura. Aura symptoms may include visual disturbance, sensory changes (i.e., paresthesia or anesthesia), speech and/or language disturbance, motor weakness, brainstem symptoms, or retinal symptoms [1]. The current Headache Classification Committee consensus for the classification and diagnosis of migraine with aura, migraine without aura, vestibular migraine, and vestibular symptoms is summarized in Table 22.1.

Table 22.1 Criteria for diagnosis of vestibular migraine (Headache Classification Committee of the International Headache Society 2013)

(A) At least five episodes fulfilling criteria C and D
(B) A current or past history of migraine without aura or migraine with aura
(C) Vestibular symptoms of moderate or severe intensity, lasting between 5 min and 72 h
(D) At least 50% of episodes are associated with at least one of the following three migrainous features:
1. Headache with at least two of the following four characteristics:
(a) Unilateral location
(b) Pulsating quality
(c) Moderate or severe intensity
(d) Aggravation by routine physical activity
2. Photophobia and phonophobia
3. Visual aura
(E) Not better accounted for by another ICHD-3 diagnosis or by another vestibular disorder

The lifetime prevalence of migraine is approximately 15–17% in women and 6% in men [4, 10]). The lifetime prevalence of vertigo (due to all causes) is approximately 7%. Epidemiologic studies suggest concurrent prevalence to be approximately 3.2%, which is higher than the 1.1% that would be expected by chance alone. Vestibular migraine is thought to account for around 10% of patients examined in dizziness clinics and at least 9% of patients examined in migraine clinics [4]. Episodic vertigo occurs in up to one-third of migraine patients, which is nearly as common as the classic visual aura [11–13].

Individuals with migraine are sensitive to lights, sounds, smells, motion, and other stimuli that are not disturbing to people without migraine. Migraineurs are extraordinarily sensitive to such stimuli during headaches, but they are typically more sensitive at baseline, as well [11]. Susceptibility to motion sickness is commonly associated with migraine; it is present in 45–70% of migraineurs, which is two to five times more common than in the general population [12–17].

Dizziness and Vertigo

Dizziness is defined as a sensation of disturbed spatial orientation [1]. Dizziness may represent vertigo, imbalance, disequilibrium, lightheadedness, or other conditions. Dizziness does not always represent a vestibular symptom. Vertigo is the illusory sensation of motion of either self or surroundings, in the absence of true motion [18]. The Bárány Society classification system for vestibular symptoms further considers vertigo as internal vertigo and external vertigo. According to this system, internal vertigo is defined as the sensation of self-motion when no self-motion is occurring or the sensation of distorted self-motion during an otherwise normal head movement, while a false sense of external motion is referred to as external vertigo or oscillopsia [19].

Vestibular symptoms are classified accordance with consensus recommendations set forth by the Committee for the Classification of Vestibular Disorders of the Bárány Society [19]. Vestibular symptoms qualifying for the diagnosis of vestibular migraine include spontaneous vertigo, positional vertigo, visually induced vertigo, head motion-induced vertigo, and head motion-induced dizziness with nausea (see Table 22.2) [1]. Spontaneous vertigo is vertigo that occurs without an obvious

Table 22.2 Vestibular symptoms, as defined by the Bárány Society's classification of vestibular symptoms, (Bisdorff et al. 2009) qualifying for a diagnosis of vestibular migraine (Headache Classification Committee of the International Headache Society 2013)

(A)	Spontaneous vertigo: vertigo that occurs without an obvious trigger
(B)	Positional vertigo: vertigo occurring after a change of head position
(C)	Visually induced vertigo: vertigo that is triggered by a complex or large moving visual stimulus
(D)	Head motion-induced vertigo: vertigo occurring during head motion
(E)	Head motion-induced dizziness with nausea

trigger. Positional vertigo is vertigo triggered by and occurring after a change of head position in space relative to gravity. Visually induced vertigo is vertigo triggered by a complex, distorted, large-field, or moving visual stimulus, including the relative motion of the visual surround associated with body movement. Head motion vertigo is vertigo occurring only during head motion (i.e., that is time locked to the head movement). It is worth noting that head motion-induced dizziness with nausea is the only form of non-vertigo dizziness that is currently included as a symptom meeting the criteria for vestibular migraine [19].

There is great variability in reports of the epidemiology of dizziness and vertigo due to inconsistencies in how these entities are defined and reported. Dizziness is one of the most common complaints in clinical medicine, affecting 11.5% of American adults within the last year [20]. The lifetime prevalence of vertigo in adults is estimated to be 7.4%, the 1-year prevalence 4.9%, and the 1-year incidence 1.4%. A 2.7:1 female-to-male preponderance was observed, and vertigo was nearly three times more common in the elderly than in young adults [21, 22].

Clinical Features of Vestibular Migraine

Vertigo, dizziness, and disequilibrium are reported by 30–50% of migraineurs at some point in time [23]. Vestibular migraine (VM) classically presents as vertigo without symptoms relating to the hearing apparatus, such as aural fullness, tinnitus, or hearing loss, though these symptoms may be observed in some patients. A personal and/or family history of migraine headaches is frequently observed in patients with vestibular migraine. In one series, migraine headaches were present before the onset of vestibular migraines in 74% of patients, and 85% of patients reported experiencing both vestibular migraine and migraine headaches within the previous year [5].

Vertigo associated with migraine may have central or peripheral features, and this may complicate diagnosis and management. The vestibular symptoms reported among migraineurs are variable, with rotational vertigo being the most common (70%), followed by intolerance of head motion (48%) and positional vertigo (42%) [3].

Nystagmus is a rapid, involuntary oscillatory movement of the eye [18]. Nystagmus with vestibular migraine is highly variable. This may be central or peripheral type, it may be spontaneous or positional, and may involve one or both eyes. Variable incidences (ranging from 29 to 100%) of positional nystagmus have been observed in vestibular migraine patients [6, 24]. Definite central-type positional nystagmus is more common, but patients may also have positional nystagmus with peripheral features [6].

The frequency and duration of episodes vary among VM patients and may vary in individual patients over time. Vertiginous episodes may last seconds (~10%), minutes (~30%), hours (~30%), or several days (~30%). Attacks may occur regularly or irregularly and may occur with anywhere from days to years between [4, 13, 14, 25, 26].

In one series [27], the vestibular symptoms of vestibular migraine were classified as spontaneous vertigo versus triggered vertigo (which included visually induced vertigo, head motion-induced vertigo, and head motion-induced dizziness with nausea) for the purpose of comparison. Spontaneous rotatory vertigo was more frequently observed in patients with migraine with aura, though the vertigo did not meet the criteria to be classified as aura (spells were either too long or too short), and visual aura was reported by these patients. Triggered vertigo was more common in migraine without aura and frequently occurred concomitantly with headaches.

Triggers for vestibular migraine are only positively identified in a minority of patients, but identification and avoidance of these triggers can be very effective in successfully managing a patient's symptoms. A wide range of triggers have been described, and these occur with variable frequency. Common triggers for vestibular migraine include stress (emotional stress, physical exertion, sleep deprivation, exposure to bright lights, and the patient's menstrual cycle), changes in weather, and dietary triggers. Dietary triggers may include caffeine (or changes in caffeine intake), alcohol, chocolate, cheese, monosodium glutamate, and nitrites, among others. Symptoms usually occur within minutes or hours of exposure to triggers, but there may be a significant delay in some cases. Maintaining a careful log of dietary intake and symptoms for several weeks can be helpful in identifying these relationships [11].

Ear-Related Symptoms with Vestibular Migraine

Auditory symptoms are common among migraine patients with dizziness. Phonophobia was reported by 66%, tinnitus by 63%, and hearing loss by 32%. In the same series, 11% reported fluctuating hearing loss with aural fullness [28]. In another series, 38% of patients with vestibular migraine had ear-related complaints (including subjective hearing loss, aural fullness, and/or tinnitus) during episodes of vertigo or headache [10]. It has been suggested that the prevalence of cochlear symptoms may increase with time. One author observed cochlear symptoms in 15% of patients at the time of initial presentation, and this increased to 49% with long-term follow-up [6]. In addition to true headaches, otalgia may be the presenting complaint in some patients with migraine (77% of patients in one series) [29].

Hearing Loss with Vestibular Migraine

Audiometry is most commonly normal in patients with vestibular migraine, but hearing loss may be observed in some patients. When present, hearing loss is a mild to moderate low-frequency sensorineural loss, and it may be unilateral or bilateral. While hearing loss tends to be fluctuating and progressive in cases of Ménière's disease, it tends to remain stable in cases of vestibular migraine [14, 30].

Mild, bilateral, symmetric, up-sloping (low-frequency), sensorineural hearing loss was observed in 18% of patients in one series [6]. Though rare, sudden sensorineural hearing loss has been observed to occur in association with migraine [31, 32]. Administration of migraine abortifacients and vasodilator medications has been observed to lead to improvement in case reports, though it is unclear if the improvement was spontaneous or the result of therapeutic intervention.

Tinnitus with Vestibular Migraine

Patients with vestibular migraine may complain of subjective tinnitus, particularly when comorbid hearing loss is present. In one series, 12% of patients with VM also had tinnitus [33]. While infrequently observed (1.9% of patients with VM), pulsatile tinnitus may be observed in the context of vestibular migraine and often resolves with standard management of the patient's VM [33].

Psychiatric Comorbidity in Vestibular Migraine

A significant number of migraine (classic migraine and vestibular migraine) patients have comorbid depression, anxiety, substance abuse, somatization disorders, and other psychiatric disorders [34]. Symptoms of depression and anxiety are frequently observed in dizzy patients [35], and anxiety and agoraphobia are even more common in patients with vestibular migraine than in patients with classic migraines [36].

Diagnosis of Vestibular Migraine

Diagnostic Criteria

The diagnosis of vestibular migraine is made in accordance with the diagnostic criteria for migraine, as established by the Bárány Society and included in the third edition of the International Classification of Headache Disorders [1].

Five criteria (designated as A through E) exist for making the diagnosis of vestibular migraine. Criteria A for making the diagnosis of vestibular migraine state that a patient must have at least five episodes fulfilling criteria C and D. To fulfill criteria B, patients must have current or past medical history of migraine without aura or migraine with aura.

Patients must have vestibular symptoms of moderate to severe intensity that last between 5 min and 72 h (criteria C). Vestibular symptoms qualifying for a diagnosis of vestibular migraine include spontaneous vertigo (may be internal or external vertigo), positional vertigo, visually induced vertigo, head motion-induced vertigo, and head motion-induced dizziness with nausea. Other forms of dizziness do not meet the criteria for diagnosis of vestibular migraine.

At least half of episodes must be associated with one of three characteristic migraine features to meet criteria D. These characteristics include (1) headache, (2) photophobia and phonophobia, and (3) visual aura. To meet these criteria, headaches must have at least two of four characteristics, including (1) unilateral location, (2) pulsating quality, (3) moderate or severe intensity, and/or (4) aggravated by routine physical activity. Lastly, criteria E states that the patient's symptoms must not be better accounted for by another ICHD-3 diagnosis or by another vestibular disorder.

Challenges in the Diagnosis of Vestibular Migraine

Identification of migraine as the cause of vertigo may be straightforward in some cases, but there is significant overlap of clinical features that may be observed with migraine and other disorders, including Ménière's disease and benign paroxysmal positional vertigo (BPPV). Beyond symptomatic overlap between vestibular migraine and BPPV, classic BPPV may be more common in patients with migraine than the general population [37].

Clinical Evaluation of Vertigo

Numerous underlying conditions may be the cause for a patient's vertigo. While most cases are due to benign conditions, some causes of vertigo are severe and life-threatening. Prompt differentiation of dangerous conditions, such as ischemic stroke, from benign causes of vertigo is a primary goal of the initial evaluation.

Patient History

The first step in evaluation of a dizzy patient is the distinction of vertigo from dizziness, which may usually be accomplished based on history alone. Vertigo is a vestibular symptom, while dizziness is not. Rotational vertigo or other illusory symptoms of motion are typical of vertigo. Symptoms such as lightheadedness, giddiness, drowsiness, or presyncope represent non-vestibular dizziness [4]. Motion sickness is commonly observed in patients diagnosed with vestibular migraine [15, 17].

Episodic vertigo, migraine, and Ménière's disease are frequently clustered in closely related individuals, including identical twins, suggestive of some heritable component to these disease entities [8, 38]. Identification of a positive family history of one or more of these can be helpful in making an accurate diagnosis.

Physical Examination

A thorough and complete physical examination is imperative in the evaluation of all patients with vertigo. Attention must be given to identify details which may be suggestive of serious underlying conditions, such stigmata of cardiovascular disease or neurologic abnormalities, even if subtle.

Imaging Studies

There are no imaging studies that are specifically useful in confirming a diagnosis of vestibular migraine. The real utility of imaging is to eliminate other possible causes for a patient's vertigo. The most common imaging studies that may be useful in the evaluation of vertigo and suspected vestibular migraine include duplex ultrasonography with Doppler, computerized tomography (CT), magnetic resonance imaging (MRI), and related technical variants of these techniques.

Ultrasonographic evaluation of the cervical carotid arteries should be considered in patients with cervical bruits noted on physical examination, history of transient ischemic attacks, and/or amaurosis fugax; patients with a strong family history of atherosclerotic disease (particularly at a young age); and older patients (especially patients with coronary artery disease, peripheral vascular disease, prothrombotic states, and/or comorbid hyperlipidemia).

CT imaging is indicated when the certain clinical features are observed in patients who present with vertigo. This modality may be useful to investigate for a cerebrovascular accident in cases of acute onset of vertigo or to evaluate for the presence of structural abnormalities of the labyrinth, such as a horizontal canal fistula from cholesteatoma or a dehiscent superior semicircular canal.

MRI modality is relatively low yield in the routine evaluation of vertiginous patients. Considering the low diagnostic efficacy and high cost of these studies, they should only be obtained for further evaluation when specifically indicated. In one series, MRIs were obtained in more than 75% of patients for the evaluation of dizziness [39].

Patients identified as having asymmetric sensorineural hearing loss with an interaural threshold difference of 10 dB or more in any three contiguous frequencies, 15 dB or more in any two contiguous frequencies, 15 dB or more difference at 3 Hz, and/or 15% or greater interaural difference in word recognition scores [40, 41] should be imaged with MRI of the internal auditory canal with and without gadolinium-based contrast, as this pattern may be observed with tumors of the cerebellopontine angle, internal auditory canal, or labyrinth. MRI studies should also be obtained in patients with stigmata of intracranial hypertension and/or persistent neural deficits to evaluate for other intracranial lesions.

Audiometry and Vestibular Testing

Audiologic assessment does not routinely provide specific diagnostic information in cases of vestibular migraine but does provide valuable information in many cases involving episodic vertigo. Audiometry should be obtained in any case involving auditory complaints, as identification of underlying hearing loss (particularly a unilateral hearing loss) is very helpful in guiding the clinician toward a diagnosis. As vestibular migraine is largely a diagnosis of exclusion, identification of hearing loss—particularly certain patterns of hearing loss—may help guide the diagnostic pursuit in the correct direction. Identification of fluctuating sensorineural hearing loss usually suggests Ménière's disease or related conditions, and serial audiometric testing is necessary to identify these cases.

Otoacoustic emission testing and reflex-evoked audiometry, such as auditory brainstem reflex testing, may be useful in the evaluation of patients when suspicion is high for retrocochlear causes of vertigo but is not routinely warranted. These tests do not offer information beyond that of behavioral audiometry in most clinical scenarios.

Routine videonystagmography (VNG) should not be obtained as part of the diagnostic pursuit in cases where history is suggestive of vestibular migraine. The most commonly observed abnormality on VNG testing is asymmetry of bithermal calorics. The reported prevalence of abnormal calorics ranges from 23 to 53% [14, 25, 26, 42]. In one series of migraine patients (with and without vertigo), 26% had canal paresis on electronystagmography, and this was observed with similar frequency in patients with and without vertigo [28]. In a comparison of caloric results between patients with migrainous vertigo and non-migraine vertigo, patients in the migraine group were observed to have nausea and emesis during caloric testing [43]. It has been suggested that some vestibular migraine patients with abnormalities on VNG testing ultimately develop Ménière's disease [25]. Migraine headaches were reported within 24 h by nearly half of a series of migraineurs after undergoing bithermal caloric testing, suggesting that vertigo can act as a trigger for migraines [44].

Electrocochleography (ECoG) may be a useful modality in some cases, but this information should be considered supplementary instead of diagnostic [43, 45, 46]. In cases of suspected Ménière's disease with failure to respond to therapeutic intervention, normal SP/AP measurements on ECoG may be suggestive of vestibular migraine as the underlying cause of episodic vertigo.

Vestibular-evoked myogenic potential (VEMP) testing may similarly be useful in certain scenarios, such as cases of suspected vestibular migraine where atypical features are present—particularly those suggestive of superior semicircular canal dehiscence syndrome, such as autophony or a positive fistula test (nystagmus provoked by pneumatic otoscopy). Abnormal cervical VEMP (cVEMP) and ocular VEMP (oVEMP) thresholds may be observed in patients with vestibular migraine and patients with Ménière's disease. To date, conflicting results [47–49] have been presented regarding the efficacy of VEMP testing in accurately differentiating vestibular migraine from Ménière's disease.

Conditions Related to Vestibular Migraine

Ménière's Disease and Vestibular Migraine

Ménière's disease may present with variable symptoms and classically comprises the triad of episodic vertigo, fluctuating hearing loss, aural fullness, and roaring, low-pitched tinnitus. Ménière's disease is diagnosed in accordance with criteria set forth by the American Academy of Otolaryngology—Head and Neck Surgery Committee [46].

Differentiation of VM from Ménière's disease (MD) may be challenging due to significant overlap of symptoms between the two disorders [7–9]. A link between vestibular migraine and Ménière's disease was suggested first by Prosper Ménière himself [50, 51]. This is further complicated by the observation of a higher prevalence of migraine in patients with Ménière's disease, as compared to the rest of the population [51] and the observation that both VM and MD may coexist in a subset of patients [4, 52].

It has been postulated that migraines may damage the inner ear over time, leading to the development of endolymphatic hydrops [8, 53]. It has been suggested that migraine-induced vasospasm and resulting ischemia may damage the stria vascularis and repetitive insults may lead to progressive endolymphatic hydrops [53]. Following this logic, some patients with vestibular migraine may experience progression to symptoms of Ménière's disease [53]. It has been suggested that some vestibular migraine patients with VNG abnormalities ultimately develop Ménière's disease [25]. This may be the result of progressive vestibular damage due to migraine, but this is uncertain due to a lack of data on the temporal evolution of these findings.

Benign Paroxysmal Vertigo of Childhood

Benign paroxysmal vertigo of childhood (BPVC) has long been considered to be a form of vestibular migraine [54]. BPVC is listed by the International Classification of Headache Disorders (ICHD) as a migraine precursor childhood periodic syndrome. The average age of onset of BPVC is approximately 3 years, and symptoms spontaneously resolve around 6 years of age, on average [55].

To make the diagnosis of BPVC, there must be five attacks meeting two criteria. First, the attacks must consist of vertigo that occurs without warning, is maximal at the time of onset, resolves spontaneously in minutes to hours, and does not involve loss of consciousness. Second, the episodes must be associated with at least one of the following: nystagmus, ataxia, vomiting, pallor, or fearfulness. A final consideration in the diagnosis of BPVC is the elimination of other possible causes, including posterior fossa tumors, seizures (i.e., must have a normal electroencephalogram), and other vestibular disorders [1].

In a case series examining long-term outcomes of benign paroxysmal vertigo [56], 100% of patients observed until at least 15 years of age went on to experience migraines. In the same series, 61.5% of affected children had at least one first degree relative with a history of migraines. Triggering factors were identified in 60% of cases. The most commonly identified factors were psychological trauma, fever, car trips, and fatigue. Associated symptoms include ataxia (100%), vegetative signs (87%), and headache (36%) [56].

Management of Vestibular Migraine

Principles of Management

A variety of stepwise algorithms for management of vestibular migraine have been described and studied. Lack of consistency in the diagnosis of vestibular migraine among practitioners, clinical trial design, and reporting of outcomes makes interpretation and comparison of efficacy among the algorithms difficult.

Strategies for medical management of vestibular migraine are similar to those for management of classic migraine [57]. In general, the first step in management of vestibular migraine involves identification and avoidance of possible triggers. In a series of 100 patients, 52% identified factors that triggered vestibular migraines. Of these patients, 61% identified mental or physical stress as a factor, 23% cited hormonal or weather changes, and 10% mentioned specific foods, such as cheese or coffee [58]. Counseling on the avoidance of typical triggering agents and the importance of stress reduction and sleep quality should be provided to all vestibular migraine patients at the time of diagnosis. Some practitioners will offer abortifacient medications to be used for symptomatic treatment of vertigo during this initial trial of lifestyle modification.

If a patient's symptoms are not sufficiently controlled with this conservative strategy, medical prophylaxis is often the next step. There are many options for migraine prophylaxis, and medications with fewer and/or less disturbing adverse effects are typically offered first. Escalation to prophylaxis with anticonvulsant medications is reserved for patients whose symptoms persist with drugs from other classes. Following this type of algorithm, complete or satisfactory control of vertigo symptoms has been achieved in 72–92% of patients [14, 59, 60].

Vestibular rehabilitation and retraining programs are sometimes offered to patients with vestibular migraine, and studies have demonstrated some benefit from this practice. In patients prescribed with vestibular suppressant medications, consideration must be given to the timing of doses to avoid interference with vestibular rehabilitation exercises [61].

Acute Symptomatic Medical Management

The acute, symptomatic management of vestibular migraine may include the use of vestibular suppressants, antiemetics, and migraine abortifacients, such as triptans. The efficacies of various migraine abortifacient medications (ergots, NSAIDs, opiates, and triptans) for the treatment of migraine-related vertigo and migraine-related non-vertigo vestibular symptoms have been observed to parallel their respective efficacies for the management of migraine headaches. In the same study, sumatriptan was found to be highly effective in improving both vertigo and headaches [62].

Pharmacologic Prophylaxis of Vestibular Migraine

When conservative management fails to control a patient's symptoms, pharmacologic prophylaxis may be offered (Table 22.3). Review of the existing literature regarding the efficacy of the various forms of pharmacologic prophylaxis is challenging due inconsistencies in diagnosis and quantification of severity of vestibular symptoms in migraine patients, as well as lack of uniformity in prescribing algorithms between authors. In one series, patients using prophylactic medications in addition to lifestyle modification had a decrease in frequency (80%), duration (65%), and intensity (68%) of episodic vertigo attacks, while only an improvement in the intensity of attacks was observed in those patients managed with lifestyle modification alone [58]. In another series, a combination of trigger avoidance and pharmacotherapy offered complete or satisfactory control of vertigo symptoms to more than 90% of patients [14].

The most appropriate choice of medication for migraine prophylaxis varies from one patient to another and depends on the patient's age, general health and functional status, history of drug reactions or adverse effects, sleeping status, and comorbidities such as depression, anxiety, or panic disorder [14].

First-line drugs for prophylaxis of classic migraines include propranolol, timolol, amitriptyline, divalproex, sodium divalproate, sodium valproate, and topiramate. Second-line options for prophylaxis include gabapentin, naproxen, timed-release dihydroergotamine mesylate (DHE-45), verapamil, metoprolol, fluoxetine, and vitamin B_2 (riboflavin), among others [64]. While there is significant therapeutic overlap between prophylactic options for classic migraine and vestibular migraine, few studies have systematically examined the efficacy of prophylactic

Table 22.3 Common pharmacologic agents for prophylaxis of vestibular migraine (UpToDate 2017 [63])

Medication	Class	Most common side effects	Notes
Nortriptyline	Tricyclic antidepressant	• Cardiac arrhythmias • Palpitations • Anticholinergic effects • Dizziness • Tinnitus • Paresthesias • Decreased libido	• US boxed warning: suicidality in children and adolescents • Serotonin syndrome may occur when combined with monoamine oxidase inhibitors (MAOi) or when an MAOi has been used within 14 days
Propranolol	β-blocker	• Bradycardia • Hypotension • Sleep disorders • Agitation • Dizziness • Fatigue	• US boxed warning: abrupt cessation may lead to angina pectoris or myocardial infarction in patients with ischemic heart disease
Metoprolol	β-blocker	• Fatigue • Bradycardia • Hypotension • Dizziness • Vertigo • Decreased libido	• US boxed warning: abrupt cessation may lead to angina pectoris or myocardial infarction in patients with ischemic heart disease
Verapamil	Calcium channel blocker	• Headache • Gingival hyperplasia • Constipation	• Caution in patients with history of cardiac arrhythmia or who take other anti-arrhythmic drugs • Contraindicated in Wolff-Parkinson-White and similar accessory conduction syndromes
Clonazepam	Long-acting benzodiazepine	• Fatigue, drowsiness • Decreased mental acuity • Ataxia • Dizziness	• US boxed warning: combination with opioids may cause profound sedation, respiratory depression, coma, and death
Topiramate	Anticonvulsant	• Paresthesia • Drowsiness • Fatigue • Dizziness • Memory impairment • Mood disorder	• Should taper dosing instead of abrupt cessation to avoid rebound effect • No additional benefit noted for doses >100 mg/day

(continued)

Table 22.3 (continued)

Medication	Class	Most common side effects	Notes
Valproic acid	Anticonvulsant	• Headache • Drowsiness • Dizziness • Insomnia • Nausea • Thrombocytopenia • Infection • Weakness	• US boxed warnings: – Hepatotoxicity – Mitochondrial disease
Fluoxetine	Antidepressant; selective serotonin reuptake inhibitor (SSRI)	• Insomnia • Headache • Drowsiness • Anxiety • Nervousness • Yawning • Nausea • Decreased libido • Weakness • Pharyngitis	• US boxed warning: suicidality and antidepressants
Venlafaxine	Antidepressant; serotonin-norepinephrine reuptake inhibitor (SNRI)	• Headache • Insomnia • Drowsiness • Dizziness • Weight loss • Nausea • Abnormal ejaculation	• Black box warning: suicidality and antidepressants

medications for vestibular migraine, specifically. Recently, a prospective randomized, controlled trial (RCT) was performed to compare the efficacy of propranolol and venlafaxine for prophylaxis of vestibular migraine symptoms. The authors found these agents to offer equal efficacy in preventing vestibular symptoms but noted venlafaxine to be more effective in managing symptoms of depression [65].

Anticonvulsant medications, including divalproex, sodium divalproate, sodium valproate, or topiramate, are usually prescribed for migraine prophylaxis in patients who have failed a trial (or trials) of another medication with fewer side effects. Topiramate has been observed to be highly effective in adequately controlling symptoms of vestibular migraine [66]. Otologists are less likely than physicians from other specialties to prescribe anticonvulsants (20% vs. 70%) for the treatment of vestibular migraine [67].

Benzodiazepines are not routinely prescribed for non-vertiginous migraine but are frequently prescribed for vestibular migraine by itself or in combination with other medications. The most commonly prescribed agent from this class is clonazepam, which is potent and long acting (half-life of 24–36 h). After oral administration, clonazepam reaches maximum blood levels in 1–2 h, making it less well suited for the management of acute episodes [14].

Specialty-Specific Opinions Surrounding Vestibular Migraine

In a survey-based study on practice patterns [67], it was observed that different perspectives exist between otologists and members of the International Headache Society (IHC; mainly neurologists but also physicians from other specialties who provide care to migraine patients) regarding clinical presentation, pathophysiology, and management of vestibular migraine. Most IHC members (73.5%) think vestibular migraine is caused by a sensory trigger, while only 30.8% of otologists held this opinion. More specifically, 60% of the IHC group believe this input is from the trigeminal nerve, compared to 9% of otologists.

Regarding symptom classification in vestibular migraine patients, significant differences also exist. IHC members were more likely (62% vs. 43%) to consider vertigo associated with vestibular migraine to be of central origin and to consider motion sickness (70% vs. 23%) to be a feature of vestibular migraine. Otologists were more likely than other physicians (56% vs. 26%) to consider hearing loss to be a symptom of migraine. Additionally, management strategies differed somewhat between groups, with IHC members being more likely to prescribe triptans (55% vs. 23%) and anticonvulsants (70% vs. 20%) for the treatment of vestibular migraine [67].

Follow-Up and Prognosis

A significant proportion of patients experience complete relief or satisfactory improvement of the symptoms of vestibular migraine with appropriate therapy. One series of 81 patients observed 16% of patients to experience adequate symptomatic relief from dietary modification alone. Following a stepwise algorithm, 31 of those patients who failed to respond adequately to dietary modification were prescribed a single prophylactic medication, which leads to significant relief in 77%. A third group of 37 patients were either treated with another medication or referred for neurology evaluation, leading to significant relief in 57% of these patients. Of patients in this series with vestibular symptoms and headaches, more than 95% reported equal improvement in both categories of symptoms. One hundred percent of patients without headaches experienced substantial relief of vertigo and disequilibrium with migraine therapy [60].

In another case series, complete or substantial control of vestibular symptoms was achieved in 68 (92%) of 74 patients with episodic vertigo, in 56 (89%) of 63 patients with positional vertigo, and in 56 (86%) of 65 patients with non-vertiginous dizziness. Aural fullness was completely resolved or substantially improved in 34 (85%) of 40 patients, ear pain in 10 (63%) of 16 patients, and phonophobia in 17 (89%) of 19 patients. Treatment leads to some symptomatic improvement in all patients [14].

While complete relief of symptoms may be achieved in many cases, many patients will still have symptoms with maximum medical therapy. The concept of satisfactory improvement remains subjective, and it is important for physicians to establish realistic expectations and effectively communicate these goals to patients.

Conclusions

Vestibular migraine represents one of the most common (if not the most common) causes of episodic vertigo. This entity presents significant diagnostic challenges due to variability in presentation, overlap with other disorders, and lack of well-defined, objective diagnostic criteria. Identification of other disorders masquerading as VM is imperative, as some potentially life-threatening conditions may present similarly. Management consists of patient education and counseling, identification and avoidance of triggers, prophylactic medical therapy, symptomatic medical therapy, and multidisciplinary specialty input, including professionals in the disciplines of general internal medicine, otology/neurotology/otolaryngology, neurology, and psychiatry, among others.

References

1. Headache Classification Committee of the International Headache Society (IHS). The International Classification of Headache Disorders, 3rd edition (beta version). Cephalalgia. 2013;33(9):629–808.
2. Dieterich M, Obermann M, Celebisoy N. Vestibular migraine: the most frequent entity of episodic vertigo. J Neurol. 2016;263(1):82–9.
3. Neuhauser H, et al. The interrelations of migraine, vertigo, and migrainous vertigo. Neurology. 2001;56(4):436–41.
4. Lempert T, Neuhauser H. Epidemiology of vertigo, migraine and vestibular migraine. J Neurol. 2009;256(3):333–8.
5. Neuhauser HK, et al. Migrainous vertigo: prevalence and impact on quality of life. Neurology. 2006;67(6):1028–33.
6. Radtke A, et al. Vestibular migraine: long-term follow-up of clinical symptoms and vestibulo-cochlear findings. Neurology. 2012;79:1607–14.
7. Ghavami Y, et al. Migraine features in patients with Meniere's disease. Laryngoscope. 2016;126(1):163–8.
8. Cha Y-H, Baloh RW. Migraine associated vertigo. J Clin Neurol. 2007;3(3):121–6.
9. Thompson TL, Amedee R. Vertigo: a review of common peripheral and central vestibular disorders. Ochsner J. 2009;9(1):20–6.
10. Neff BA, et al. Auditory and vestibular symptoms and chronic subjective dizziness in patients with Ménière's disease, vestibular migraine, and Ménière's disease with concomitant vestibular migraine. Otol Neurotol. 2012;33(7):1235–44.
11. Cherchi M, Hain TC. Migraine-associated vertigo. Otolaryngol Clin North Am. 2011;44(2):367–75.
12. Baloh RW. Neurotology of migraine. Headache J Head Face Pain. 1997;37(10):615–21.
13. Kayan A, Hood JD. Neuro-otological manifestations of migraine. Brain. 1984;107(4):1123–42.
14. Johnson GD. Medical management of migraine-related dizziness and vertigo. Laryngoscope. 1998;108(S85):1–28.

15. Golding JF. Motion sickness susceptibility questionnaire revised and its relationship to other forms of sickness. Brain Res Bull. 1998;47(5):507–16.
16. Aromaa M, et al. Childhood headache at school entry: a controlled clinical study. Neurology. 1998;50(6):1729–36.
17. Murdin L, Chamberlain F, Cheema S. Motion sickness in migraine and vestibular disorders. J Neurol Neurosurg Psychiatry. 2015;86(5):585–7.
18. Bhattacharyya N, et al. Clinical practice guideline: benign paroxysmal positional vertigo (update) executive summary. Otolaryngol Head Neck Surg. 2017;156(3):403–16.
19. Bisdorff A, et al. Classification of vestibular symptoms: towards an international classification of vestibular disorders. J Vestib Res. 2009;19:1–13.
20. Lin HW, Bhattacharyya N. Impact of dizziness and obesity on the prevalence of falls and fall-related injuries. Laryngoscope. 2014;124(12):2797–801.
21. Neuhauser HK. The epidemiology of dizziness and vertigo. Handb Clin Neurol. 2016;137:67–82.
22. Neuhauser HK, et al. Epidemiology of vestibular vertigo: a neurotologic survey of the general population. Neurology. 2005;65(6):898–904.
23. Stolte B, et al. Vestibular migraine. Cephalalgia. 2015;35(3):262–70.
24. Polensek SH, Tusa RJ. Nystagmus during attacks of vestibular migraine: an aid in diagnosis. Audiol Neurootol. 2010;15(4):241–6.
25. Cutrer FM, Baloh RW. Migraine-associated dizziness. Headache J Head Face Pain. 1992;32(6):300–4.
26. Dieterich M, Brandt T. Episodic vertigo related to migraine (90 cases): vestibular migraine? J Neurol. 1999;246(10):883–92.
27. Pereira CB, et al. Vestibular migraine: vestibular symptom may identify different subgroups. Otol Neurotol. 2016;37(3):281–3.
28. Dash AK, et al. Migraine and audiovestibular dysfunction: is there a correlation? Am J Otolaryngol. 2008;29(5):295–9.
29. Teixido M, et al. Otalgia associated with migraine. Otol Neurotol. 2011;32(2):322–5.
30. Battista RA. Audiometric findings of patients with migraine-associated dizziness. Otol Neurotol. 2004;25(6):987–92.
31. Viirre ES, Baloh RW. Migraine as a cause of sudden hearing loss. Headache J Head Face Pain. 1996;36(1):24–8.
32. Lipkin AF, Jenkins HA, Coker NJ. Migraine and sudden sensorineural hearing loss. Arch Otolaryngol Head Neck Surg. 1987;113(3):325–6.
33. Weinreich HM, Carey JP. Prevalence of pulsatile tinnitus among patients with migraine. Otol Neurotol. 2016;37(3):244–7.
34. Radat F, Swendsen J. Psychiatric comorbidity in migraine: a review. Cephalalgia. 2005;25(3):165–78.
35. Kim SK, et al. Clinical analysis of dizzy patients with high levels of depression and anxiety. J Audiol Otol. 2016;20(3):174–8.
36. Kutay Ö, et al. Vestibular migraine patients are more anxious than migraine patients without vestibular symptoms. J Neurol. 2017;107(5):1123.
37. Teixido M, Baker A, Isildak H. Migraine and benign paroxysmal positional vertigo: a single-institution review. J Laryngol Otol. 2017;131(6):1–6.
38. Cha YH, Kane MJ, Baloh RW. Familial clustering of migraine, episodic vertigo, and Ménière's disease. Otol Neurotol: Official. 2008;29(1):93–6.
39. To-Alemanji J, Ryan C, Schubert MC. Experiences engaging healthcare when dizzy. Otol Neurotol. 2016;37(8):1122–7.
40. Hojjat H, et al. To image or not to image? A cost-effectiveness analysis of MRI for patients with asymmetric sensorineural hearing loss. Laryngoscope. 2017;127(4):939–44.
41. Ahsan SF, et al. Clinical predictors of abnormal magnetic resonance imaging findings in patients with asymmetric sensorineural hearing loss. JAMA Otolaryngol Head Neck Surg. 2015;141(5):451–6.

42. Aragones JM, et al. Migraine: an alternative in the diagnosis of unclassified vertigo. Headache J Head Face Pain. 1993;33(3):125–8.
43. Vitkovic J, Paine M, Rance G. Neuro-otological findings in patients with migraine- and nonmigraine-related dizziness. Audiol Neurootol. 2008;13(2):113–22.
44. Murdin L, Davies RA, Bronstein AM. Vertigo as a migraine trigger. Neurology. 2009;73(8):638–42.
45. Boyev KP. Meniere's disease or migraine?: the clinical significance of fluctuating hearing loss with vertigo. Arch Otolaryngol Head Neck Surg. 2005;131(5):457–9.
46. Committee on Hearing and Equilibrium. Committee on hearing and equilibrium guidelines for the diagnosis and evaluation of therapy in Meniere's disease. Otolaryngol Head Neck Surg. 1995;113(3):181–5.
47. Zuniga MG, et al. Can vestibular-evoked myogenic potentials help differentiate Ménière disease from vestibular migraine? Otolaryngol Head Neck Surg. 2012;146(5):788–96.
48. Taylor RL, et al. Vestibular evoked myogenic potentials to sound and vibration: characteristics in vestibular migraine that enable separation from Meniere's disease. Cephalalgia. 2012;32(3):213–25.
49. Inoue A, et al. Vestibular evoked myogenic potentials in vestibular migraine. Ann Otol Rhinol Laryngol. 2016;125(11):931–7.
50. Moshtaghi O, et al. A historical recount: discovering Ménière's disease and its association with migraine headaches. Otol Neurotol. 2016;37(8):1199–203.
51. Rassekh CH, Harker LA. The prevalence of migraine in Ménière's disease. Laryngoscope. 1992;102(2):135–8.
52. Neuhauser H, Lempert T. Vestibular migraine. Neurol Clin. 2009;27(2):379–91.
53. Lee H, et al. Can migraine damage the inner ear? Arch Neurol. 2000;57(11):1631–4.
54. Basser LS. Benign paroxysmal vertigo of childhood (a variety of vestibular neuronitis). Brain. 1964;87(3):141–52.
55. Batuecas-Caletrío Á, et al. Is benign paroxysmal vertigo of childhood a migraine precursor? Eur J Paediatr Neurol. 2013;17(4):397–400.
56. Krams B, et al. Benign paroxysmal vertigo of childhood: long-term outcome. Cephalalgia. 2011;31(4):439–43.
57. Fotuhi M, et al. Vestibular migraine: a critical review of treatment trials. J Neurol. 2009;256(5):711–6.
58. Baier B, Winkenwerder E, Dieterich M. Vestibular migraine: effects of prophylactic therapy with various drugs. J Neurol. 2009;256(3):436–42.
59. Mikulec AA, Faraji F, Kinsella LJ. Evaluation of the efficacy of caffeine cessation, nortriptyline, and topiramate therapy in vestibular migraine and complex dizziness of unknown etiology. Am J Otolaryngol. 2012;33(1):121–7.
60. Reploeg MD, Goebel JA. Migraine-associated dizziness: patient characteristics and management options. Otol Neurotol. 2002;23(3):364–71.
61. Vitkovic J, et al. Vestibular rehabilitation outcomes in patients with and without vestibular migraine. J Neurol. 2013;260(12):3039–48.
62. Bikhazi P, Jackson C, Ruckenstein MJ. Efficacy of antimigrainous therapy in the treatment of migraine-associated dizziness. Am J Otol. 1997;18(3):350–4.
63. UpToDate, 2017. Medication Reference. [online] UpToDate. www.uptodate.com. Accessed 1 Mar 2017.
64. Modi S, Lowder DM. Medications for migraine prophylaxis. Am Fam Physician. 2006;73(1):72–8.
65. Salviz M, et al. Propranolol and venlafaxine for vestibular migraine prophylaxis: a randomized controlled trial. Laryngoscope. 2016;126(1):169–74.
66. Carmona S, Bruera O. Prophylactic treatment of migraine and migraine clinical variants with topiramate: an update. Ther Clin Risk Manag. 2009;5:661–9.
67. Millen SJ, Schnurr CM, Schnurr BB. Vestibular migraine: perspectives of otology versus neurology. Otol Neurotol. 2011;32:330–7.

Chapter 23
Peripheral Nerve Stimulation for Head and Face Pain

Shannon W. Clark, Ashwini Sharan, and Chengyuan Wu

Introduction

Neuromodulation has emerged as a potentially promising therapeutic modality for many headache and facial pain disorders. Electrical stimulation of a peripheral nerve (PNS) is a mode of neuromodulation that can be used to treat not only neuropathic pain that manifests in dermatomal patterns, but also primary headache disorders that affect a region of maximal pain not correlating with one specific dermatome. Common PNS strategies for head and face pain include implantation of subcutaneous electrodes to various named nerves such as occipital nerve stimulation (ONS), supraorbital nerve stimulation (SONS), sphenopalatine ganglion (SPG) stimulation, and vagal nerve stimulation (VNS).

The technique of PNS was first described in 1966 by Wall and Sweet [1] and further popularized as a treatment option by the description by Weiner and Reed [2] as a percutaneous PNS technique in 1999 when it was used in a series of patients with occipital neuralgia. Such methods offered less invasive alternatives to the open exploration of a nerve and direct application of an electrode resulting in easier trial for patients [3]. Currently, this percutaneous technique is employed by various specialties including neurosurgeons, otolaryngologists, plastic surgeons, physiatrists, and interventional pain management specialists to treat medically refractory craniofacial pain syndromes [4].

S. W. Clark · A. Sharan · C. Wu (✉)
Department of Neurological Surgery, Thomas Jefferson University, Philadelphia, PA, USA
e-mail: Ashwini.sharan@jefferson.edu

J. Y. Suen, E. Petersen (eds.), *Diagnosis and Management of Head and Face Pain*, https://doi.org/10.1007/978-3-319-90999-8_23

Peripheral nerve field stimulation (PNfS), also known as subcutaneous neurostimulation, is a key concept that broadens the indication of ONS and SONS from neuropathic pain to primary headache disorders [5]. Field stimulation produces paresthesia along a diffuse painful area that may not correlate with one specific dermatome or otherwise be well-defined [3]. Body regions rather than nerves are used to describe indications for PNfS; hence the documented efficacy of PNfS for holohemispheric headaches such as migraine allowed larger patient population to benefit from the therapy [6].

In this chapter, we focus the discussion on ONS with and without SONS, SPG stimulation, and noninvasive vagal nerve stimulation (nVNS)—as these are the most commonly utilized PNS modalities for head and face pain with promising evidence-based efficacy.

Occipital Nerve Stimulation

ONS provides a minimally invasive, reversible, and effective treatment for a number of intractable headache disorders. The technique is thought to work by inhibiting central nociceptive impulses by stimulation of the peripheral extensions of the trigeminocervical complex, the nerve branches of C2 and C3 [7]. One hypothesis by which PNS reduces centrally transmitted pain is based upon the gate control theory as described by Melzack and Wall [8], which suggests that there is an inverse relationship between activity in small diameter nociceptive afferents and large diameter nerve fibers. As a result, stimulation of large diameter fibers leads to suppression of small diameter fiber nociceptive input and elevation of pain thresholds.

Indications

ONS has been used successfully in the treatment of occipital neuralgia and many primary headache disorders such as migraine [2, 6, 9, 10], cluster headache [11–13], and hemicrania continua [11]. Reports have also suggested its efficacy in secondary headache disorders such as cervicogenic headache [14], C2-mediated headaches [15], posttraumatic headaches [11], and postsurgical headaches [16].

Surgical Technique

The procedure can be performed with local anesthetic and conscious sedation, monitored anesthesia care, or general anesthesia. In some centers, ultrasound is used as adjunct to identify occipital nerves and occipital arteries to ensure optimal electrode positioning [17]. In our institution, a small vascular Doppler ultrasound is used to mark out the occipital artery, which is then used as a guide to estimate the greater occipital nerve (GON). Careful identification of the region of pain guides the appropriate placement of electrodes especially in cases of PNfS. Marking the region based on the patient report before electrode placement facilitates the optimal position at the site of maximal pain. The number of leads implanted may vary based on the location and dimension of painful area.

Either cylindrical electrodes or narrow steerable paddle electrodes may be introduced percutaneously. Cylindrical electrodes have a concentric electric field in all directions, which permits ease of placement, but are more prone to migrate and consume more current than paddle electrodes [18].

Trial Electrode Implantation

- Preoperative Considerations
  In case of ONS, the stimulator lead can be directed medially from a lateral entry point (medial and inferior to the mastoid process) or laterally from a midline entry point. The authors prefer a lateral point entry in unilateral cases since the patient can be placed in the lateral decubitus position, which may also allow for concurrent implantation of a SONS electrode. The midline point entry, however, is more appropriate in bilateral ONS cases when the patient is positioned prone. Midline placement also offers a stronger foothold for anchors at the midline nuchal ligament [6]. If the plan is to place combined ONS and SONS electrodes to cover holohemispheric headache, we suggest either placing ONS with SONS unilaterally or placing bilateral ONS for the trial period so that the patient can compare the therapeutic benefit to the non-treated side/area.
- Patient Positioning
  In case of unilateral lead placement, patients are placed in lateral decubitus position on a horseshoe headrest. In case of bilateral lead placement, patients are placed prone on a horseshoe headrest. Pillows can be placed under the chest to augment the neck flexion. For trial lead placement, monitored anesthesia care is often administered to facilitate a wake up test for proper paresthesia coverage if necessary.
  After positioning, a small handheld Doppler is used to identify the path of the occipital artery, which runs parallel to both occipital nerves. Once identified, the arterial path is marked with a surgical marker (Fig. 23.1).
  Standard surgical preparation and draping are performed with the entire planned path of the electrode visible in the field (Fig. 23.2).
- Surgical Steps
  Step 1: The occiput C1–C2 interspace is palpated to identify the starting point for needle entry. The skin is infiltrated with local anesthetic at the entry point, and a small entry incision is made with a 15 blade.
  Step 2: A Tuohy needle is advanced subcutaneous space overlying the nerve in the occiput C1–C2 interspace. The needle is inserted to the distance from the midline insertion point to the mastoid tip (Fig. 23.1).

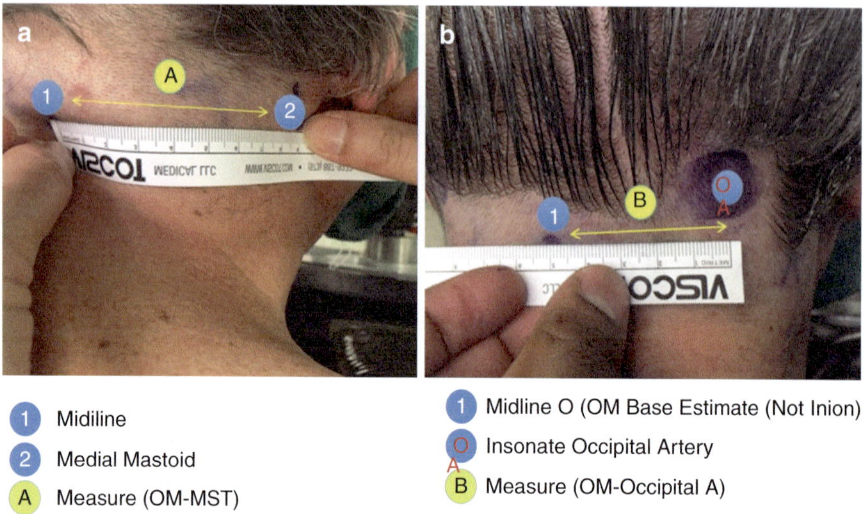

Fig. 23.1 (**a**) The distance between the midline insertion point 1 to the mastoid point 2 is noted with A. (**b**) The distance between the midline insertion point1 to the insonated occipital artery (OA) is noted with B. Tip of implanted ONS electrode should come between the length of A and B (shorter than from midline to mastoid but longer than from midline to insonated occipital artery distance)

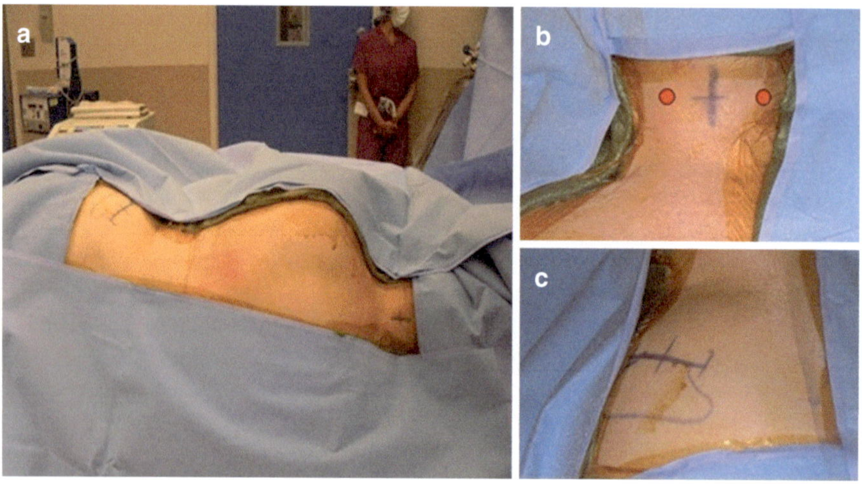

Fig. 23.2 (**a**) Patient prepped and draped in right lateral decubitus position with battery site planned at the left gluteal location. (**b**) Cross mark is made on C1–C2 interspace in the midline. Red dots denote insonated occipital arteries, and these are the directions of tunneling the electrodes. (**c**) Battery side should be sufficiently lower than the belt line to prevent discomfort

Step 3: The inner stylet of the Tuohy needle is withdrawn, and an eight-contact cylindrical lead marked the same length as the tunneled length of Tuohy needle is inserted into the needle until the marking is reached. The inner wire stylet of the electrode is removed, and the Tuohy needle is withdrawn while taking care not to pull the electrode back as well.
Step 4: The electrode is stitched in place to the skin over the entry site using 2-0 silk suture, and relaxing loops are made before placement of bacitracin and occlusive dressing. The externalized trial electrodes are connected to the trial stimulator system. Further programming of the stimulator is performed postoperatively.
Step 5: Intraoperative fluoroscopic imaging or a postoperative skull X-ray is performed to confirm the proper placement of electrodes before patient discharge. The patient is discharged with oral antibiotics to be taken during the entire trial period.

- Operative Pearls

  – The level and depth of lead placement are crucial for a successful ONS trial. Placing the lead too superficially risks failure of nerve stimulation and lead erosion through the skin [19]. Patients tend to experience unpleasant burning sensation with shallow leads. On the contrary, leads placed too deep risk stimulating posterior neck muscles and causing unpleasant muscle spasms [20]. In the case of deeply placed paddle leads, stimulation may be directed superficially thereby targeting the greater occipital nerve. Therefore, we recommend operative ultrasound guidance for visualizing occipital nerve in cases of paddle leads placement as described by Deer and Hayek [20].
  – Intraoperatively, the patient's sedation may be lightened to enable testing. If the patient reports paresthesia is perceived in the area of pain, then lead placements are optimal. Alternatively, stimulation parameters can be changed to see if the coverage area becomes optimal. However, the wake up test is not necessary if the occipital artery path is identified properly.
  – Hayek et al. [20] have recommended positioning the stimulator lead subcutaneously at the level of nuchal line where GON is superficial rather than the originally described method of placing over the C1 level by Weiner and Reed [2]. At the level of C1, the trapezius and semispinalis capitis muscles lie over the GON, therefore placing the lead further from the nerve and increases the chance for inducing muscle spasms. Our preference is to insert the lead to a more rostral position as described by Hayek.

- Postoperative Care
  The trial period lasts 5–7 days on average. Periodic adjustment of the stimulator settings may be required to achieve optimal relief of pain. Externalized cables should be kept dry, and as such, patients are advised not to wash hair or take a bath during the course of the trial. A trial is typically considered successful if a patient experiences more than 50% improvement of pain severity. Only patients with a successful trial and satisfaction with the trial therapy should proceed with permanent stimulator and battery placement.

Permanent Stimulator Placement

The steps for implantation of the permanent system are similar to the trial except that this procedure is typically performed under general anesthesia to prevent pain associated with tunneling the leads subcutaneously and implantation of the implantable pulse generator (IPG). If desired, intraoperative fluoroscopic guidance can facilitate identical placement to the trial leads.

Steps 1 through 3 along with positioning and draping are the same with the trial procedure.

Step 4: The electrode is anchored to the fascia. This step can be performed using a nonabsorbable stitch or with anchors provided in the stimulator kit. A strain relief loop should be created to minimize the risk of lead migration. We recommend 1–2 anchors per lead.

Step 5: An additional incision is made at the cervical-thoracic level. And an additional loop is created at this point. The superior loop likely mitigates the motion at occiput C1–C2, while the inferior loop likely protects from the translational, flexion extension forces at the cervical-thoracic junction (Fig. 23.3). The addition of this loop has resulted in decreased migrations [21].

Step 6: A subcutaneous pocket approximately 2cm deep from the skin is prepared for the battery. We typically place a flank or gluteal IPG, particularly when the patient is positioned prone, as doing so has the benefit of not having to reposition the patient for IPG implantation. Similarly, if the patient was positioned in a lateral decubitus position, either infraclavicular or axillary sites may be considered for purposes of proximity.

Step 7: The leads are tunneled from the anchor site to the IPG pocket. Extension cables are frequently required for IPGs in the flank or gluteal locations. The leads, with or without extensions, are then connected to the IPG.

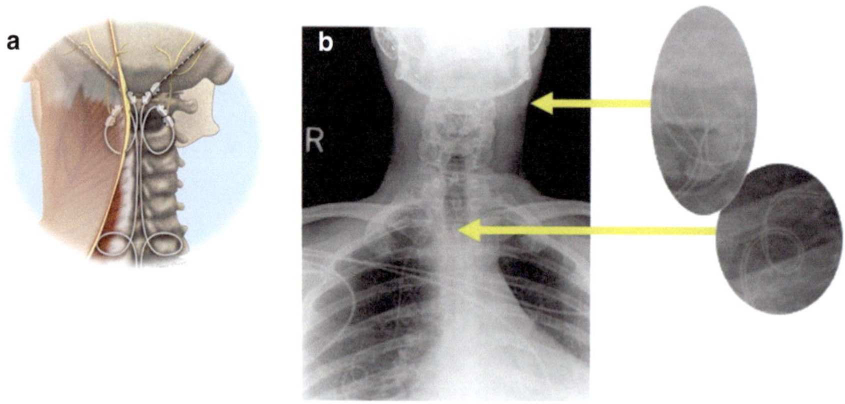

Fig. 23.3 (**a**) Schematic drawing of two strain relief loops placed at the incision made in the midline (along nuchal line) for needle incision site as well as at the cervicothoracic junction. (**b**) Postoperative X-ray demonstrating the actual strain relief loops. In our experience, the second strain relief loop at this very mobile location of the neck greatly reduced the pullout rate of electrodes

Step 8: An impedance check is performed on the system to assess technical function of the entire system.
Step 9: All wounds are irrigated with antibiotic-impregnated solution, and the incisions are closed.

- *Complications*
  The major complication with ONS (and SONS) is lead migration. The incidence of lead migration was reported to be 24–60% within the first year and 100% after 3 years of implantation [10, 22, 23]. As a result some practitioners [20] have used self-anchoring leads in ONS with encouraging preliminary results. In a case series of patients implanted in this manner, none of 12 patients required a surgical revision for lead migration for a mean follow-up period of 13 months [20]. For SONS electrodes, forehead muscles and skin tend to move more than that of the occipital area due to facial expressions. Hence, lead migrations and erosions are more common in the facial leads, not to mention cosmetic concerns in this area. The details of SONS are described in the next section.

Clinical Results in the ONS Literature

1. *Occipital Neuralgia*
   Occipital neuralgia (ON) is a disorder characterized by sharp, electrical, paroxysmal pain, occasionally throbbing in quality, originating from the occiput and extending along the posterior scalp, in the distribution of the greater, lesser, and/or third occipital nerve [24]. The initial use of ONS in craniofacial pain was its application for treatment of ON by Weiner and Reed [2]. Though use of spinal cord stimulator as ONS for any craniofacial pain including ON is not approved by FDA, numerous studies (Table 23.1) have shown its efficacy for ON. In fact the Congress of Neurological Surgeons (CNS) published the evidence-based guideline [24] for use of ONS for medically refractory ON in 2015, recommending it as a mainstay surgical treatment for ON.
2. *Chronic Migraine*
   There have been numerous case series documenting the efficacy of ONS as therapy for medically refractory chronic migraine (CM) since the late 1990s. Their efficacies range from 50 to 100%. Table 23.2 summarizes the major early clinical results reported.
   Given these promising results, randomized controlled trials (RCT) of ONS for CM have recently been undertaken. Three trials have been performed and are summarized in Table 23.3. Subjects in the ONSTIM (Occipital Nerve Stimulation for the Treatment of Chronic Migraine Headache) study included patients who were diagnosed with medically refractory CM for an average of 10 years with approximately 23 headache days per month [33]. Three-month responder rates were 39% for adjustable stimulation group, 6% for sham stimulation group, and 0% for medical management group. Lead migration occurred in 12 of 51 (24%) subjects.

Table 23.1 Clinical results of ONS for ON

Author	N	Results	Complications
Weiner and Reed, 1999 [2]	13	All patients with >50% pain relief at the last follow-up (mean 2 years, range 1.5–5.5 years)	Lead infection, breakage, and migration (8%)
Oh et al., 2004 [25]	10	Nine of ten patients with >75% relief at 6 months (length of follow-up was only 6 months)	Worsened cervical pain (10%)
Kapural et al., 2005 [9]	6	Significant decrease in VAS from 8.7 to 2.5 at 3 months as well as pain disability index from 49.8 to 14.0	Allergic reaction over battery (10%)
Slavin et al., 2006 [26]	10	Seven patients had 60–90% reduction of pain at mean follow-up of 22 months (range, 5–32 months)	Infection (10%)
Johnstone et al., 2006 [27]	8	Reduction in VAS in five patients at mean follow-up of 25 months (range 6–47 months) and two acquired employment	Migration (10%) Infection (29%)
Melvin et al., 2007 [15]	11	Mean of 64% improvement in SF-MPQ compared with baseline and 67% decrease in VAS at 3 months	Lead migration and reoperation (18%)
Magown et al., 2009 [28]	7	Mean reduction of 96% on the VAS at mean of 17 months (range, 2–30)	Infection (14%)
Palmisani et al., 2013 [29]	3	All three patients reported >50% reduction in pain intensity and frequency at 28–31 months	Reposition of battery (33%)
Abhinav et al., 2013 [30]	4	Median VAS pre- and postoperatively was 9 and 0	None

Table 23.2 Early case series reporting clinical results of ONS for CM

Author	N	Results	Complications
Weiner and Reed, 1999 [2]	12	80% response rate	NA
Popenoy et al., 2003 [31]	25	HA reduced from 76/90 to 38/90 days with responder rate 88%	Nine migrations, one infection
Oh et al., 2004 [25]	10	90% relief in 7 patients (f/u 6 months)	Two infections
Schwedt et al., 2007 [10]	15	HA reduced from 90/90 to 60/90 days and severity decreased from 6.75 to 4.5; plus reduction of depression score	Three migrations
Matharu et al., 2004 [32]	8	PET study of ONS showing pain center modulated by ONS. 6 patients had >75% and 2 patients had >50% relief	Three migrations

In another prospective randomized multicenter double-blind controlled study, 125 subjects with CM were implanted with a neurostimulation system and randomized to an active or control group for 12 weeks [34], after which patients were followed in an open-label phase. Reduction in the number of headache (HA) days was recorded. Although there was not a significant group difference in the number of patients with a 50% reduction on the visual analogue scale (VAS)

Table 23.3 Prospective RCTs of PNS for migraine

Author		N	Result	Complications
Saper et al., 2011 [33]	ONSTIM	75	39% responder rate to adjustable ONS	24% lead migrations
Silberstein et al., 2012 [34]		125	Reduction in headache days and MIDAS score with ONS	70% complications of which 40.7% required surgical intervention
Lipton et al., 2009 [35]	PRISM	139	No statistically significant reduction in HA days with ONS vs. sham	6.8% revision surgery and 15.1% required explanation due to complications

Table 23.4 Case series reporting clinical results of ONS for CH

Author	N	f/u	Results
Burns et al., 2007 [12]	14	17.5 months	10/14 improved (3 had >90%, 3 had >40%, 4 had 20–30%)
Magis et al., 2007 [13]	15	36.8 months	80% had 90% reduction in frequency, 10% did not respond. 29% reduced prophylaxis medication
Lainez et al., 2008 [36]	5	24 months	3/5 had excellent response, 1 had partial, and 1 did not respond
Fontaine et al., 2011 [37]	13	14 months	Attack frequency and intensity reduced by 68% and 49%. 10 responders, prophylactic medication decrease in 8
Mueller et al., 2013 [38]	27	20 months	93% response. 21 patients satisfied with treatment

(primary endpoint), there was a significant group difference at 30% ($p < 0.05$), which has still been considered to be clinically significant. In the active and control groups, number of HA days decreased by 7.0 and 2.7, respectively; total migraine disability assessment (MIDAS) scores improved by 72.9 and 27.2, respectively; and a 30% reduction in VAS was achieved in 36.4% and 13.5% of patients, respectively. The authors concluded that these results provide evidence to support the safety and efficacy of ONS for management of chronic migraine.

In a 52-week outcome analysis of the study, headache days were significantly reduced by 6.7 days in the intention to treat population ($p < 0.001$). The percentages of patients who achieved a 30% and 50% reduction in headache days and/or pain intensity were 59.5% and 47.8%, respectively. However, a total of 70% of patients experienced adverse events such as 11 infections, 29 lead migrations and breakages, and 38 persistent pains at surgical sites, of which 8.6% required hospitalization and 40.7% required surgical revision.

In a third prospective, double-blinded, randomized controlled, multicenter trial, 139 patients were randomized to receive either active stimulation or sham stimulation. The full study results are only available in abstract form [35].ONS did not produce statistically significant benefits in relation to sham stimulation for the primary endpoint of change from baseline migraine days per month.

3. *Cluster Headache*

A number of observational studies have demonstrated promising efficacy of ONS for the management of chronic cluster headache (CH). Table 23.4 summarizes the results of the main studies ($n > 5$) reported in recent years. The efficacy ranges from 60 to 90% in these reported series with similar complication profiles as reports for CM.

Supraorbital Nerve Stimulation

Since the distribution of pain may either be isolated to the anterior head region or present both anteriorly and posteriorly, the potential for bilateral supraorbital nerve stimulation (SONS) in combination with ONS was explored in more recent years. There have been several case series documenting promising efficacy of combined stimulations especially for primary headaches such as CM and CH.

Surgical Steps for Implanting SONS

Step 1: After prepping and draping the ipsilateral forehead, neck, and chest, the incision site and needle insertion site are marked. For one SONS lead, an incision is made in the lateral forehead just behind the hairline (approximately 1.5 cm superolateral to the tip of eyebrow) for the ON-Q® T-peel introducer needle with over the needle catheter (i.Flow*). We use ON-Q system (6 inch × 17 GA needle) for SONS because it is more malleable as opposed to the stiff Tuohy needles. It can also be used for ONS placements. Another incision is made in the right temporal region, to which the distal SONS wire is tunneled.

Note: Trial lead placement for SONS is similar to the step 1, only the stab incision behind the hairline is made, and the trial electrode is anchored to the scalp with 2-0 silk sutures at the entry site without being tunneled. Place bacitracin ointment and occlusive dressing on top. Patients are advised to not wash their hair for the duration of trials (approximately 5 days) to prevent electrodes pullout.

Step 2: The ON-Q needle with catheter is prebent to the curvature of the forehead. The direction is chosen in such a way that the electrode contacts are positioned perpendicular to the course of the supraorbital nerves. After the ON-Q is in position, the inner needle is pulled out leaving the plastic sheath in place. A standard electrode (four-contact or eight-contact) is passed into the epifascial plane, and the tip of the electrode is buried and anchored with a 4-0 neurolon suture subperiosteally via a small nick incision made in the forehead crease to hold the tip down and reduce lead migration (or later sticking out at the forehead).

Step 3: After removing the guide sheath, the electrode is tunneled back to the incision in the right temporal region, and a titanium dog bone–shaped plate is used to anchor the electrode to the cranium at the temporal incision (Fig. 23.4).

Step 4: A strain relief loop is created at the temporal incision, and the distal wire is further tunneled down to the neck behind the ear. Another incision is typically

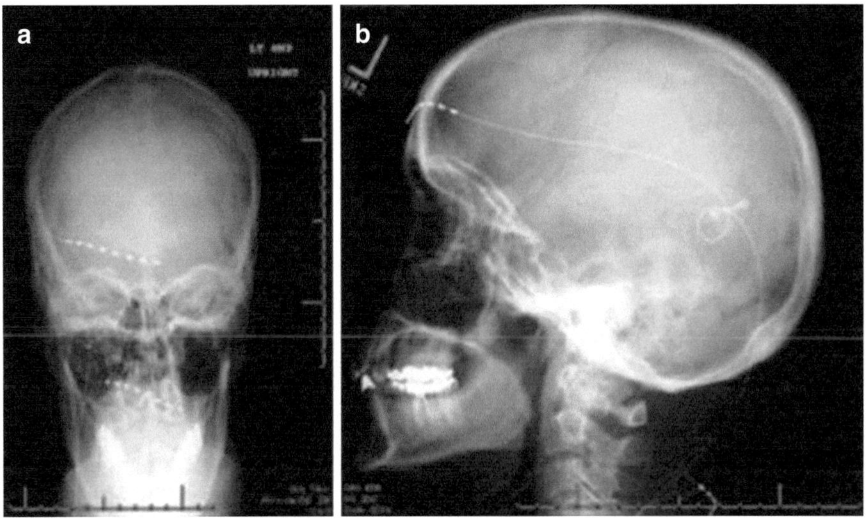

Fig. 23.4 (a) Postoperative A–P view X-ray of right-sided SONS and ONS. (b) Lateral view shows that the supraorbital lead is anchored to the skull with a dog bone-shaped titanium plate

made behind the neck medial to the scapula to connect extension cord as well as to create another strain relief loops to prevent leads from pulled out on flexion and extension of the neck and back.

Subsequent tunneling and battery implantations are the same as the ONS procedure.

Clinical Results in SONS Literature

There are limited data available regarding the efficacy of SONS for the treatment of headaches. Initial investigations in its use were predominantly for trigeminal autonomic cephalgias (TACs) given the predominant frontal localization of the pain [39]. Since then, many centers started to use combined SONS and ONS to cover holohemispheric pain and are now believed to have higher HA control rate with combined stimulation than SONS or ONS alone [6]. Table 23.5 summarizes the clinical studies published in recent years regarding the use of SONS for craniofacial pain.

In treating craniofacial pain, the variables that are predictive of the need for SONS in addition to ONS are unclear. The question of whether ONS can effectively ameliorate anterior pain was investigated in a study by Yancy et al. [40]. Thirty-three patients who had undergone implantation of unilateral or bilateral ONS leads for the treatment of medically resistant chronic craniofacial pain showed 26 patients with more than 50% improvement in pain severity. Of the responders, nine reported ONS was more effective for the posterior pain, while 15 considered ONS equally effective for both anterior and posterior pain. Therefore, while posterior pain was preferentially improved in one-third of patients, two-thirds experienced significant and equal relief of both anterior and posterior pain. The authors concluded that these results support a role for central inhibition of sensory trigeminal pathways from peripheral ONS.

Sphenopalatine Ganglion Stimulation

The sphenopalatine ganglion (SPG), which contains parasympathetic efferents destined for meningeal blood vessels, lacrimal gland, and nasal mucosa, has been implicated in the pathogenesis of the headache and cranial autonomic features associated with CH and other TACs. Cranial autonomic symptoms reflect activation of an increase outflow from parasympathetic efferents within the SPG. Since Sluder [46] first described the application of cocaine or alcohol to the SPG for treatment of headache, the SPG has been the target of a variety of surgical and nonsurgical interventions of the treatment of headaches, including percutaneous alcohol injection [47], lidocaine or corticosteroid application [48], radiofrequency lesioning [49], and neuromodulation [50].

In a recent review of SPG stimulation, Khan and colleagues [51] speculated that SPG stimulation may work by either interrupting SPG parasympathetic outflow by interfering with preganglionic superior salivatory nucleus to SPG efferents, or by interfering with postganglionic outflow, or by modulating the sensory processing in trigeminal nucleus caudalis (TNC) via slow neuromodulatory changes to the pain processing structures of the brain stem.

The SPG Microstimulator Device

Currently, a CE-marked SPG stimulator device from Autonomic Technologies™ is undergoing clinical trials in the USA for its efficacy in CH. The Pulsante microstimulator system provides a novel, non-systemic therapy designed to deliver patient controlled, real-time stimulation of the SPG. The microstimulator is a miniaturized implantable device including the device body, an integral lead with six stimulating electrodes, and an integral fixation plate (Fig. 23.5). The device is implanted such that the electrodes are positioned within the pterygopalatine fossa (PPF) on the side of the patients most prevalent CH, with the body positioned on the lateral posterior maxilla medial to the zygomatic arch and anchored to the zygomatic process of the maxilla using the fixation plate. The stimulator is inserted transorally using an incision to the outer gingiva, with the aid of custom surgical tools and intraoperative fluoroscopy. It is powered and controlled by a handheld rechargeable remote controller held to the patient's cheek [52].

Table 23.5 Clinical studies of SONS and combined SONS and ONS for craniofacial pain

Author	Types of HA	N	Mode of stimulation	Results	Complications
Slavin et al., 2006 [41]	Neuropathic craniofacial pain	30	SONS, ONS, and infraorbital stimulation	15 patients had either partial or complete pain relief and were satisfied	Three had reoperation due to migration or infection
Narouze et al., 2007 [42]	CCH	1	SONS only	Complete resolution of HA attacks after 2 months	None
Reed et al., 2010 [43]	CCH	7	Combined SONS and ONS	100% had >50% decreased severity	14% lead migration
Reed et al., 2011 [6, 44]	CM	44	Combined SONS and ONS	Frequency of HA decreased by 81% and 50% had near elimination of HA	Not reported
Hann et al., 2013 [6]	CM	14	Combined SONS and ONS	71% had >50% decrease in severity	Lead migration (42.8%), lead allodynia (21%)
Vaisman et al., 2014 [45]	TACs	5	SONS only	VAS decreased from 8.9 to 1.6 and 60% weaned off opiate use	Two lead migrations requiring surgery

Surgical Planning

A preoperative maxillofacial CT with 0.5–1.9 mm slice thickness is obtained to evaluate the patient's anatomy of the PPF and pterygomaxillary fissure (PMF). A minimum PMF width of 1.2 mm is required for surgical eligibility as the integral lead diameter of the neurostimulator is 1 mm. Dental or gum disease on ipsilateral side of the treatment may predispose implant infection and is also a contraindication for surgery.

Once surgical eligibility is established, custom surgical planning is performed with the assistance of the manufacturer, and a recommendation for microstimulator length and target positioning is provided based on patient-specific anatomy. Four lengths are available ranging from 3.6 to 6.0 cm. The stimulating electrode target location is the putative location of the SPG, typically located between the vidian canal and the foramen rotundum. Based on the preoperative thin cut CT, a 3D patient-specific anatomical rendering with digitally placed microstimulator is created (Fig. 23.6). A 2D representation is also created at the same time to be used for intraoperative direct comparison with the live fluoroscopic images.

1. *Surgical Steps*

   Step 1: Preoperative antibiotics appropriate for oral surgery, such as IV clindamycin, is given. Oral decontamination prior to surgery is necessary and should include both a mouth rinse with chlorhexidine solution (0.12% solution) and a scrub of the mucosa with iodine swabs.

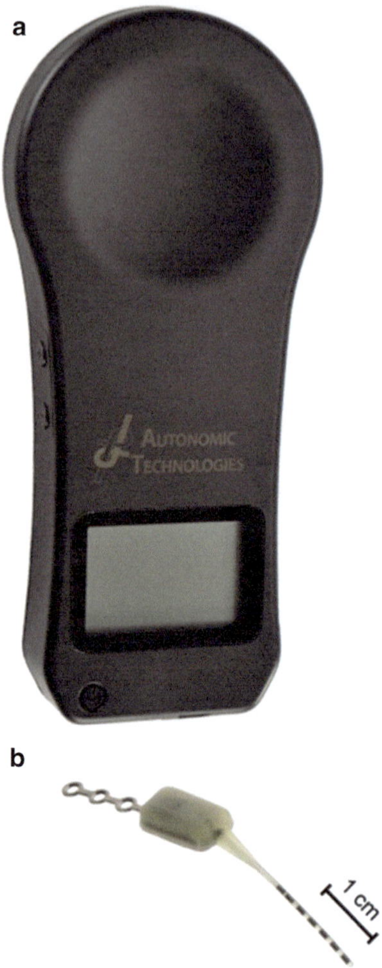

Fig. 23.5 (**a**) The handheld remote controller inductively powers and controls the microstimulator. (**b**) The insertable Pulsante microstimulator with six electrodes attached to a body (battery) with fixation plate

Step 2: The patient is placed under general anesthesia with the oral intubation tube positioned on the opposite side of the oral cavity. Nasal intubation is not recommended, as fluoroscopic images may be more difficult to assess. The patient is placed supine on a fluoroscopy compatible table with chin slightly elevated for easier access to the oral cavity.

Step 3: After injection of xylocaine 1% with 1:100,000 epinephrine, an incision of 2 cm is made in gingival crevice over the posterior maxillary buttress along the molars, leaving an inferior cuff of mucosa to allow suture closure. A limited subperiosteal tissue dissection of the lateral and posterior maxilla is then performed.

Step 4: After this initial subperiosteal elevation dissection, a procedure-specific curved subperiosteal elevator is used to continue the dissection and to identify

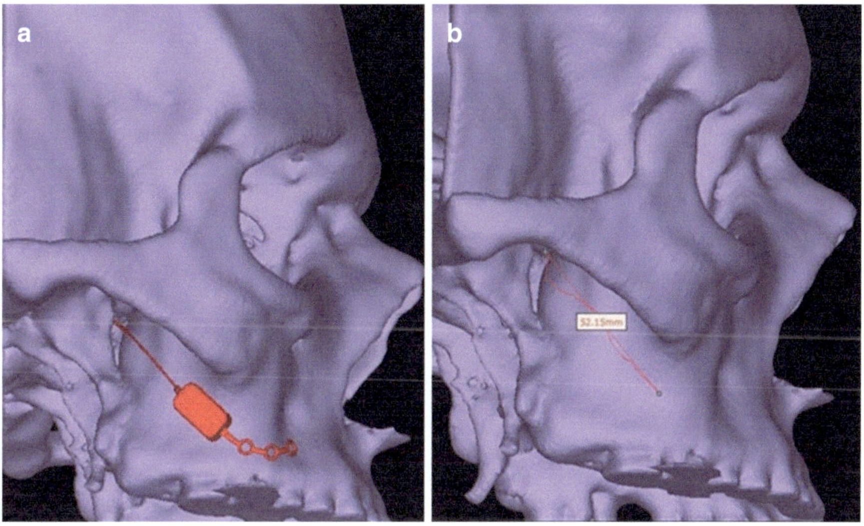

Fig. 23.6 (**a**) 3D reconstruction of thin cut facial bone CT demonstrating where the Pulsante microstimulator should be placed. (**b**) Demonstrates the measurement of the device size

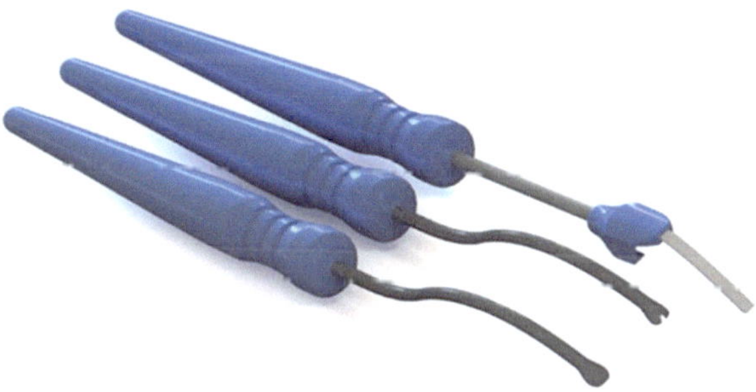

Fig. 23.7 Dissectors and introducers for the microstimulator. The two on the left are both subperiosteal dissectors specifically designed to create corridors to fit the electrodes. While the right one is used to place the microstimulator

the PMF. This instrument allows for blunt atraumatic subperiosteal dissection, while maintaining close contact to the posterior wall of the maxillary tuberosity to avoid trauma to the surrounding tissues. Periodic fluoroscopy image guidance is recommended to verify appropriate surgical introducer location.

Step 5: The dissection is completed once the instrument is positioned at the entrance to the PPF and aimed toward the superomedial aspect of the PPF. The device is then inserted with the aid of a shielded surgical introducer (Fig. 23.7). Prior to insertion, the fixation plate must be bent appropriately to the anatomy of the posterior lateral and zygomatic processes of the maxilla.

Step 6: The microstimulator is anchored to the maxilla using the most distal fixation plate hole using a standard craniofacial screw. Placement is confirmed with

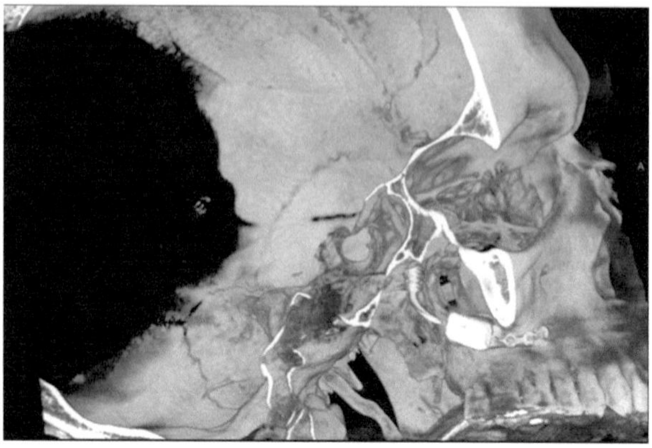

Fig. 23.8 Postoperative thin cut CT with 3D reconstruction demonstrating microstimulator being placed in sphenopalatine fossa

fluoroscopic images while comparing it with the preoperatively rendered 2D planning imaging. Electrode impedance testing should be performed to ensure proper functionality before closing wound with 4-0 resorbable sutures.

2. *Postoperative Care*
   Patent should avoid undue pressure to the surgical area, smoking, and gum chewing and maintain a soft diet and proper oral hygiene. Any postoperative wound infections should be treated by surgical wound debridement, possible removal of the implant, and antibiotics as appropriate.
   On the first postoperative day, a thin cut facial bone CT should be taken to confirm proper placement of the microstimulator (Fig. 23.8). If location revision is needed, the microstimulator should be removed and replaced within the first days after the initial procedure to achieve ideal placement.

Clinical Results in the SPG Stimulation Literature

A small, open-label study using Pulsante microstimulator system indicated that this modality may be effective in patients with chronic CH [53]. SPG stimulation resulted in complete resolution of headache in 11 of 18 CH attacks with partial improvement (>50% improvement in VAS) in three others. Pain relief was noted within several minutes of stimulation. SPG stimulation has also been attempted in ten migraine patients during attacks triggered by alcohol and odors [50]; but unfortunately, one patient responded to sham stimulation, making it difficult to interpret the response. Two patients had complete pain relief within 3 min of SPG stimulation, three had reduction in pain, and five had no response. As in the CH study, accurate placement of the stimulation needle and electrode was the most important predictor of clinical success.

In a recent multicenter randomized, sham-controlled study [54] performed in Europe, 32 CH patients were implanted with the Pulsante microstimulator system.

Twenty-eight patients completed the study, and 67.1% of the attacks treated with full stimulation resulted in pain relief compared to 7.4% of sham-treated attacks ($p < 0.0001$). In addition, 36% of patients experienced a ≥50% decrease in attack frequency. Overall, 68% of patients experienced a clinically significant improvement during the study by achieving pain relief of at least 50% in intensity and 50% reduction in attack frequency.

In the USA, a multicenter randomized, sham-controlled, prospective study to evaluate the use of an implanted SPG neurostimulator for the treatment of migraine headache intensity, symptoms, and frequency in chronic migraineurs (NCT01540799) is active but no longer recruiting. In addition, a US multicenter randomized sham-controlled study evaluating an implanted SPG neurostimulator for the treatment of CH is currently recruiting subjects (NCT02168764).

Vagal Nerve Stimulation

Stimulation of the vagus nerve (VNS) has received increasing interest as a treatment for head and face pain, primarily for migraine and cluster headaches. VNS was first approved by FDA in 1997 for partial-onset seizures refractory to antiepileptic medications. Subsequently, it was approved as a therapy for medically refractory depression in 2005. Thus far, in several case series in epilepsy and depression cohorts, chronic use of implanted VNS was associated with headache relief. In early 2000, Kirchner et al. and Sadler et al. each reported a case where headache improved significantly following VNS implantation [55, 56]. However, the evidence thus far is sparse, retrospective, and mainly derived from patients who had undergone placement of a vagal nerve stimulator treatment of refractory epilepsy.

A new preclinical investigation of VNS on an animal model of trigeminal pain (pretreated with dural noxious inflammatory soups) showed that a single dose of VNS (1–2 s of electrical stimulation directly applied to a dissected vagal nerve of an anesthetized rat) suppressed ongoing spontaneous and noxious dural-evoked trigeminocervical neuronal firing. Two doses of VNS (second stimulation given 3 min after the first one) also suppressed superior salivatory nucleus-evoked trigeminocervical neuronal responses. VNS had no effect on normal somatosensory cutaneous facial responses throughout [57]. This study provides a mechanistic rationale for the observed benefits of VNS in the abortive treatment of trigeminal pain and primary headaches.

Given the concern for surgical risks associated with VNS implantation, evaluation of the nociceptive benefit of chronic VNS in headache sufferers has been undertaken with noninvasive VNS (nVNS). In three retrospective studies of nVNS with small numbers of patients, at least 50% reported a substantial (>50%) reduction in migraine frequency after at least 6 months of stimulation [58, 59]. Table 23.6 summarizes the recent results of nVNS for craniofacial pain in RCTs and cases series.

Noninvasive VNS has been studied in several primary headache disorders. To date, most headache-related nVNS clinical studies utilized the transcervical VNS

Table 23.6 Clinical study of nVNS for headaches

Author	Type of HA	Type of study	N	Result
Silberstein et al., 2017 ACT1 study [62]	CH	RCT	133	No significant difference for nVNS and sham for primary endpoint of being pain-free at 15 min after treatment. However, on subgroup analysis, episodic CH patients had significantly higher response rate in nVNS group
Silberstein et al., 2017 the EVENT study [63]	CM	RCT	59	No significant difference between the reduction in HA days per month during blind phase (−1.4 days for stim group and −0.2 days for sham group), but during open-label phase, nVNS resulted in −7.9 HA after 8 months of treatment
Nesbitt et al., 2015 [61]	CH	Case series	19	Among 11 chronic and 8 episodic cluster patients, 15 reported overall improvements (47% had complete resolution of pain within 11 min of stimulation)
Goadsby et al., 2014 [60]	Acute migraine	Case series	30	80 acute migraine attacks were treated with 90-s session of nVNS. 22% of moderate to severe attacks were aborted at assessment 2 h after stimulation

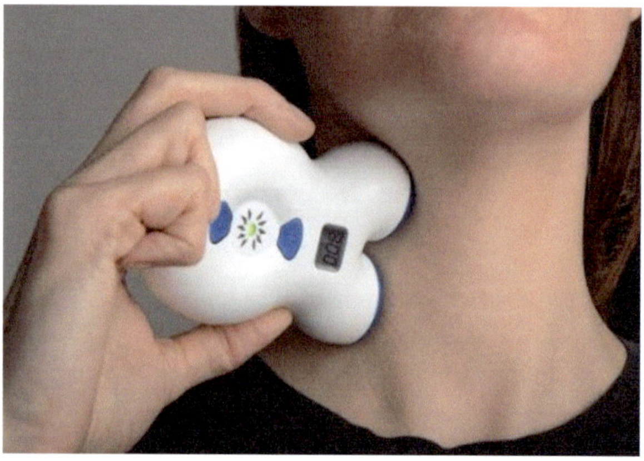

Fig. 23.9 gammaCore® percutaneous VNS system in use over the cervical vagal nerve

device from gammaCore® (Fig. 23.9). gammaCore is the first nVNS therapy applied at the neck for acute treatment of CH approved by the FDA in 2017.

In one of the first open-label, single-arm studies evaluating the efficacy and safety of an nVNS for the acute treatment of migraine with and without aura, 27 subjects were treated for 80 painful migraine attacks with two 90-s doses, at 15-min intervals; stimulation was delivered to the right cervical branch of the vagus nerve. Minor adverse events were reported in 13 patients, including neck twitching, hoarseness of voice, and redness at the device site. No unanticipated serious or severe adverse events were reported. For the first moderate to severe migraine attack treated (total of 19), the pain-free rate assessed at 2 h after the stimulation was 21% (4 out of 19). For all the moderate to severe attacks treated (total of 54), the pain-free rate at 2 h after stimulation was 22% (23 out of 54) [60].

External vagal nerve stimulation was also reported as being effective in an open-label, observational cohort study [61] in 19 CH patients (11 chronic, 8 episodic). Fifteen patients reported an overall improvement in their condition. Of all attacks treated, 47% were terminated within an average of 11 min of commencing stimulation. Ten patients reduced their acute use of high flow oxygen by 55%, and nine patients reduced triptan use by 48%. Prophylactic use of the device resulted in a substantial reduction in estimated mean attack frequency from 4.5/24 h to 2.6/24 h ($p < 0.0005$) posttreatment.

Most recently, Silberstein et al. have published a double-blinded RCT for episodic and chronic CH known as the ACT1 study involving 133 patients which have failed to observe significant difference between the stimulation and sham group for the primary endpoint of being pain-free at 15 min after stimulation (26.7% of nVNS and 15.1% of sham; $P = 0.1$). However, in their subgroup analysis breaking down to episodic and chronic cohorts, episodic CH patients had significantly higher proportions of improvement over the sham group (nVNS, 34.2%; sham, 10.6%; $P = 0.008$). Authors concluded that this is a promising treatment for patients with episodic CH with no significant adverse effect [62].

In a separate prospective, multicenter, double-blind, sham-controlled study, Silberstein et al. investigated the use of nVNS on preventing attacks of CM (the *Event* study). In it, 59 patients were studied during the blind phase (2 months) and found that there was no difference in the reduction in HA days between the stimulation and sham group (−1.4 in nVNS and −0.2 in sham; $\Delta = 1.2$; $p = 0.56$). However, in the following open-label phase (8 months), when all were placed in stimulation group, the HA day reduction was −7.9 days per month, suggesting potential prophylactic benefit in persistent use [63].

Early studies demonstrated the potential of invasive VNS and nVNS in the management of distinct types of headache disorders. VNS may be effective for both acute and prophylactic treatment of headache [61, 64]. As with other forms of neuromodulation, chronic use of VNS seems to be associated with a better outcome, which improves over time [65]. Nevertheless, a clearly effective double-blinded, sham-controlled study that has a strongly positive primary endpoint for various types of headache is still needed. With a good safety profile and the strong suggestion of efficacy in previous trials, nVNS may constitute an effective headache and facial pain treatment.

Conclusion

Over the past decade, the evidence that PNS may be effective for the acute and preventative management of head and facial pain disorders has accumulated from investigators around the world. The response to the initial efficacy reports has been measured, and the results of observational studies from different investigators have been very similar. Sham-controlled studies that have been performed for ONS show early promise.

The ability to blind several of these modalities has proven to be uniquely challenging, as has finding sensitive outcome measures that capture the improvements seen at the bedside, particularly in the most highly disabled and medically intractable patient populations. In addition adverse events—especially lead migration, battery failure, and infection—were relatively high in early studies. Nevertheless, continuing developments and more robustly designed randomized controlled trials are underway.

Cost and surgical risk will likely continue to be concerns for PNS modalities used to treat chronic pain. Noninvasive PNS such as nVNS will have advantage in adoptability by general public due to low cost and low adverse event from the therapy. Cost-effectiveness studies will be necessary if pivotal phase III studies confirm the efficacy and long-term safety of implantable neurostimulation devices.

For patients who are disabled and suffer intensely and have failed to respond to conventional and evidence-based pharmacologic and non-drug therapies, the emergence of PNS offers hope for a safe and effective long-term strategy to reduce the suffering associated with intractable headache and craniofacial pain.

References

1. Wall PD, Sweet WH. Temporary abolition of pain in man. Science (New York, NY). 1967;155:108–9.
2. Weiner RL, Reed KL. Peripheral neurostimulation for control of intractable occipital neuralgia. Neuromodulation. 1999;2:217–21.
3. Petersen EA, Slavin KV. Peripheral nerve/field stimulation for chronic pain. Neurosurg Clin N Am. 2014;25:789–97.
4. Deogaonkar M, Machado AG, Sharan A. Pain management, an issue of neurosurgery clinics of North America, E-Book. Philadelphia, PA: Elsevier; 2014.
5. Levy RM. Differentiating the leaves from the branches in the tree of neuromodulation: the state of peripheral nerve field stimulation. Neuromodulation. 2011;14:201–5.
6. Hann S, Sharan A. Dual occipital and supraorbital nerve stimulation for chronic migraine: a single-center experience, review of literature, and surgical considerations. Neurosurg Focus. 2013;35:E9.
7. Goadsby PJ, Bartsch T, Dodick DW. Occipital nerve stimulation for headache: mechanisms and efficacy. Headache. 2008;48:313–8.
8. Melzack R, Wall PD. Evolution of pain theories. Int Anesthesiol Clin. 1970;8:3–34.
9. Kapural L, Mekhail N, Hayek SM, Stanton-Hicks M, Malak O. Occipital nerve electrical stimulation via the midline approach and subcutaneous surgical leads for treatment of severe occipital neuralgia: a pilot study. Anesth Analg. 2005;101:171–4, table of contents.
10. Schwedt TJ, Dodick DW, Hentz J, Trentman TL, Zimmerman RS. Occipital nerve stimulation for chronic headache—long-term safety and efficacy. Cephalalgia. 2007;27:153–7.
11. Schwedt TJ, Dodick DW, Trentman TL, Zimmerman RS. Occipital nerve stimulation for chronic cluster headache and hemicrania continua: pain relief and persistence of autonomic features. Cephalalgia. 2006;26:1025–7.
12. Burns B, Watkins L, Goadsby PJ. Treatment of medically intractable cluster headache by occipital nerve stimulation: long-term follow-up of eight patients. Lancet (London, England). 2007;369:1099–106.

13. Magis D, Allena M, Bolla M, De Pasqua V, Remacle JM, Schoenen J. Occipital nerve stimulation for drug-resistant chronic cluster headache: a prospective pilot study. Lancet Neurol. 2007;6:314–21.
14. Rodrigo-Royo MD, Azcona JM, Quero J, Lorente MC, Acin P, Azcona J. Peripheral neurostimulation in the management of cervicogenic headache: four case reports. Neuromodulation. 2005;8:241–8.
15. Melvin EA Jr, Jordan FR, Weiner RL, Primm D. Using peripheral stimulation to reduce the pain of C2-mediated occipital headaches: a preliminary report. Pain Physician. 2007;10:453–60.
16. Ghaemi K, Capelle HH, Kinfe TM, Krauss JK. Occipital nerve stimulation for refractory occipital pain after occipitocervical fusion: expanding indications. Stereotact Funct Neurosurg. 2008;86:391–3.
17. Skaribas I, Alo K. Ultrasound imaging and occipital nerve stimulation. Neuromodulation. 2010;13:126–30.
18. Kinfe TM, Schu S, Quack FJ, Wille C, Vesper J. Percutaneous implanted paddle lead for spinal cord stimulation: technical considerations and long-term follow-up. Neuromodulation. 2012;15:402–7.
19. Hayek SM, Levy R, Deer TR, editors. Neurostimulation for the treatment of chronic pain. Philadelphia, PA: Elsevier/Saunders; 2012.
20. Hayek SM, Jasper JF, Deer TR, Narouze SN. Occipital neurostimulation-induced muscle spasms: implications for lead placement. Pain Physician. 2009;12:867–76.
21. Falowski S, Wang D, Sabesan A, Sharan A. Occipital nerve stimulator systems: review of complications and surgical techniques. Neuromodulation. 2010;13:121–5.
22. Eldabe S, Buchser E, Duarte RV. Complications of spinal cord stimulation and peripheral nerve stimulation techniques: a review of the literature. Pain Med (Malden, Mass). 2016;17:325–36.
23. Schwedt TJ, Green AL, Dodick DW. Occipital nerve stimulation for migraine: update from recent multicenter trials. Prog Neurol Surg. 2015;29:117–26.
24. Sweet JA, Mitchell LS, Narouze S, et al. Occipital nerve stimulation for the treatment of patients with medically refractory occipital neuralgia: congress of neurological surgeons systematic review and evidence-based guideline. Neurosurgery. 2015;77:332–41.
25. Oh MY, Ortega J, Bellotte JB, Whiting DM, Alo K. Peripheral nerve stimulation for the treatment of occipital neuralgia and transformed migraine using a c1-2-3 subcutaneous paddle style electrode: a technical report. Neuromodulation. 2004;7:103–12.
26. Slavin KV, Nersesyan H, Wess C. Peripheral neurostimulation for treatment of intractable occipital neuralgia. Neurosurgery. 2006;58:112–9; discussion 112–9.
27. Johnstone CS, Sundaraj R. Occipital nerve stimulation for the treatment of occipital neuralgia-eight case studies. Neuromodulation. 2006;9:41–7.
28. Magown P, Garcia R, Beauprie I, Mendez IM. Occipital nerve stimulation for intractable occipital neuralgia: an open surgical technique. Clin Neurosurg. 2009;56:119–24.
29. Palmisani S, Al-Kaisy A, Arcioni R, et al. A six year retrospective review of occipital nerve stimulation practice—controversies and challenges of an emerging technique for treating refractory headache syndromes. J Headache Pain. 2013;14:67.
30. Abhinav K, Park ND, Prakash SK, Love-Jones S, Patel NK. Novel use of narrow paddle electrodes for occipital nerve stimulation—technical note. Neuromodulation. 2013;16:607–9.
31. Popeney CA, Alo KM. Peripheral neurostimulation for the treatment of chronic, disabling transformed migraine. Headache. 2003;43:369–75.
32. Matharu MS, Bartsch T, Ward N, Frackowiak RS, Weiner R, Goadsby PJ. Central neuromodulation in chronic migraine patients with suboccipital stimulators: a PET study. Brain. 2004;127:220–30.
33. Saper JR, Dodick DW, Silberstein SD, McCarville S, Sun M, Goadsby PJ. Occipital nerve stimulation for the treatment of intractable chronic migraine headache: ONSTIM feasibility study. Cephalalgia. 2011;31:271–85.
34. Silberstein SD, Dodick DW, Saper J, et al. Safety and efficacy of peripheral nerve stimulation of the occipital nerves for the management of chronic migraine: results from a randomized, multicenter, double-blinded, controlled study. Cephalalgia. 2012;32:1165–79.

35. Lipton RGP, Cady R, et al. PRISM study: occipital nerve stimulation for treatment-refractory migraine. Cephalalgia. 2009;29(Suppl. 1):S30.
36. Lainez M. Clinical benefits of early triptan therapy for migraine. Cephalalgia. 2004;24(Suppl 2):24–30.
37. Fontaine D, Christophe Sol J, Raoul S, et al. Treatment of refractory chronic cluster headache by chronic occipital nerve stimulation. Cephalalgia. 2011;31:1101–5.
38. Mueller O, Diener HC, Dammann P, et al. Occipital nerve stimulation for intractable chronic cluster headache or migraine: a critical analysis of direct treatment costs and complications. Cephalalgia. 2013;33:1283–91.
39. Goldberg SW, Nahas SJ. Supratrochlear and supraorbital nerve stimulation for chronic headache: a review. Curr Pain Headache Rep. 2015;19:26.
40. Yancy HM, Trentman TL, Dodick DW. The effect of occipital nerve stimulation on anterior pain in primary headache disorders. Headache. 2013;52(5):897–8.
41. Slavin KV, Colpan ME, Munawar N, Wess C, Nersesyan H. Trigeminal and occipital peripheral nerve stimulation for craniofacial pain: a single-institution experience and review of the literature. Neurosurg Focus. 2006;21:E5.
42. Narouze SN, Kapural L. Supraorbital nerve electric stimulation for the treatment of intractable chronic cluster headache: a case report. Headache. 2007;47:1100–2.
43. Reed KL, Black SB, Banta CJ 2nd, Will KR. Combined occipital and supraorbital neurostimulation for the treatment of chronic migraine headaches: initial experience. Cephalalgia. 2010;30:260–71.
44. Reed KL, Will KR, Chapman J, Richter E. Combined occipital and supraoprbital neurostimulation for chronic migraine headaches: an extended case serise (abstract). Berlin, Germany: Cephalgia; 2011. p. 98–9.
45. Vaisman J, Lopez E, Muraoka NK. Supraorbital and supratrochlear stimulation for trigeminal autonomic cephalalgias. Curr Pain Headache Rep. 2014;18:409.
46. Sluder G. The role of the sphenopalatine (or Meckle's) ganglion in nasal headaches. N Y Med J. 1908:989–90.
47. Devoghel JC. Cluster headache and sphenopalatine block. Acta Anaesthesiol Belg. 1981;32:101–7.
48. Kudrow L, Kudrow DB, Sandweiss JH. Rapid and sustained relief of migraine attacks with intranasal lidocaine: preliminary findings. Headache. 1995;35:79–82.
49. Narouze S, Kapural L, Casanova J, Mekhail N. Sphenopalatine ganglion radiofrequency ablation for the management of chronic cluster headache. Headache. 2009;49:571–7.
50. Tepper SJ, Rezai A, Narouze S, Steiner C, Mohajer P, Ansarinia M. Acute treatment of intractable migraine with sphenopalatine ganglion electrical stimulation. Headache. 2009;49:983–9.
51. Khan S, Schoenen J, Ashina M. Sphenopalatine ganglion neuromodulation in migraine: what is the rationale? Cephalalgia. 2014;34:382–91.
52. Assaf AT, Hillerup S, Rostgaard J, et al. Technical and surgical aspects of the sphenopalatine ganglion (SPG) microstimulator insertion procedure. Int J Oral Maxillofac Surg. 2016;45:245–54.
53. Ansarinia M, Rezai A, Tepper SJ, et al. Electrical stimulation of sphenopalatine ganglion for acute treatment of cluster headaches. Headache. 2010;50:1164–74.
54. Schoenen J, Jensen RH, Lanteri-Minet M, et al. Stimulation of the sphenopalatine ganglion (SPG) for cluster headache treatment. Pathway CH-1: a randomized, sham-controlled study. Cephalalgia. 2013;33:816–30.
55. Kirchner A, Birklein F, Stefan H, Handwerker HO. Left vagus nerve stimulation suppresses experimentally induced pain. Neurology. 2000;55:1167–71.
56. Sadler RM, Purdy RA, Rahey S. Vagal nerve stimulation aborts migraine in patient with intractable epilepsy. Cephalalgia. 2002;22:482–4.
57. Akerman S, Simon B, Romero-Reyes M. Vagus nerve stimulation suppresses acute noxious activation of trigeminocervical neurons in animal models of primary headache. Neurobiol Dis. 2017;102:96–104.

58. Lenaerts ME, Oommen KJ, Couch JR, Skaggs V. Can vagus nerve stimulation help migraine? Cephalalgia. 2008;28:392–5.
59. Mauskop A. Vagus nerve stimulation relieves chronic refractory migraine and cluster headaches. Cephalalgia. 2005;25:82–6.
60. Goadsby PJ, Grosberg BM, Mauskop A, Cady R, Simmons KA. Effect of noninvasive vagus nerve stimulation on acute migraine: an open-label pilot study. Cephalalgia. 2014;34:986–93.
61. Nesbitt AD, Marin JC, Tompkins E, Ruttledge MH, Goadsby PJ. Initial use of a novel noninvasive vagus nerve stimulator for cluster headache treatment. Neurology. 2015;84:1249–53.
62. Silberstein SD, Mechtler LL, Kudrow DB, et al. Non-invasive vagus nerve stimulation for the acute treatment of cluster headache: findings from the randomized, double-blind, sham-controlled ACT1 study. Headache. 2016;56:1317–32.
63. Silberstein SD, Calhoun AH, Lipton RB, et al. Chronic migraine headache prevention with noninvasive vagus nerve stimulation: the EVENT study. Neurology. 2016;87:529–38.
64. Gaul C, Magis D, Liebler E, Straube A. Effects of non-invasive vagus nerve stimulation on attack frequency over time and expanded response rates in patients with chronic cluster headache: a post hoc analysis of the randomised, controlled PREVA study. J Headache Pain. 2017;18:22.
65. Kinfe TM, Pintea B, Muhammad S, et al. Cervical non-invasive vagus nerve stimulation (nVNS) for preventive and acute treatment of episodic and chronic migraine and migraine-associated sleep disturbance: a prospective observational cohort study. J Headache Pain. 2015;16:101.

Chapter 24
Neuromodulation for Trigeminal Autonomic Cephalalgias

Tsinsue Chen, Manjit Matharu, and Ludvic Zrinzo

Introduction

Trigeminal autonomic cephalalgias (TAC) refer to a group of strictly unilateral primary headache syndromes with cranial autonomic features and include cluster headache (CH), short lasting unilateral neuralgiform headaches with autonomic symptoms (SUNHA), paroxysmal hemicrania and hemicrania continua; SUNHA is further subdivided into short-lasting unilateral neuralgiform headache attacks with conjunctival injection and tearing (SUNCT) and short-lasting unilateral neuralgiform headache attacks with cranial autonomic features (SUNA). These syndromes are thought to be caused by dysfunction in the pain matrix involving the hypothalamic region and trigeminocervical complex as well as the trigemino-parasympathetic

T. Chen
Victor Horsley Department of Neurosurgery, National Hospital of Neurology and Neurosurgery, London, UK

Division of Neurosurgery, Barrow Neurological Institute, St. Joseph's Hospital and Medical Center, Phoenix, AR, USA
e-mail: tsinsue.chen@barrowbrainandspine.com

M. Matharu
Department of Neurology, National Hospital of Neurology and Neurosurgery, London, UK

UCL Institute of Neurology and The National Hospital for Neurology and Neurosurgery, Headache Group, London, UK
e-mail: m.matharu@uclmail.net

L. Zrinzo (✉)
Victor Horsley Department of Neurosurgery, National Hospital of Neurology and Neurosurgery, London, UK

Unit of Functional Neurosurgery, Department of Movement Disorders, UCL Institute of Neurology, University College London, London, UK
e-mail: l.zrinzo@ucl.ac.uk

J. Y. Suen, E. Petersen (eds.), *Diagnosis and Management of Head and Face Pain*, https://doi.org/10.1007/978-3-319-90999-8_24

reflex. Peripheral neuromodulation methods target the trigeminocervical complex and the trigemino-parasympathetic reflex via extracranial stimulation of the occipital nerve or sphenopalatine ganglion, respectively, while the central neurostimulation methods target the posterior hypothalamic region and spinal dorsal columns via deep brain stimulation and spinal cord stimulation [1, 2].

Peripheral Neuromodulation Techniques

Sphenopalatine Ganglion Stimulation and Lesioning

Mechanism and Use of SPG stimulation

The sphenopalatine ganglion (SPG) lies in the pterygopalatine fossa and receives trigeminal sensory inputs as well as cranial parasympathetic outflow from the superior salivary nucleus. Meningeal vessels and facial structures are innervated by post-ganglionic SPG fibres, and neurotransmitters released by these fibres activate trigeminal nociceptors and thus the trigeminal system. This positively feeds back on the parasympathetic outflow and forms the trigemino-parasympathetic reflex [3]. Modulation of the SPG via stimulation or lesioning of the SPG via radiofrequency ablation is thought to work by disrupting this trigemino-parasympathetic reflex. Acute attacks are terminated by a direct effect on the trigeminal inflow and/or parasympathetic output, and attack prevention may be mediated by changes in neurotransmitter production over time [4].

Sphenopalatine ganglion stimulation involves implanting a small neurostimulator device into the pterygopalatine fossa via a small transoral incision through the gum above the upper premolar teeth, overlying the maxilla. The stimulator delivers an electrical current by induction from a remote held over the cheek by the patient in both abortive and preventive contexts. After the procedure, the patient is initially evaluated every 1–2 weeks to ensure that optimal stimulation settings result in comfortable soft palate paraesthesias. At the initiation of an attack, the patient activates the device by placing the remote on the cheek over the implant and stimulates for a least 15 min. If the attack persists, stimulation is turned off and rescue medication used. The device can also be used prophylactically by stimulating for 15 min one to two times per week. Ongoing studies are currently assessing the optimal regimen for both abortive and preventive control [4].

Evidence for SPG Stimulation and Lesioning

Recently, a multicentre trial of 28 chronic cluster headache (CCH) patients treated with SPG stimulation demonstrated a significant difference in number of attacks reported as showing pain relief at 15 min between stimulation and sham groups (67.1% vs. 7.3%, $p < 0.0001$) as well as number of attacks reported as demonstrating pain freedom at 15 min between the stimulation vs. sham groups (34.1% vs. 1.6%, $p < 0.0001$). After 2 months of therapy, acute rescue medications were only being used in 31% of cluster attacks in the stimulation group vs. 77.4% of CH attacks in the sham group ($p < 0.0001$). Complications encountered included infection (6%), lead misplacement or migration (15%) and transient sensory deficits in the maxillary nerve distribution (81%) [5].

In a recent series of 33 CCH patients treated with SPG stimulation, Barloese et al. reported ten patients (30%) who experienced at least one remission period lasting at least 1 month, with an average remission period of 134 ± 86 days. All ten patients were taking triptans preoperatively, and at 24 months post-operatively, 60% were not using triptans and 30% were not using any acute medications [6]. To our knowledge, there have been no reports of SPG stimulation for the treatment of TACs other than cluster headache.

Expert consensus published in 2014 recommended SPG stimulation for patients with unilateral chronic cluster headache who have failed all medical therapies. The device may be especially effective in patients with a high number of daily attacks and those who are nonresponsive to or cannot tolerate triptans [7]. Given its minimally invasive nature and potential to serve as both a preventive and abortive treatment, SPG stimulation may be considered as a possible first-line option for medically refractory CH patients. The device does, however, require patient cooperation to turn it on and off during acute attacks, and this must be emphasized since clinical improvement may only occur after weeks or months of stimulation.

Various lesioning methods of the SPG including Gamma Knife, anaesthetic blocks and alcohol injections have been explored as treatment options for TACs [8]. In 1997, Sanders et al. reported 30% complete relief in 10 chronic cluster headache patients and 60.7% complete relief in 56 episodic cluster headache patients undergoing radiofrequency (RF) lesioning [9]. Narouze's group subsequently reported a 48.8% average reduction in attack frequency at 18-month follow-up in 15 patients undergoing percutaneous RF ablation for chronic cluster headache. In this series, approximately 50% of patients (7 of 15) reported transient paraesthesias in the upper cheek and gums, which resolved by 3–6 weeks post-procedure. One patient experienced permanent loss of sensation over the cheek area [10]. Recently, Bendersky et al. reported a failed initial attempt at pain relief with pulsed radiofrequency in three CCH patients; however, after continuous radiofrequency ablation was used, all patients became pain-free through 8–11 months follow-up [11].

Occipital Nerve Stimulation (ONS)

Mechanism and Clinical Use of ONS

Occipital nerve stimulation (ONS) has been used to treat medically refractory chronic cluster headache and involves implanting one or two electrodes at the craniocervical junction to stimulate the greater occipital nerve [12, 13]. Electrodes are connected to an internal pulse generator, typically in the subclavicular area. After implantation, the neurostimulator is programmed to achieve tolerable levels of paraesthesia in the greater occipital nerve distribution and used as a preventive therapy for TACs. Implantation of bilateral leads is recommended given the reports of conversion from unilateral to bilateral symptoms after initiating unilateral stimulation. Symptom improvement may not be seen for up to 3 months post-implantation; however, there is unlikely to be clinical benefit after 1 year of clinical unresponsiveness [4].

While the exact mechanism of occipital nerve stimulation for trigeminal autonomic cephalalgias is unclear, it likely involves non-specific modulatory effects on descending pain-control systems. Although the paraesthesia induced by stimulation follows the occipital nerve distribution, the therapeutic goal is to mimic the "extra-occipital" effects that were initially seen in glucocorticoid injection studies for primary headache prevention [14–16]. Early animal studies demonstrated anatomical convergence of somatic, cervical and trigeminovascular afferents on trigeminocervical complex nociceptors [17, 18], which serve as an important relay for head and facial pain to higher centres of pain processing in the thalamus, hypothalamus and brainstem. These animal studies were later supported by fluorodeoxyglucose positron emission tomography (FDG-PET) imaging in drug-resistant cluster headache patients who were treated with occipital nerve stimulation. Hypermetabolism in several pain areas normalized after 3–6 months of stimulation, whereas hypermetabolism in the untreated ipsilateral hypothalamus remained unchanged [19].

Evidence for ONS

To date, outcomes on 199 patients undergoing ONS for chronic cluster headache have been published in ten major studies, with reported efficacies ranging from 52.9 to 100% [12, 13, 19–26]. In these studies, a positive therapeutic response was defined as patients who have achieved ≥50% improvement in headache attack frequency and/or severity compared to baseline. Recently, Fontaine et al. reported a 59% responder rate in 44 CCH patients being treated with ONS at 12 months [23]; Miller et al. demonstrated a response rate of 52.9% in 51 CCH patients with mean follow-up of 39.2 months (range, 2–81) [25], and Leone's group reported 66.7% response rate in 35 CCH patients with a median follow-up of 6.1 years (range, 1.6–10.7) [24].

Reports of ONS for the treatment of SUNHA and hemicrania continua are limited to smaller case series. In 2007, Schwedt et al. reported near resolution of pain at 3 months in a hemicrania continua patient treated with ONS [27]. One year later, Burns et al. reported a 66.7% response rate in six hemicrania continua patients after 6–21 months of microstimulation of the occipital nerve using the Bion device [28]. Recently, Lambru et al. reported an 89% response rate (eight of nine patients) at a median follow-up of 38 months (range, 24–55) in three SUNA and six SUNCT patients treated with ONS. Four of these patients became pain-free, and the remaining four had >80% improvement [29]. Adverse events encountered can include electrode migration (18.8%), hardware malfunction (9.4%) [24], hardware erosion through the skin (3.9%) and infection (2%) [25].

Central Neuromodulation Techniques

Cervical Spinal Cord Stimulation (SCS)

Mechanism and Use of SCS

Application of high cervical spinal cord stimulation (SCS) to treat trigeminal autonomic cephalalgias is based on clinical data from studies using spinal cord stimulation to treat other chronic pain conditions, in particular chronic back pain [30–32]. In animal spinal cord models, afferent nociceptive inputs have been found to be inhibited by modulating a wide range of neuronal activity. For example, in chronic pain states, wide dynamic range (WDR) neurons are frequently hyperactive. Preclinical models have demonstrated that stimulation of these neurons at high frequency results in desensitization and decreased neuronal output, subsequently restoring them closer to their preinjury condition [30].

Operative Technique

SCS implantation for TACs is similar to the techniques used for chronic back pain. Patients initially undergo a test stimulation phase for 7–14 days, where either one or two octad leads are placed in the epidural space. Fluoroscopy is used to determine the appropriate entry point on the skin, based on accessing the upper thoracic spine (usually the T2–3 interspace). After local anaesthetic is injected, a small incision is made under conscious sedation. Using fluoroscopic guidance, a 14-gauge Tuohy needle is inserted into the T2–T3 interspace and advanced cranially into the dorsal epidural space. Epidural placement is confirmed using a saline probe with loss of resistance technique.

Electrode(s) are advanced cranially in the dorsal epidural space until the distal lead tip reaches the area between the occiput and the C2 vertebral body. For normal frequency stimulation, intraoperative test stimulation is performed to confirm the presence of ipsilateral paraesthesia over the neck, occipital, parietal and frontal scalp areas as well as the facial areas encompassing the C2 root sensory supply and V1–V2 trigeminal division. Test stimulation is not performed for high-frequency, paraesthesia-free stimulation systems.

Leads are anchored by suturing them to the supraspinal ligament, and temporary extensions are connected and tunnelled under the skin surface. The extensions are then connected to an external stimulator during the trial period. High-frequency stimulation targets the dorsal columns at the C2–C3 level, with parameters performed at 10 kHZ frequency, 30 μs pulse width and 1.4–4 mA. If test stimulation is successful, permanent extensions and an internal pulse generator are implanted, typically in the gluteal region [2, 33].

Evidence for SCS

Two small series evaluating SCS for treatment of TACs both involve high-frequency, paraesthesia-free stimulation at 10 Kz and low-frequency stimulation with induced paraesthesia (Table 24.1). Wolter et al. treated seven medication-resistant chronic cluster headache patients with low-frequency SCS and followed them for a mean of 23 months (range, 3–78). Continuous stimulation was used in all cases but one, where intermittent stimulation was used. Stimulation settings were as follows: frequency, 40–110 Hz; pulse width, 100–500 μs; and amplitude, 2.0–25.5 mA. Six patients (85.7%) achieved at least 50% or more reduction in attack frequency and/or intensity, and one patient achieved pain freedom. Baseline mean frequency of attacks decreased from 6 attacks/day to 1.4 attacks/day. Five patients (71.4%) were able to discontinue triptan use, and the remaining two were able to reduce triptan dosages. Four patients were completely medication free. All seven patients state they would recommend the treatment to other patients, and six of seven would undergo the procedure again if given the option. Adverse events included one lead fracture requiring revision and two lead migrations requiring revision [33].

Table 24.1 Major studies of high cervical spinal cord stimulation for the treatment of medication-resistant trigeminal autonomic cephalalgias

Study	Diagnosis	No. of patients implanted (*n*)	Follow-up: average months	Pain-free patients (*n*)	Improvement of at least 50% in intensity and/ or frequency	Medication-free at follow-up	Adverse events
Wolter, 2011 [33]	Cluster headache	7	23 (3–78)	1	5	4	Dislocated lead requiring revision [2], lead fracture requiring revision [1]
Lambru, 2016 [2]	SUNA	2	35	1	1	1	None
	Cluster headache	1	11	0	0	0	Lead migration requiring revision

SUNA short-lasting unilateral neuralgiform headache attacks with autonomic symptoms

Recently, Lambru et al. treated four chronic migraine, two SUNA and one chronic cluster headache patient with high-frequency SCS. Average follow-up was 25.3 months (range, 12–40), and continuous stimulation was used in all cases. Of the two SUNA patients, one reported near complete pain resolution at 42 months, and the other reported 70% improvement at 28 months follow-up and has discontinued preventive medications. The one cluster headache patient treated reported 50% improvement in attacks at 9 months [2].

Deep Brain Stimulation (DBS)

Mechanism and Use of DBS

Initial functional neuroimaging studies in chronic cluster headache patients demonstrated activation of the ipsilateral posterior hypothalamic area during acute cluster headache attacks [34]. This led to the first successful DBS electrode implantation for TAC in a chronic cluster headache patient in 2001, with lead placement in the ipsilateral posterior inferior hypothalamic area. The patient experienced complete resolution of symptoms within 48 h of initiating stimulation and remained pain-free at 13-month follow-up [35]. Since then, there have been over 100 patients implanted with DBS for the treatment of TACs (Table 24.2), with the majority being treated for cluster headache [36–47], and a few small series and case reports of DBS for SUNCT, SUNA and paroxysmal hemicrania continua [48–52]. The target used in DBS for TACs was initially called "the posterior hypothalamus"; however, the area between the mammillothalamic tract and red nucleus is more accurately referred to as the ventral tegmental area [53].

After implantation, stimulators are programmed at 60 μs, 180–185 Hz, and the voltage is titrated based on clinical benefit and side effect profiles. The stimulation is delivered chronically, and patients are not typically given adjustable parameters, as it is sometimes done during therapy for movement disorders such as Parkinson's disease or essential tremor. Patients are usually evaluated more frequently in the initial 2–3 months. Similar to occipital nerve stimulation, if there has been no improvement after 6–12 months of stimulation, it is unlikely that stimulation will provide any clinical benefit [4].

Potential DBS candidates should be evaluated at a specialized DBS centre by a multidisciplinary team consisting of neurologists, neurosurgeons and a neuropsychologist. In large-volume DBS centres, overall risks of the procedure can be as lower than 1% for intracranial haemorrhage [54–56] and 2% for hardware infection [55, 57]. Other potential complications include seizure, hardware discomfort and hardware failure. Seizures are rare and typically transient, occurring only in the immediate post-operative period. Transient side effects associated with stimulation in the hypothalamic and ventral tegmental area may include vertical diplopia, dizziness, vertigo and emotional disturbances (i.e. panic, anxiety) [47, 58].

Table 24.2 Major studies of deep brain stimulation for the treatment of medication-resistant trigeminal autonomic cephalalgias

Study	Patients (*n*)	Follow-up (months): average (range, if available)	Pain-free patients (*n*)	Improvement of at least 50% in intensity and/or frequency	No. of patients who are medication-free at follow-up	Surgical or device-related adverse events
Cluster headache						
Leone, 2001 [35]	1	13	1 (100%)	0	NR	NR
Franzini, 2003 [36]	5	10.2 (2–22)	5 (100%)	0	2	None
Schoenen, 2005 [5]	6	14.5 ± 1.5 (12–17)	2	1	NR	Fatal intracranial haemorrhage [1], aborted procedure due to intraoperative panic attack [1]
Leone, 2006 [38]	16	23 (1–52)	10	0	13	Asymptomatic ventricular haemorrhage [1]
Starr, 2007 [39]	4	12	0	2	0	Transient ischemic attack 5 min after intraoperative stimulation [1]
Owen, 2007 [40]	1	8	1	0	NR	None
Bartsch, 2008 [41]	6	17 (9–24)	2	1	1	Hardware discomfort over connection cable requiring revision [1]
Bartsch, 2009 [42]	2	48	0	0		None
Fontaine, 2010 [44]	11	12 (12)	3	3	2	Subcutaneous infection requiring hardware removal [1]
Hiding, 2011 [43]	1	NR	0	0	0	Constant dull headache, high-frequency tremor [1]

Seijo, 2011 [45]	5	2.8	2	3	1	Breakage of intracranial electrode requiring replacement [1]
Akram, 2016 [47]	21	18 (4–60)	0	11	0	Superficial infection resolved with antibiotics [1]
Chabardes, 2016 [46]	7	12	2	3	NR	None
SUNCT/SUNA						
Leone, 2005 [49]	1	17	1	0	0	None
Lyons, 2009 [50]	1	12	0	1	0	None
Bartsch, 2011 [48]	1	15	0	1	0	NR
Miller, 2016 [51]	11	Median 29 (7–63)	0	9	4	IPG "flipping" in the chest pocket requiring surgical repositioning [1], wound infection requiring hardware removal [1], wound dehiscence without infection [1]
Paroxysmal hemicrania						
Walcott, 2009 [52]	1	27	1	0	1	None

SUNCT short-lasting unilateral neuralgiform headache attacks with conjunctival injection and tearing, *SUNA* short-lasting unilateral neuralgiform headache attacks with autonomic symptoms, *NR* not reported

Operative Technique

DBS leads can be implanted with myriad stereotactic techniques and utilizing magnetic resonance imaging (MRI)-guided techniques or MRI-computerized tomography (CT) fusion. Most studies for TACs use frame-based (Leksell) stereotaxy with intraoperative microelectrode recording and test stimulation. Many centres target the posterior hypothalamus using atlas coordinates based on the midcommisural point (MCP). Target location varied between 2–6 mm posterior to the MCP, 0–2 mm lateral to the MCP and 1–3 mm below the midcommissural plane. The procedure is performed under conscious sedation, and the electrode is introduced in a rigid cannula, 10 mm to target. Intraoperative test stimulation is performed typically at 60 μs, 180 or 185 Hz. Side effects seen with higher-voltage macrostimulation of the posterior hypothalamus include diplopia, subjective mood changes (i.e. feelings of anxiety, fear and/or panic), vertigo and changes in blood pressure or pulse rate [35–42, 44, 45].

Our institution has adopted a MRI-guided, MRI-verified approach, without microelectrode recording, utilizing frame-based stereotaxy (Leksell frame model G) under general anaesthesia. This technique has been previously published for other DBS targets used in movement disorders [59, 60] and was used in our recent reports of chronic cluster headache and SUNA patients treated with ventral tegmental area (VTA) DBS. The most distal contact on the Medtronic 3389 lead is placed in the ventral tegmental area, which is visualized on a 1.5T T2-weighted axial MRI sequence at a level immediately superior to the mammillary bodies, anteromedial to the red nucleus and posterolateral to the mammillothalamic tract (Fig. 24.1). An immediate post-implantation stereotactic iMRI is obtained for patients without

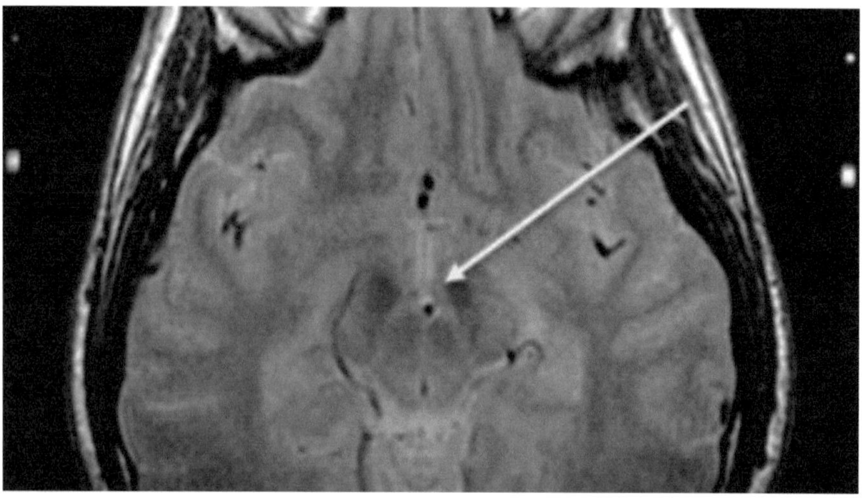

Fig. 24.1 An axial T2-weighted 1.5T MRI through the midbrain following right ventral tegmental area DBS. The lead artefact can be seen in between the hypointense red nucleus and mammillothalamic tract

ONS implants to confirm lead positioning (Fig. 24.1), and a stereotactic computerized tomography scan (CT) is obtained for patients with existing ONS hardware. Internal pulse generators are implanted in the infraclavicular area either in the same procedure or within a week after surgery [47].

Evidence for DBS

There have been 18 published studies (excluding abstracts) on 101 patients undergoing DBS for TAC, with the majority of patients being treated for chronic cluster headache (13 studies, 86 patients), followed by those with SUNCT or SUNA (4 studies, 14 patients) and paroxysmal hemicrania (1 case report) (Table 24.2). Amongst the 86 chronic cluster headache patients treated, there was a 60.5% response rate ($n = 52$) at 2.8–60-month follow-up, and 32.6% of patients ($n = 28$) achieved a pain freedom [35–47]. Amongst the SUNCT and SUNA patients, there was an 85.7% response rate ($n = 11$) at 7–63-month follow-up, and 7.1% ($n = 1$) achieved pain freedom [48–51]. There has only been one case report of a patient with paroxysmal hemicrania continua being treated with posterior hypothalamic DBS who achieved pain freedom after 27 months [52].

The only placebo-controlled trial for DBS was a multicentre study led by Fontaine and colleagues, randomizing 11 chronic cluster headache patients to receive active versus sham stimulation over a 1-month period. There were no differences in primary and secondary outcome measures during the blinded sham versus active stimulation phase. However, this may have been related to the relatively short duration of the randomized phase, given that it is now established that 3–6 months may be needed to develop a response to DBS. After an additional 10 months of open label stimulation in all patients, 54.5% ($n = 6$) achieved >50% improvement in frequency of attacks, and three of these patients were pain-free [44].

Our institution recently published the two largest prospective open-label series of patients treated with ventral tegmental deep brain stimulation for chronic cluster headache ($n = 21$) and SUNHA ($n = 11$). In the CCH study, at median follow-up of 18 months (range, 4–60), 76% of patients had at least a 50% reduction in headache load (a composite score accounting for severity, frequency and attack duration). Overall headache frequency improved significantly by 60%, headache severity improved by 30%, and headache load improved by 68%. Seventy-six percent of patients had at least a 50% reduction in headache load. Significant improvements were also observed in quality of life, disability and mood scales. There were four nonresponders (19%), of which three had also previously failed ONS treatment [47]. In the SUNHA study, at median follow-up of 29 months (range, 7–63), 82% of patients ($n = 9$) demonstrated a positive response. Overall, there was a 78% reduction in median attack frequency and 99% median reduction in headache load. The median time to achieve 50% clinical improvement was 1 month (range, 1–2 months) [51].

Summary

Neuromodulation for TACs includes stimulation of both peripheral and central targets and should be considered in patients who have failed all conservative therapies. Our centre recommends SPG stimulation or ONS as initial therapeutic options in compliant patients. Given that SPG stimulation is a minimally invasive implantation technique and can be used in both an abortive and preventive therapy, it is an attractive first-line therapy in CCH patients. Though used only as a preventive therapy, ONS can also be considered given its low risk of adverse events and well-established efficacy. Should peripheral neuromodulation strategies fail or be contraindicated, central neuromodulation methods can be considered. The response rates of DBS thus far appear comparable to ONS, though the therapy is associated with slightly different risks, albeit low, given the intracranial nature of the procedure. DBS can be considered as an alternative therapy for those who have failed SPG and/or ONS or those in whom peripheral modulation is contraindicated. High cervical spinal cord stimulation has recently emerged as an alternate central modulation technique although current evidence is limited to small case series, and larger cohort and randomized placebo-controlled trials will be needed. Thorough patient evaluation by a multidisciplinary team at a specialist centre is necessary to determine the most appropriate treatment modality for the unique symptoms and clinical needs of each individual patient.

References

1. Magis D, Schoenen J. Advances and challenges in neurostimulation for headaches. Lancet Neurol. 2012;11(8):708–19.
2. Lambru G, Trimboli M, Palmisani S, Smith T, Al-Kaisy A. Safety and efficacy of cervical 10 kHz spinal cord stimulation in chronic refractory primary headaches: a retrospective case series. J Headache Pain. 2016;17(1):66.
3. May A, Goadsby PJ. The trigeminovascular system in humans: pathophysiologic implications for primary headache syndromes of the neural influences on the cerebral circulation. J Cereb Blood Flow Metab. 1999;19(2):115–27.
4. Miller S, Sinclair AJ, Davies B, Matharu M. Neurostimulation in the treatment of primary headaches. Pract Neurol. 2016;16(5):362–75.
5. Schoenen J, Jensen RH, Lanteri-Minet M, Lainez MJ, Gaul C, Goodman AM, et al. Stimulation of the sphenopalatine ganglion (SPG) for cluster headache treatment. Pathway CH-1: a randomized, sham-controlled study. Cephalalgia. 2013;33(10):816–30.
6. Barloese MC, Jurgens TP, May A, Lainez JM, Schoenen J, Gaul C, et al. Cluster headache attack remission with sphenopalatine ganglion stimulation: experiences in chronic cluster headache patients through 24 months. J Headache Pain. 2016;17(1):67.
7. Jurgens TP, Schoenen J, Rostgaard J, Hillerup S, Lainez MJ, Assaf AT, et al. Stimulation of the sphenopalatine ganglion in intractable cluster headache: expert consensus on patient selection and standards of care. Cephalalgia. 2014;34(13):1100–10.
8. Devoghel JC. Cluster headache and sphenopalatine block. Acta Anaesthesiol Belg. 1981;32(1):101–7.
9. Sanders M, Zuurmond WW. Efficacy of sphenopalatine ganglion blockade in 66 patients suffering from cluster headache: a 12- to 70-month follow-up evaluation. J Neurosurg. 1997;87(6):876–80.

10. Narouze S, Kapural L, Casanova J, Mekhail N. Sphenopalatine ganglion radiofrequency ablation for the management of chronic cluster headache. Headache. 2009;49(4):571–7.
11. Bendersky DC, Hem SM, Yampolsky CG. Unsuccessful pulsed radiofrequency of the sphenopalatine ganglion in patients with chronic cluster headache and subsequent successful thermocoagulation. Pain Pract. 2015;15(5):E40–5.
12. Burns B, Watkins L, Goadsby PJ. Treatment of medically intractable cluster headache by occipital nerve stimulation: long-term follow-up of eight patients. Lancet. 2007;369(9567):1099–106.
13. Magis D, Allena M, Bolla M, De Pasqua V, Remacle JM, Schoenen J. Occipital nerve stimulation for drug-resistant chronic cluster headache: a prospective pilot study. Lancet Neurol. 2007;6(4):314–21.
14. Afridi SK, Shields KG, Bhola R, Goadsby PJ. Greater occipital nerve injection in primary headache syndromes—prolonged effects from a single injection. Pain. 2006;122(1–2):126–9.
15. Ambrosini A, Vandenheede M, Rossi P, Aloj F, Sauli E, Pierelli F, et al. Suboccipital injection with a mixture of rapid- and long-acting steroids in cluster headache: a double-blind placebo-controlled study. Pain. 2005;118(1–2):92–6.
16. Anthony M. Headache and the greater occipital nerve. Clin Neurol Neurosurg. 1992;94(4):297–301.
17. Bartsch T, Goadsby PJ. Stimulation of the greater occipital nerve induces increased central excitability of dural afferent input. Brain. 2002;125(Pt 7):1496–509.
18. Bartsch T, Goadsby PJ. Increased responses in trigeminocervical nociceptive neurons to cervical input after stimulation of the dura mater. Brain. 2003;126(Pt 8):1801–13.
19. Magis D, Bruno MA, Fumal A, Gerardy PY, Hustinx R, Laureys S, et al. Central modulation in cluster headache patients treated with occipital nerve stimulation: an FDG-PET study. BMC Neurol. 2011;11:25.
20. Burns B, Watkins L, Goadsby PJ. Treatment of intractable chronic cluster headache by occipital nerve stimulation in 14 patients. Neurology. 2009;72(4):341–5.
21. de Quintana-Schmidt C, Casajuana-Garreta E, Molet-Teixido J, Garcia-Bach M, Roig C, Clavel-Laria P, et al. Stimulation of the occipital nerve in the treatment of drug-resistant cluster headache. Rev Neurol. 2010;51(1):19–26.
22. Fontaine D, Christophe Sol J, Raoul S, Fabre N, Geraud G, Magne C, et al. Treatment of refractory chronic cluster headache by chronic occipital nerve stimulation. Cephalalgia. 2011;31(10):1101–5.
23. Fontaine D, Blond S, Lucas C, Regis J, Donnet A, Derrey S, et al. Occipital nerve stimulation improves the quality of life in medically-intractable chronic cluster headache: Results of an observational prospective study. Cephalalgia. 2017;37(12):1173–9.
24. Leone M, Proietti Cecchini A, Messina G, Franzini A. Long-term occipital nerve stimulation for drug-resistant chronic cluster headache. Cephalalgia. 2017;37(8):756–63.
25. Miller S, Watkins L, Matharu M. Treatment of intractable chronic cluster headache by occipital nerve stimulation: a cohort of 51 patients. Eur J Neurol. 2017;24(2):381–90.
26. Mueller O, Diener HC, Dammann P, Rabe K, Hagel V, Sure U, et al. Occipital nerve stimulation for intractable chronic cluster headache or migraine: a critical analysis of direct treatment costs and complications. Cephalalgia. 2013;33(16):1283–91.
27. Schwedt TJ, Dodick DW, Hentz J, Trentman TL, Zimmerman RS. Occipital nerve stimulation for chronic headache—long-term safety and efficacy. Cephalalgia. 2007;27(2):153–7.
28. Burns B, Watkins L, Goadsby PJ. Treatment of hemicrania continua by occipital nerve stimulation with a bion device: long-term follow-up of a crossover study. Lancet Neurol. 2008;7(11):1001–12.
29. Lambru G, Shanahan P, Watkins L, Matharu MS. Occipital nerve stimulation in the treatment of medically intractable SUNCT and SUNA. Pain Physician. 2014;17(1):29–41.
30. Van Buyten JP, Al-Kaisy A, Smet I, Palmisani S, Smith T. High-frequency spinal cord stimulation for the treatment of chronic back pain patients: results of a prospective multicenter European clinical study. Neuromodulation. 2013;16(1):59–65; discussion 65–6.
31. Al-Kaisy A, Van Buyten JP, Smet I, Palmisani S, Pang D, Smith T. Sustained effectiveness of 10 kHz high-frequency spinal cord stimulation for patients with chronic, low back pain: 24-month results of a prospective multicenter study. Pain Med. 2014;15(3):347–54.

32. Al-Kaisy A, Palmisani S, Smith T, Harris S, Pang D. The use of 10-kilohertz spinal cord stimulation in a cohort of patients with chronic neuropathic limb pain refractory to medical management. Neuromodulation. 2015;18(1):18–23.
33. Wolter T, Kiemen A, Kaube H. High cervical spinal cord stimulation for chronic cluster headache. Cephalalgia. 2011;31(11):1170–80.
34. May A, Bahra A, Buchel C, Frackowiak RS, Goadsby PJ. Hypothalamic activation in cluster headache attacks. Lancet. 1998;352(9124):275–8.
35. Leone M, Franzini A, Bussone G. Stereotactic stimulation of posterior hypothalamic gray matter in a patient with intractable cluster headache. N Engl J Med. 2001;345(19):1428–9.
36. Franzini A, Ferroli P, Leone M, Broggi G. Stimulation of the posterior hypothalamus for treatment of chronic intractable cluster headaches: first reported series. Neurosurgery. 2003;52(5):1095–9; discussion 9–101.
37. Schoenen J, Di Clemente L, Vandenheede M, Fumal A, De Pasqua V, Mouchamps M, et al. Hypothalamic stimulation in chronic cluster headache: a pilot study of efficacy and mode of action. Brain. 2005;128(Pt 4):940–7.
38. Leone M, Franzini A, Broggi G, Bussone G. Hypothalamic stimulation for intractable cluster headache: long-term experience. Neurology. 2006;67(1):150–2.
39. Starr PA, Barbaro NM, Raskin NH, Ostrem JL. Chronic stimulation of the posterior hypothalamic region for cluster headache: technique and 1-year results in four patients. J Neurosurg. 2007;106(6):999–1005.
40. Owen SL, Green AL, Davies P, Stein JF, Aziz TZ, Behrens T, et al. Connectivity of an effective hypothalamic surgical target for cluster headache. J Clin Neurosci. 2007;14(10):955–60.
41. Bartsch T, Pinsker MO, Rasche D, Kinfe T, Hertel F, Diener HC, et al. Hypothalamic deep brain stimulation for cluster headache: experience from a new multicase series. Cephalalgia. 2008;28(3):285–95.
42. Bartsch T, Paemeleire K, Goadsby PJ. Neurostimulation approaches to primary headache disorders. Curr Opin Neurol. 2009;22(3):262–8.
43. Hidding U, May A. Mere surgery will not cure cluster headache—implications for neurostimulation. Cephalalgia. 2011;31(1):112–5.
44. Fontaine D, Lazorthes Y, Mertens P, Blond S, Geraud G, Fabre N, et al. Safety and efficacy of deep brain stimulation in refractory cluster headache: a randomized placebo-controlled double-blind trial followed by a 1-year open extension. J Headache Pain. 2010;11(1):23–31.
45. Seijo F, Saiz A, Lozano B, Santamarta E, Alvarez-Vega M, Seijo E, et al. Neuromodulation of the posterolateral hypothalamus for the treatment of chronic refractory cluster headache: experience in five patients with a modified anatomical target. Cephalalgia. 2011;31(16):1634–41.
46. Chabardes S, Carron R, Seigneuret E, Torres N, Goetz L, Krainik A, et al. Endoventricular deep brain stimulation of the third ventricle: proof of concept and application to cluster headache. Neurosurgery. 2016;79(6):806–15.
47. Akram H, Miller S, Lagrata S, Hyam J, Jahanshahi M, Hariz M, et al. Ventral tegmental area deep brain stimulation for refractory chronic cluster headache. Neurology. 2016;86(18):1676–82.
48. Bartsch T, Falk D, Knudsen K, Reese R, Raethjen J, Mehdorn HM, et al. Deep brain stimulation of the posterior hypothalamic area in intractable short-lasting unilateral neuralgiform headache with conjunctival injection and tearing (SUNCT). Cephalalgia. 2011;31(13):1405–8.
49. Leone M, Franzini A, D'Andrea G, Broggi G, Casucci G, Bussone G. Deep brain stimulation to relieve drug-resistant SUNCT. Ann Neurol. 2005;57(6):924–7.
50. Lyons MK, Dodick DW, Evidente VG. Responsiveness of short-lasting unilateral neuralgiform headache with conjunctival injection and tearing to hypothalamic deep brain stimulation. J Neurosurg. 2009;110(2):279–81.
51. Miller S, Akram H, Lagrata S, Hariz M, Zrinzo L, Matharu M. Ventral tegmental area deep brain stimulation in refractory short-lasting unilateral neuralgiform headache attacks. Brain. 2016;139(Pt 10):2631–40.
52. Walcott BP, Bamber NI, Anderson DE. Successful treatment of chronic paroxysmal hemicrania with posterior hypothalamic stimulation: technical case report. Neurosurgery. 2009;65(5):E997; discussion E.

53. Matharu MS, Zrinzo L. Deep brain stimulation in cluster headache: hypothalamus or midbrain tegmentum? Curr Pain Headache Rep. 2010;14(2):151–9.
54. Zrinzo L, Foltynie T, Limousin P, Hariz MI. Reducing hemorrhagic complications in functional neurosurgery: a large case series and systematic literature review. J Neurosurg. 2012;116(1):84–94.
55. Chen T, Mirzadeh Z, Chapple K, Lambert M, Ponce FA. Complication rates, lengths of stay, and readmission rates in "awake" and "asleep" deep brain simulation. J Neurosurg. 2017;127(2):360–9.
56. Fenoy AJ, Simpson RK Jr. Risks of common complications in deep brain stimulation surgery: management and avoidance. J Neurosurg. 2014;120(1):132–9.
57. Patel DM, Walker HC, Brooks R, Omar N, Ditty B, Guthrie BL. Adverse events associated with deep brain stimulation for movement disorders: analysis of 510 consecutive cases. Neurosurgery. 2015;11(Suppl 2):190–9.
58. Leone M, Franzini A, Cecchini AP, Bussone G. Efficacy of hypothalamic stimulation for chronic drug-resistant cluster headache. Cephalalgia. 2012;32(4):267–8.
59. Holl EM, Petersen EA, Foltynie T, Martinez-Torres I, Limousin P, Hariz MI, et al. Improving targeting in image-guided frame-based deep brain stimulation. Neurosurgery. 2010;67(2 Suppl Operative):437–47.
60. Foltynie T, Zrinzo L, Martinez-Torres I, Tripoliti E, Petersen E, Holl E, et al. MRI-guided STN DBS in Parkinson's disease without microelectrode recording: efficacy and safety. J Neurol Neurosurg Psychiatry. 2011;82(4):358–63.

Part IV
Representative Clinical Cases

Chapter 25
Clinical Case of Type I Trigeminal Neuritis

James Y. Suen and John Diaz Day

Representative Case

J. W. is a 29-year-old white male with sudden onset of pain in his right jaw over a year ago. The pain is severe, electric-like, and intermittent. It can be triggered by eating or talking. When the pain is intense, he cannot stay still and cries in agony (Fig. 25.1). The pain has been so severe that he lost his job and had to quit college. He had tried on anticonvulsants, tricyclic antidepressants, and pain medications, which helped slightly but did not control his pain. A brain MRI at an outside facility was said to be normal. He was referred by his neurologist to Dr. Suen for other suggestions.

Overview

Trigeminal neuritis can be divided into the classic type I or atypical trigeminal neuritis. Type I TN is a condition where an artery is adjacent to the trigeminal nerve as it exits the pons and pulsates against the nerve which stimulates it and causes severe pain [1]. To diagnose type I trigeminal neuritis, a special MRI scan which focuses

J. Y. Suen (✉)
Department of Otolaryngology—Head and Neck Surgery, University of Arkansas for Medical Sciences, Little Rock, AR, USA
e-mail: suenjamesy@uams.edu

J. D. Day
Department of Neurosurgery, University of Arkansas for Medical Sciences, Little Rock, AR, USA
e-mail: jdday@uams.edu

J. Y. Suen, E. Petersen (eds.), *Diagnosis and Management of Head and Face Pain*, https://doi.org/10.1007/978-3-319-90999-8_25

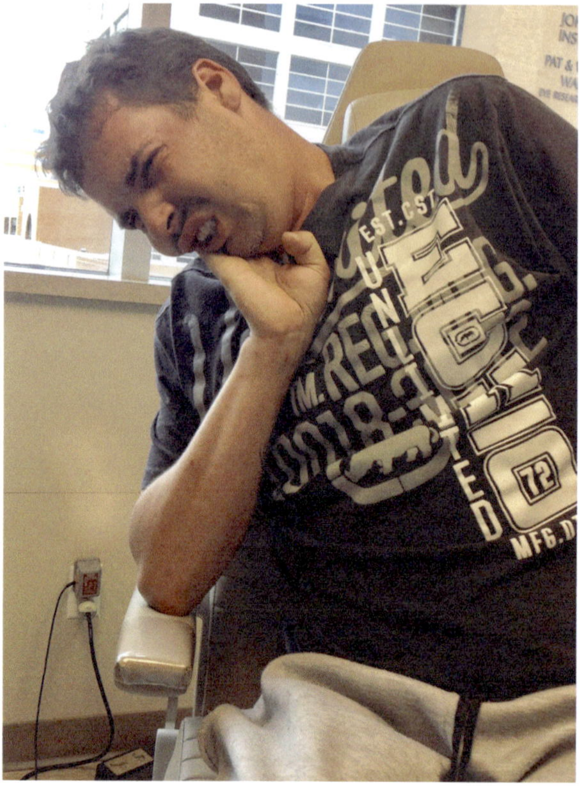

Fig. 25.1 Patient with severe, electric-like pain. Unable to stay still or talk

on the root of the nerve must be done and the artery must be looked for. This condition can be corrected with surgical decompression by placing a Teflon pad between the artery and nerve [2].

The most common branch of the trigeminal nerve involved in type I is the third division or mandibular division.

Representative Case Management

This patient presented with severe, electric-like pain which was intermittent and debilitating. Because he was not responding to medical management and his MRI was said to be normal, he was referred to Dr. Suen for consideration of nerve blocks. His history and exam pinpointed his pain to the third division of his trigeminal nerve. Diagnostic nerve blocks of his right inferior alveolar nerve where it enters the mandible on the medial surface of the ascending ramus of his mandible were performed using xylocaine and bupivacaine. He would get immediate relief, but the relief would only last about 1–2 days. Because the nerve blocks were not lasting long enough, an indwelling catheter was placed percutaneous, so that the tip of the catheter was adjacent to the inferior alveolar nerve where it enters the mandible. When the bupivacaine was injected, his pain would stop, and so the patient was instructed to give the bupivacaine through the catheter as needed.

The catheter would be effective for several weeks at a time, but because he had such severe pain when the anesthetic would wear off, we recommended another MRI scan to focus on the root of the trigeminal nerve. This MRI revealed an artery touching the trigeminal nerve at its origin, and the patient was referred for microvascular decompression. Postoperative relief of pain was rapid; when the patient awoke from his surgery, he stated the severe pain was gone. The patient has been followed for over 2 years with no further pain and is back working and was able to finish college.

Differential Diagnosis

- Dental infections can cause severe pain but is not usually electric-like nor intermittent.
- Sinus infection of the maxillary sinus usually has pain over the midface.
- Cervical plexus pain is frequently in the jaw and ear area.

Diagnostic Tests

- An MRI with special focus on the root of the trigeminal nerve must be performed to rule out type I trigeminal neuritis (see Chap. 6 on imaging). It is not uncommon for vascular compression of the trigeminal nerve to be missed on a "routine MRI."
- Dental evaluation with appropriate X-rays.
- A good history to rule out history of herpes zoster, trauma, or history of cancer.
- A good physical exam to rule out tumors or cancer.

Key Points

- The appropriate MRI scan must be performed to diagnose the vascular compression of the trigeminal nerve at its origin.
- If a previous MRI scan has been performed and said to be negative, but the pain is consistent with type I trigeminal neuritis, another scan should be considered.
- Even in the absence of imaging findings, classic clinical presentation may lead a surgeon to recommend microvascular decompression to good effect.
- Pain in the jaw area can be from the mandibular division of the trigeminal nerve or can be from the upper cervical plexus and must be differentiated.

References

1. Zakrzewska JM, McMillan R. Trigeminal neuralgia: the diagnosis and management of this excruciating and poorly understood facial pain. Postgrad Med J. 2011;87:410–6.
2. Chakravarthi PS, Ghanta R, Kattimani V. Microvascular decompression treatment for trigeminal neuralgia. J Craniofac Surg. 2011;22:894–8.

Chapter 26
Representative Clinical Cases: Atypical Trigeminal Neuralgia, Type 2

Byron Hills and Jonathan P. Miller

Representative Case History

The patient is a 44-year-old woman with a history of migraine headache presenting with a 3-year history of pain in the face, described as a primary constant, dull, burning ache with superimposed periods of sharp, electric shock-like sensation predominantly in the V1 distribution unilaterally. The patient states that although she experiences mostly pain in the face, there are also periods of intermittent hypesthesia. The pain is not triggerable by light touch but is made worse by showering, washing her hair, and brushing her teeth. Shortly after the pain started, she experienced pain-free intervals of up to a few weeks, but for the last year, it has been present constantly. There is no history of multiple sclerosis, facial trauma, herpes zoster, or previous surgical treatment for facial pain. Neurological examination is normal with intact cranial nerves, no evidence of facial sensory loss, and normal temporomandibular joint mobility. Carbamazepine is prescribed which produces moderate but incomplete relief. However, she continues to have severe pain.

B. Hills
Department of Neurosurgery, University Hospitals Cleveland Medical Center, University Heights, OH, USA
e-mail: Byron.hills@uhhospitals.org

J. P. Miller (✉)
Department of Neurological Surgery, University Hospitals Cleveland Medical Center, Case Western Reserve University, Cleveland, OH, USA
e-mail: jonathan.miller@uhhospitals.org

J. Y. Suen, E. Petersen (eds.), *Diagnosis and Management of Head and Face Pain*, https://doi.org/10.1007/978-3-319-90999-8_26

Overview

Trigeminal neuralgia (TN) is a specific type of chronic pain that affects the trigeminal nerve [1]. The condition can be very debilitating to patients, affecting every aspect of life. According to the Burchiel's classification, idiopathic trigeminal neuralgia can be categorized into two different classes, Type 1 and Type 2, based on whether lancinating or constant pain predominates [2]. Type 1, the classic and more common form, involves episodes of electrical shock-like sensations that usually lasts for only seconds with relatively mild or no pain between attacks. Type 2 TN involves primarily constant pain, although shock-like pain is sometimes superimposed. Both types can be further subdivided: Type 1a refers to exclusively lancinating pain with no pain whatsoever between attacks, Type 1b is mostly lancinating pain with minor constant pain, Type 2a is constant pain with superimposed lancinating pain, and Type 2b is constant pain only [3]. It is possible that the spectrum of pain from Type 1a to Type 2b represents a continuum from neuralgia to neuropathic pain [4]. Because of the constant nature of the pain, Type 2 TN is sometimes confused with other craniofacial pain syndromes, including headaches, disorders of the temporomandibular joint, or musculoskeletal disease. Common clinical characteristics of TN including trigger points, memorable onset, pain-free intervals, and antiepileptic response may be present in Type 2 TN but are more common in Type 1 [3]. Patients with Type 2 TN can experience altered facial sensation, are less likely to have a neurovascular compression, and are less likely to respond to both conservative and surgical treatments [5]. For example, type of TN is the single most important predictor of long-term outcome after microvascular decompression for trigeminal neuralgia. At 3 years postoperatively, approximately 2/3 of patients with Type 1 TN are pain-free off medications, compared with 1/3 of Type 2 TN patients, and the likelihood of excellent outcome is correlated with the amount of lancinating pain experienced by the patient [3].

Differential Diagnosis

Many facial pain syndromes can mimic Type 2 TN (Table 26.1). Non-neuropathic causes of facial pain include sinusitis, dental disease, orbital disease, facial trauma, cancer, temporal arteritis, cavernous sinus syndromes, and autonomic cephalalgias such as cluster headache, petrous apicitis, temporomandibular joint pathology, and primary headache syndromes such as migraine [1]. If there is a history of incidental or intentional injury to the trigeminal nerve, the pain syndrome is called trigeminal neuropathic pain or trigeminal deafferentation pain, respectively. TN in the presence of multiple sclerosis is called symptomatic trigeminal neuralgia, and neuropathic pain after herpes zoster is called postherpetic neuralgia. Finally, pain that is confirmed by psychological testing to be psychogenic in origin is called atypical facial pain [1].

Table 26.1 Common causes of facial pain

Extraoral	
Headache	Tension headache, cluster headache, migraines
Musculoskeletal	TMJ disorders
Neuropathic	TGN, posttraumatic trigeminal pain, glossopharyngeal neuralgia, postherpetic neuralgia
Vascular	Giant cell arteritis, malignancy
Atypical	Persistent idiopathic facial pain
Oral	
Dental	Caries, pulpitis, periapical disease, cracked tooth, alveolar osteitis, periodontal disease
Non-dental	Salivary gland disorders, sinusitis, cancer, mucosal disorders, atypical odontalgia

Diagnostic Work-Up

A detailed clinical history is essential for accurate diagnosis of Type 2 TN. It is important to determine the distribution and the characteristics of the pain including chronicity, aggravating or alleviating factors, and efficacy of conservative management options [6]. A thorough physical examination should be performed to access for facial tenderness, scarring from previous surgeries in the region of interest, basic dental exam, and detailed cranial nerve exam. MR imaging should also be performed to rule out other causes of pain such as tumors, vascular malformations, or multiple sclerosis. In addition, high-resolution balanced fast-field echo sequences can allow for assessment of neurovascular compression of the trigeminal nerve [5].

Treatment Options

As with all pain syndromes, a trial of nonsurgical treatment should be attempted prior to consideration of surgery (Table 26.2). A substantial proportion of patients with Type 2 TN will experience pain relief using antiepileptic medication such as carbamazepine. Medically intractable patients with Type 2 TN and neurovascular compression often improve with microvascular decompression, with 32% of patients having complete resolution of pain and 68% exhibiting substantial improvement [3]. Rhizolysis techniques such as radio frequency, glycerol injection, balloon compression, stereotactic radiosurgery, or open internal neurolysis can be effective if there is no evidence of neuropathic pain. Finally, neuromodulation approaches such as trigeminal nerve stimulation, motor cortex stimulation, and high cervical intrathecal drug delivery have been used with some success in refractory cases [1].

Table 26.2 Conservative therapies for trigeminal neuralgia

Drug	Class	Major side effects
First line		
Carbamazepine	Anticonvulsant	Aplastic anemia, SIADH, CYP450 inducer
Oxcarbazepine	Anticonvulsant	Skin rash (potentially fatal)
Second line		
Lamotrigine	Anticonvulsant	Skin rash (potentially fatal)
Baclofen	Muscle relaxant	Drowsiness, respiratory depression

Case Management

This patient had a 3-year history of constant, aching, burning pain in the V1 distribution with occasional lancinating electrical shock-like pain that is less severe than the constant pain. She is diagnosed with Type 2a TN. MRI showed neurovascular compression of a branch of the SCA into the root entry zone of the trigeminal nerve. Treatment options were discussed with the patient, and she elected to proceed with microvascular decompression. After the procedure, she experienced substantial relief. At 3 years after the operation, she has occasional pain that is well controlled using a small dose of gabapentin.

Alternative Management Options

- Conservative management including pain medications, especially antiepileptic agents
- Microvascular decompression in cases of vascular compression of the trigeminal nerve on imaging and no response to conservative therapy
- Neuromodulation approaches including neurostimulators or intrathecal pumps
- Rhizolysis procedures including internal neurolysis, radio frequency, glycerol injection, balloon compression, and stereotactic radiosurgery

Key Points

- Type 2 trigeminal neuralgia refers to idiopathic neuropathic facial pain syndrome that involves primarily constant rather than intermittent lancinating pain.
- A careful assessment of clinical history and physical examination is essential for accurate diagnosis of Type 2 TN.
- MRI is needed to rule out any other lesions causing facial pain.
- Conservative therapy with medications is the initial treatment option.
- Surgical results for Type 2 TN patients are inferior to those with Type 1 TN. In patients with Type 2 TN undergoing MVD, 1/3 will experience complete relief, 1/3 incomplete relief, and 1/3 no change in pain after surgery.
- If MRI does not show vascular compression, rhizolysis or neuromodulation techniques may be efficacious in the appropriate patient population.

References

1. Burchiel K. Surgical management of pain. 2nd ed. New York: Thieme; 2015.
2. Burchiel KJ. A new classification for facial pain. Neurosurgery. 2003;53:1164–7.
3. Miller JP, Acar F, Burchiel KJ. Classification of trigeminal neuralgia: clinical, therapeutic, and prognostic implications in a series of 144 patients undergoing microvascular decompression. J Neurosurg. 2009;111(6):1231–4.
4. Miller JP, Magill ST, Acar F, Burchiel KJ. Predictors of long-term success after microvascular decompression for trigeminal neuralgia. J Neurosurg. 2009;110(4):620–6.
5. Zacest AC, Magill ST, Miller JP, Burchiel KJ. Preoperative magnetic resonance imaging in type 2 trigeminal neuralgia. J Neurosurg. 2010;113(3):511–5.
6. Barker FG, Jannetta PJ, Bissonette DJ, Larkins MV, Jho HD. The long-term outcome of microvascular decompression for trigeminal neuralgia. NEJM. 1996;334:1077–83.

Chapter 27
Trigeminal Nerve Pain, V1 Distribution: Representative Case

James Y. Suen and Chelsey Smith

Representative Case History

The patient is a 34-year-old white female with a history of an auto accident 4 years previously, who sustained a non-displaced fracture of her orbital rim. Since that injury she has had severe pain in her supraorbital and supratrochlear nerves. Her pain was constant, and she required daily narcotic pain medications to make the pain tolerable.

Overview

The supraorbital and supratrochlear nerves are the terminal branches of the ophthalmic division of the trigeminal nerve or V1. These nerves innervate the ipsilateral forehead up to the vertex of the scalp. It also innervates the upper eyelid. Pain in these nerves are not uncommon and is frequently associated with "migraine" headaches. It is usually unilateral and may have various etiologies. It can be the trigger point for migraine headaches or generalized headaches. It is commonly called a sinus headache. There is a connection of the trigeminal nerve with the upper cervical nerve roots called the *trigeminocervical complex* [1]. This can explain bidirectional relay of sensation between the trigeminal nerve and the occipital nerves. Trigeminal pain in V1 can trigger off occipital headaches and vice versa.

J. Y. Suen (✉)
Department of Otolaryngology—Head and Neck Surgery, University of Arkansas for Medical Sciences, Little Rock, AR, USA
e-mail: suenjamesy@uams.edu

C. Smith
ENTcare, Dothan, AL, USA
e-mail: chelseyjsmith5@gmail.com

J. Y. Suen, E. Petersen (eds.), *Diagnosis and Management of Head and Face Pain*, https://doi.org/10.1007/978-3-319-90999-8_27

Differential Diagnosis

- Trauma—can compress nerves or cause neuromas.
- Compression within the supraorbital foramen or the notch.
- Herpes zoster involving V1. About 10% will have chronic pain.
- Skin cancer involvement with perineural invasion.
- Entrapment from reconstruction titanium plates and screws after craniotomy or fracture repair.
- Frontal sinus infections—history and scans can rule out this possibility.
- Brain tumors—imaging scans can rule this possibility out.
- Classic trigeminal neuralgia from vascular compression at the origin of the trigeminal nerve.
- Congenital malformations involving the orbit can cause V1 pain. This includes lymphatic, venous, and arteriovenous malformations.
- Migraine headaches.
- Supraorbital neuralgia of unknown etiology.

Diagnostic Workup

The history is important to determine how long the pain has been present and if they have had previous trauma or surgery near the supraorbital or supratrochlear nerves or have a history of herpes zoster or skin cancers in the forehead. It is important to ask if the pain seems to originate in the eyebrow or forehead area and if that is the trigger point for more generalized headaches, including occipital headaches.

A physical exam should be done to check for tenderness over the supraorbital or supratrochlear nerves, which can be very sensitive. One should look for scars from previous skin cancer excisions or feel for titanium plates or screws in the forehead. Look for vascular malformations involving the orbit or periorbital structures.

With regard to tests, an MRI/MRA scan can be performed to rule out vascular compression of classic trigeminal neuralgia, brain tumors, aneurysms, and sinusitis.

Representative Case Management

This patient had a history of trauma to the orbital rim and has had chronic daily pain which started after her injury. Her previous CT scan did not show any displaced fracture of her orbit or signs of sinusitis. She did not have an MRI to rule out vascular compression because of this history. She was tried on numerous medications, including anticonvulsants and amitriptyline, but could not tolerate most of these drugs because of side effects. She required hydrocodone, six to eight tablets per day, in order to make the pain tolerable.

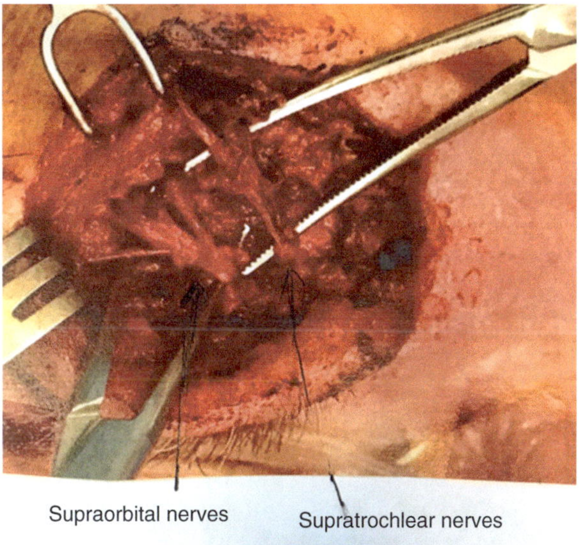

Fig. 27.1 Supraorbital and supratrochlear nerves prior to excision

Because she had localized pain in her left forehead and it was sensitive to touch, she was treated with nerve blocks [2] of the supraorbital and supratrochlear nerves using lidocaine 1% with epinephrine (3 mL) and 3 mL of 0.5% bupivacaine [2]. This would give her good relief of her head pain for 1½ to 2 weeks. When Kenalog, 0.3 mL (40 mg/mL), was added, she would get 3–5 extra days of relief.

After about 18 months of these nerve blocks about once a month, it was recommended to her that those nerves be resected. We resected both the supratrochlear and supraorbital nerves. The nerves appeared enlarged but no compression or neuroma was noted (Fig. 27.1). She obtained immediate relief and has not had any significant pain in the 12 months since surgery. The numbness of her forehead has not bothered her, because she is so grateful to be pain-free. She was able to taper off of her pain medications.

Alternative Management Options

- A decompression procedure of her supratrochlear and supraorbital nerves could be tried as a first option. This would include identifying both nerves and following them from where they exited the orbit and freeing the nerves from any adhesions or compression while removing the accompanying blood vessels with the nerve.
- Medical treatment using the commonly used anticonvulsants or amitriptyline and, if necessary, pain medications starting with the nonsteroidal anti-inflammatory drugs or various narcotics.

- Ablation using alcohol or radio-frequency techniques would be another option. Alcohol ablation can be very painful.

Key Points

- Medical therapy is commonly the initial treatment.
- If the patient can identify the supraorbital and supratrochlear nerves as the trigger points or where the pain is primarily present, then we prefer to do nerve blocks of those nerves. It is helpful if the patient is having pain at the time when the nerve blocks are performed, because if the pain goes away after the nerve blocks, then there is a good chance the nerve blocks can be effective.
- It is common to repeat several nerve blocks before longer pain relief can be obtained.
- We have found that 1% lidocaine with epinephrine, 2–3 mL for the initial injection, is less painful. If the lidocaine stops the pain, then we follow it with the same amount of 0.5% Marcaine. If this turns out to be effective for several weeks, we may not use Kenalog. If the pain relief only lasts a few days, we add the Kenalog (0.5 mL of 40 mg/mL) to the local anesthetics.
- In superficial areas, the steroids can cause tissue atrophy which is usually noticeable.

If the nerve blocks are effective, but the pain continues to recur, then we discuss ablation of the nerves as a more permanent solution.

References

1. Bartsch T, Goadsby PJ. Increased responses in trigeminocervical nociceptive neurons to cervical input after stimulation of the dura mater. Brain. 2003;126:1801–13.
2. Levin M. Nerve blocks in the treatment of headache. Neurotherapeutics. 2010;7:197–203.

Chapter 28
Representative Clinical Case: Trigeminal Nerve Pain—V-2 Distribution

James Y. Suen and Chelsey Smith

Representative Case

History

The patient is a 37-year-old white female with a history of pain in her left midface for more than 20 years. She initially thought it was related to her teeth, and the dentist did root canals and eventually extracted one molar tooth with no pain relief. She had no history of trauma , shingles, or other pathologies. Her pain progressed and became severe and chronic. Sinus X-rays and an MRI to rule out vascular compression of her trigeminal nerve were negative. She was referred to us for evaluation by a neurosurgeon who did not feel he could help her pain.

Overview

The second division of the trigeminal nerve has several branches which should be known. The main trunk of V-2 leaves the skull through the foramen rotundum and then passes through the inferior orbital fissure at the back of the orbit. Before entering the fissure, it gives off a branch which curves around the posterior-lateral wall of the maxillary sinus and enters the bone and supplies the posterior maxillary teeth

J. Y. Suen (✉)
Department of Otolaryngology—Head and Neck Surgery, University of Arkansas for Medical Sciences, Little Rock, AR, USA
e-mail: suenjamesy@uams.edu

C. Smith
ENTcare, Dothan, AL, USA
e-mail: chelseyjsmith5@gmail.com

J. Y. Suen, E. Petersen (eds.), *Diagnosis and Management of Head and Face Pain*, https://doi.org/10.1007/978-3-319-90999-8_28

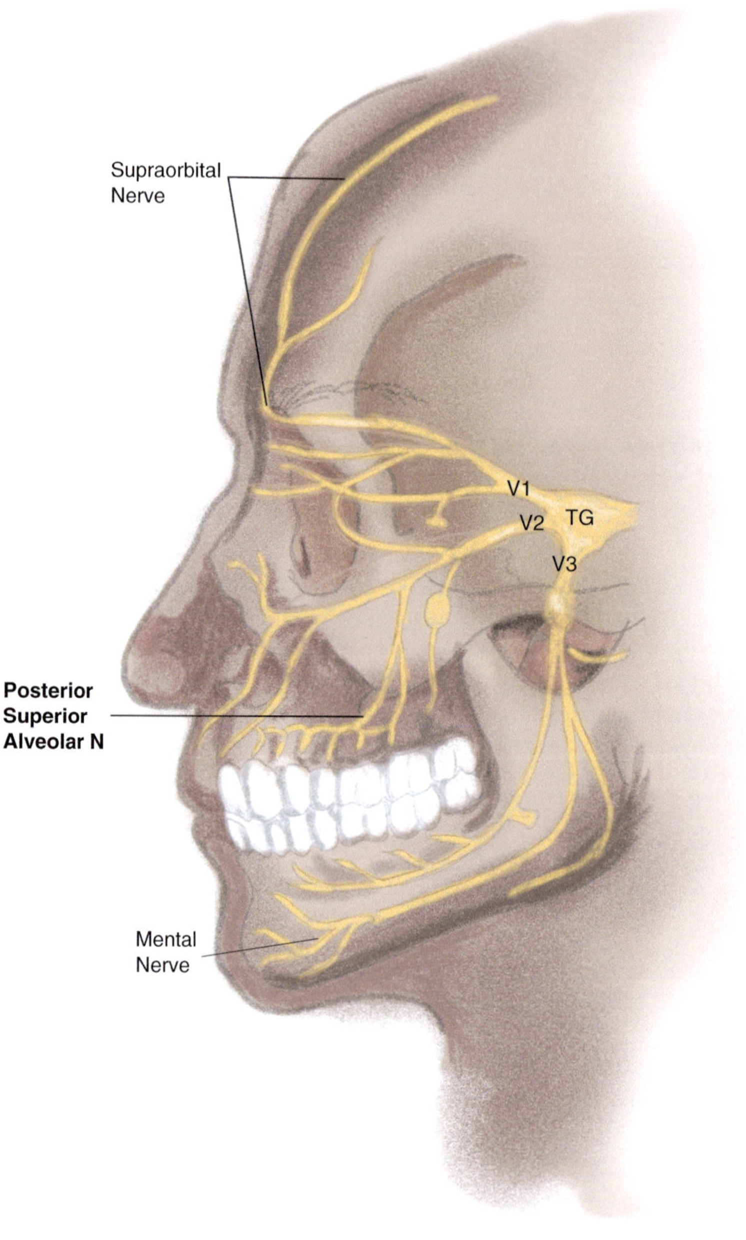

Fig. 28.1 Area innervated by the maxillary division of the trigeminal nerve

(Fig. 28.1). This branch is called the *posterior superior alveolar nerve*. Pain can originate from this nerve only and should be known for nerve block purposes.

Also a branch comes off while in the infraorbital canal in the floor of the orbit and exits through the zygoma to supply the zygoma and anterior temple area. It is called the *zygomaticotemporal nerve* [1] and can be involved with migraine or tension headaches. This nerve can be the source of pain in this area and can respond to nerve blocks for pain relief.

The main nerve branch of V-2 is the *infraorbital* nerve, which supplies the ipsilateral cheek dermatome, including the lateral nose, the lip, and the midface. The lower eyelid is also supplied by this nerve.

Pain located in this area is commonly treated as dental or sinus in origin but often times is not related. It is possible that dental procedures on the maxillary teeth may initiate pain in this area. The pain is usually unilateral and may involve only one branch of V-2 but can trigger pain in the rest of the dermatome and even in adjacent dermatomes.

Differential Diagnosis

- Trauma can compress nerves or cause neuromas.
- Nerve compression within the infraorbital foramen, the zygomaticotemporal nerve in the zygoma, or the posterior superior alveolar nerve in the lateral maxilla bony wall.
- Dental pathology.
- Skin cancer with perineural invasion.
- Entrapment from reconstructive plates or screws.
- Maxillary sinusitis.
- Classic trigeminal neuralgia from vascular compression at the origin of the trigeminal nerve.
- Infraorbital neuralgia of unknown etiology.

Diagnostic Workup

History and physical exam are paramount in the workup of pain in this area. Oftentimes pain can start after having a dental procedure, but with a careful history, it may reveal that the dental procedure was performed because of the pain. It is important to distinguish the specific nerves involved. The pain may involve only one branch or all of them. Having the patient point to the location of the pain is important. Pain in the infraorbital branch is located in the anterior midface and includes the side of the nose, anterior cheek, and upper lip. Pain in the posterior superior alveolar nerve is usually located in the face just above the premolar and molar maxillary teeth. Pain in the zygomaticotemporal branch of the V-2 will be mostly in the temple area just above the zygoma and lateral orbital rim. This can direct where the nerve blocks will be most effective.

The oral cavity should be examined carefully for dental or other oral problems, such as a malignancy.

Imaging may be helpful to look for sinonasal problems.

Representative Case Management

This patient did not have any inciting events to her knowledge that may have caused her pain. Initially she thought she had a toothache, and she had a root canal with no improvement, so one molar tooth was extracted with no relief of pain. Her MRI 1 year ago was negative for vascular compression of her trigeminal nerve.

Medications tried for pain relief included anticonvulsants, tramadol, steroids, amitriptyline, and hydrocodone. The medications did not stop her pain but helped some.

After referral to us, we recommended nerve blocks [2] and found that 1% lidocaine with 1:100,000 epinephrine injected into the mucosa where the posterior superior alveolar nerve was located and the infraorbital nerve would stop her pain. We then followed that with 0.5% bupivacaine. Her pain control would last from 1 to 2 weeks and then recur.

Because of inadequate prolonged pain relief from the nerve block, we recommended surgery of the nerves we felt were involved: the posterior superior alveolar nerve and the infraorbital nerves.

We decompressed the infraorbital foramen and destroyed the infraorbital artery. Then, with a coarse diamond burr, we removed the bone of the lateral wall of the maxilla where the posterior superior alveolar nerve innervates the molars and premolars (Fig. 28.1).

The surgery was performed under general anesthesia as an outpatient procedure.

After surgery, she did well, with no pain for 3 months. Then the pain recurred in her left cheek area where the infraorbital nerve innervates. We had decompressed the nerve and caused it to be numb for several months, and when the nerve recovered, her pain recurred. We have seen this temporary pain relief with decompression only and feel that nerve resection is more permanent. We took her back to surgery and resected the nerve and expect her pain should be relieved indefinitely.

Alternative Management Options

- Medical treatment which was tried and had minimum pain relief.
- Ablation of V-2 at the trigeminal ganglion or at the foramen rotundum using alcohol or radio-frequency techniques.
- Resection of the involved nerve could have been done initially.

Key Points

- Nerve blocks of the involved V-2 nerves using lidocaine with epinephrine as a diagnostic test, and if pain is relieved then add the bupivacaine for prolonged effects. This can be easily performed in the clinic setting.
- Repeat nerve blocks may increase the pain relief intervals.

- The posterior superior alveolar nerve is within the bone of the lateral wall of the maxillary sinus just above the upper premolar and molar teeth, so that bone must be removed to remove the nerve.
- If pain becomes intolerable and the nerve blocks only provide temporary relief, then surgical decompression or resection of the involved nerves should be considered.

References

1. Totonchi A, Pashmini N, Guyuron B. The zygomaticotemporal branch of the trigeminal nerve: an anatomical study. Plast Reconstr Surg. 2005;115:273–7.
2. Blumenfeld A, Ashkenazi A, Napchan U, Bender SD, Klein BC, B erliner R, Ailani J, Schim J, Friedman DI, Charleston L IV, Young WB, Robertson CE, Dodick DW, Silberstein SD, Robbins MS. Expert consensus recommendations for the performance of peripheral nerve blocks for headaches-a narrative review. Headache. 2013;53(3):437–46.

Chapter 29
V-3 Pain: Representative Clinical Case

James Y. Suen and Chelsey Smith

Representative Case History

This patient is a 54-year-old male who was diagnosed with multiple sclerosis, which had progressed to the point that the patient was a quadriplegic with only head and face movement. He could talk and had normal mental function.

About 10 years before, he was seen by us; he developed severe right jaw pain which he described as severe and electric-like. It was almost constant and was incapacitating to him. Talking and eating would trigger the severe pain. He had an MRI which did not show any vascular compression of the takeoff of his trigeminal nerve. His neurologist tried multiple medications, but they sedated him too much and did not stop his pain. He underwent Gamma Knife radiosurgery treatment to his trigeminal nerve which helped for about 8 weeks, but then the pain recurred and was as severe as before.

Because he was paralyzed and difficult to move and transport to emergency rooms, his neighbor (a dentist) did transoral nerve blocks of his right inferior alveolar nerve, using lidocaine, that would stop the pain for several hours. The dentist even taught the patient's wife how to do the nerve blocks, because the patient's pain would be so severe. Her nerve blocks would only help for about 30–60 min.

The patient was referred by his neurologist to see if we had anything to offer for his pain.

J. Y. Suen (✉)
Department of Otolaryngology—Head and Neck Surgery, University of Arkansas for Medical Sciences, Little Rock, AR, USA
e-mail: suenjamesy@uams.edu

C. Smith
ENTcare, Dothan, AL, USA
e-mail: chelseyjsmith5@gmail.com

J. Y. Suen, E. Petersen (eds.), *Diagnosis and Management of Head and Face Pain*, https://doi.org/10.1007/978-3-319-90999-8_29

Overview

The third division of the trigeminal nerve (V-3), the mandibular division, has both sensory and motor function. The motor function is to the masticatory muscles. The main branches of the sensory innervation are to the tongue (*lingual nerve*), mandible and teeth with the terminal branch going to the ipsilateral chin and lip (*inferior alveolar and mental nerves*), and the *auriculotemporal nerve* which exits behind the temporomandibular joint and supplies the temple area above the ear.

It is important to differentiate pain coming from the jaw and teeth (inferior alveolar nerve) compared to the skin of the lower ear and jawline which is superficial and not in the jaw (upper cervical plexus nerves) because the origin of the pain is different (Fig. 29.1).

The auriculotemporal nerve innervates the temporal area and can be a frequent cause of migraine or tension headaches.

The lower mandibular teeth are supplied by the inferior alveolar nerve and commonly present as a toothache resulting in dental extractions, but the pain in the jaw persists.

The mandibular division of the trigeminal nerve is the most common to be involved with the classic type I trigeminal neuritis. An MRI with emphasis on the takeoff of the trigeminal nerve from the pons should be performed to rule out this etiology.

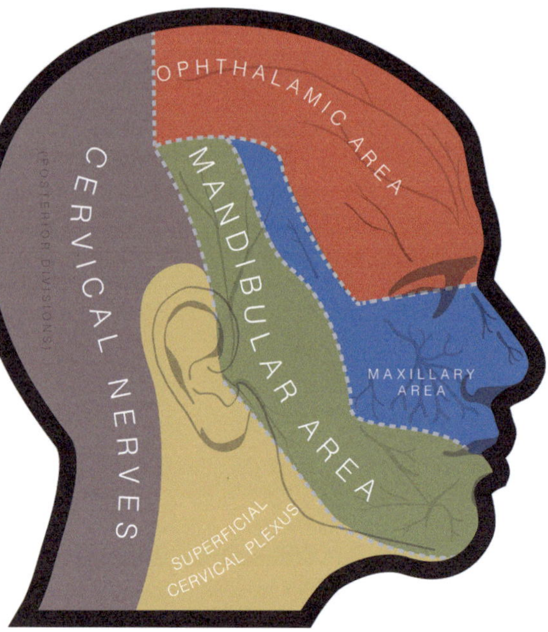

Fig. 29.1 Trigeminal nerve with its three divisions. The mandibular division, V-3, is shown with the branches

Differential Diagnosis

- Trauma, such as mandible fractures or dental extractions or root canals, can injure the inferior alveolar nerve.
- Compression within the inferior alveolar canal or mental foramen.
- Skin or jaw cancers with perineural invasion.
- Entrapment from reconstructive plates or screws.
- Classic trigeminal neuritis from vascular compression at the root entry zone of the trigeminal nerve.
- Multiple sclerosis.
- Inferior alveolar nerve or mental nerve neuralgia of unknown etiology.

Diagnostic Workup

Gathering a pertinent history from the patient allows knowledge of the location, severity, time course, and precipitating or alleviating factors for their pain. Inciting events could include previous surgeries, including dental procedures, trauma, infections, and previous radiation.

A comprehensive head and neck exam, coupled with palpation, is also of utmost importance, because underlying pathology can exist externally or intraorally.

Always obtain information about trigger points and the origin of pain.

Palpate the overlying skin and the TMJ for pain as well as the gingiva and teeth. Close attention can reveal underlying dental pathology, masses, reconstructive apparatus, or vascular malformations.

With regard to imaging, CT, MRI, and MRA can all be of utility depending on likelihood of diagnosis.

Representative Case Management

This patient had been treated for over 10 years with different medications, but none helped his pain, and the medications kept him sedated most of the time. He was referred to us for evaluation and treatment. He is a quadriplegic from multiple sclerosis. He described his pain as being in the distribution of the right inferior alveolar nerve—the right mandible and chin. A nerve block of the inferior alveolar nerve was recommended to him as a diagnostic test. [1] We blocked the nerve where it enters the medial mandible just below the condylar notch using a transoral approach, the same as what the dentist uses to block the mandibular teeth (Fig. 29.2). Four mL of 1% lidocaine with 1:100,000 epinephrine was used to inject the nerve. The block stopped his pain completely, so we followed the lidocaine with 4 mL of 0.5% bupivacaine which can cause numbness for up to 4–5 h.

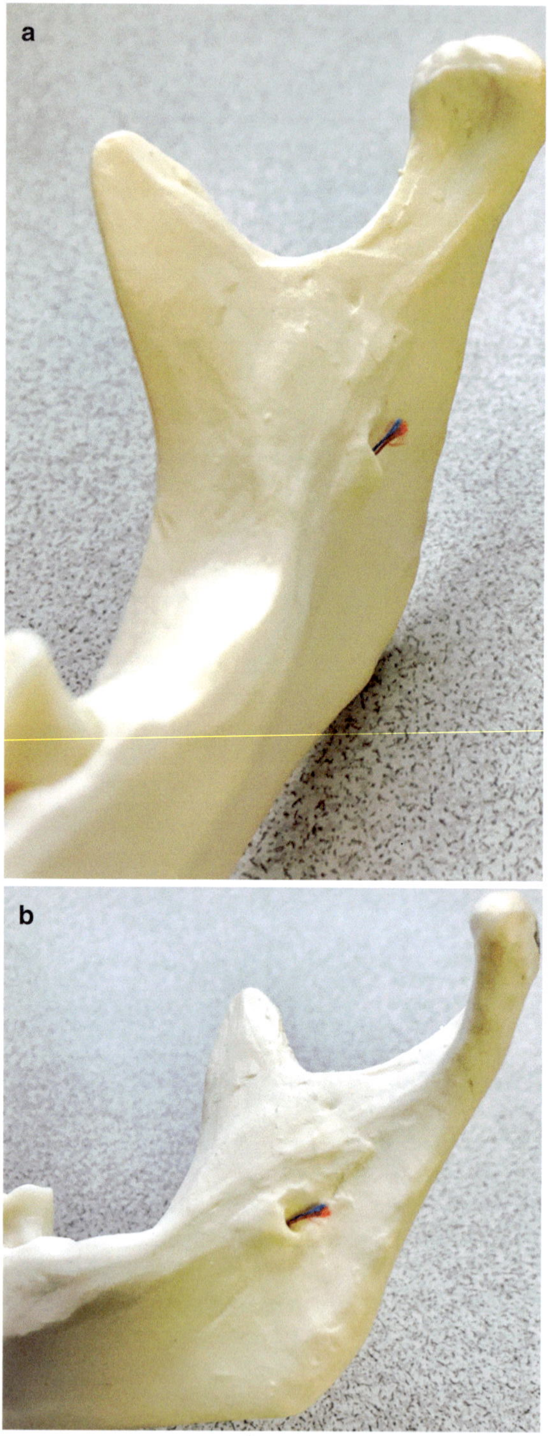

Fig. 29.2 (**a**) and (**b**) are two different views of the inferior alveolar nerve and entering the mandible at the level of the lower teeth and about 2–2.5 cm posterior to the anterior edge of the ascending mandibular ramus. When doing the injection, the 25 Ga needle is curved laterally to go around the prominence just anterior to the nerve foramen

He was seen 2 weeks later and reported that the pain relief lasted almost the full 2 weeks, which had never happened before. The nerve blocks were repeated at 2- to 3-week intervals for several months, and then we were able to extend the intervals of nerve blocks to 7–8 weeks. We did add 0.5 mL of Kenalog (40 mg/mL) after several injections, and it seemed to prolong the duration of the pain relief. The patient has gone over 2½ years with no pain, but we do the nerve blocks every 8 weeks to prevent pain. He and his wife state that the nerve blocks have "given him his life back."

His multiple sclerosis has remained stable for the past 2 years.

Alternative Management Options

- Medical therapy using anticonvulsants, tricyclic antidepressants, and pain medications were tried, and none were helpful.
- Ablation of the V-3 nerve in the foramen ovale using alcohol or radio-frequency techniques can be tried but have variable success rates.
- Gamma Knife to the main trigeminal nerve may give some relief but has a high relapse rate.
- Nerve decompression procedures may have some success but is difficult for V-3 because of the location entering the mandible and its course.

Key Points

- Medical therapy is commonly the first-line of treatment; however, if we can pinpoint the nerve involved, we will do a nerve block as a diagnostic test. It is better if the patient is having pain, and after the block, if the pain resolves, it is an indication that that nerve is the cause of the pain.
- Patients are seen about 1–2 weeks after the initial nerve block, and if the pain has recurred, another nerve block is performed. Adding 0.5–1 mL of Kenalog (40 mg/mL) can prolong the duration of pain relief.
- We will tell patients that we cannot tell how long the nerve blocks will last because every patient is different.
- Repeat nerve blocks are done as needed and may prolong the duration of the pain relief.
- We have done repeated nerve blocks every few weeks to few months for several years with continued pain relief, so they can be done indefinitely as long as they help.

Reference

1. Tsui BCH, Dullane D, Funicane BT. Neural blockade for the surgery to the head and neck. Chronic pain. In: Cousins MJ, et al., editors. Cousins and Bridenbaugh's neural blockade in clinical anesthesia and pain medicine. 4th ed. Philadelphia: LWW; 2009. p. 486–91.

Chapter 30
Temporomandibular Pain Case Presentation

John K. Jones and James Y. Suen

A 23-year-old female presents with a 4-week complaint of pain in the right pre-auricular/auricular area and limited range of mandibular motion. She has no previous history of similar discomfort. She denies any significant blunt trauma to the face or mandible. By history she was eating a bagel when she had acute pain and a sensation of instability in her right jaw joint. She has noticed a slight change in her occlusion with an inability to make her right posterior teeth touch (posterior open bite). Over time she has noticed that she has slowly regained some of her range of motion, but she still has significant pain especially with opening her mouth. Upon careful history taking, she does have a history of occasional "clicking" of her jaw joints. The noise was not accompanied by any pain or limited range of motion. She specifically denies any parafunctional habits such as clenching or bruxism. She did not seek any treatment until now. She has tried OTC analgesics with limited success in pain relief. She is very concerned about her limited range of motion. In addition the pain that she is experiencing is resulting in lost productivity.

J. K. Jones
Department of Otolaryngology/Head and Neck Surgery/Oral and Maxillofacial Surgery, University of Arkansas for Medical Sciences, Little Rock, AR, USA
e-mail: jjones353f@uams.edu

J. Y. Suen (✉)
Department of Otolaryngology—Head and Neck Surgery, University of Arkansas for Medical Sciences, Little Rock, AR, USA
e-mail: suenjamesy@uams.edu

J. Y. Suen, E. Petersen (eds.), *Diagnosis and Management of Head and Face Pain*, https://doi.org/10.1007/978-3-319-90999-8_30

Overview

Temporomandibular pain complaints are very common. The pain can be due to intra-articular changes (internal derangement), extra-articular muscle and ligamentous pain, or a combination. Temporomandibular disorders can also manifest with other symptoms such as malocclusion, otalgia, tinnitus, a sensation of ear fullness, dizziness, as well as adnexal muscular pain and cephalalgia [1]. Because of the variety of presentations, it can be a diagnostic challenge. Evaluation by a dental professional with interest and experience in the management of temporomandibular disorders should be considered if a temporomandibular disorder is suspected.

Differential Diagnosis

Internal derangement right temporomandibular joint
Temporomandibular arthralgia
Local muscle soreness right temporomandibular joint
Impacted third molar teeth
Primary rheumatologic disease
Acute otitis media
Otitis externa
Maxillary sinusitis
Referred pain from odontogenic (dental) source

Diagnostic Work-Up

The work-up begins with careful history taking to include onset, duration, and quality of pain as well as any relieving or exacerbating factors. Problems with other articulations should be investigated. The trends since the onset of pain are also important. Past history of similar pain, joint noise, or limited range of motion should be investigated as should a history of any significant trauma to the head and neck [2]. Examination consists of otologic examination for evidence of disease, auscultation of both temporomandibular joints, and a recording of the mandibular range of motion in maximal opening, protrusion, and right and left lateral excursions. Intraoral examination should include an inspection of the occlusion especially the relative stability as well as any excessive attrition or fractures to the teeth. Possible dental sources of pain can be identified by obvious decay, gingivitis, tooth mobility, or very heavily restored teeth. The muscles of mastication should be palpated to determine tenderness. The preauricular area should be examined for edema and tenderness to palpation.

Initial imaging is ideally accomplished with a panoramic radiograph to evaluate joint position as well as screen for any osseous changes consistent with arthritis. The panoramic radiograph also allows one to screen for maxillary sinusitis and dental disease. If internal derangement is suspected, an open/closed mouth MRI may be helpful in determining meniscal mobility and position as well as condition. CT scanning is less efficacious due to the inability to examine the meniscus but can be useful especially if osseous pathology is suspected.

Case Management

After taking a careful history, examination was accomplished. The external auditory canal was clear, and the tympanic membrane was intact and without any evidence of otitis media. Palpation to the right preauricular region elicited point tenderness over the right temporomandibular joint. Auscultation revealed no crepitus or clicks. Palpation of the muscles of mastication revealed significant tenderness on the right side particularly the right lateral pterygoid muscle on intraoral palpation. Inspection of the occlusion revealed a well-maintained adult dentition without evidence of parafunctional wear. The occlusion appeared very stable with very good interdigitation of the teeth when together. Maximal interincisal opening was 29 mm. Protrusion resulted in pain and a deviation of the chin to the right. Left lateral excursion was minimal and accompanied by pain. Right lateral excursion was 7 mm. Base on the history and examination, a diagnosis of internal derangement of the right temporomandibular joint was strongly suspected. Given the acute onset, limited mobility and lack of improvement over time, the working diagnosis was anteriorly dislocated right temporomandibular meniscus without reduction.

A panorex radiograph was obtained which revealed a healthy dentition without the presence of impacted third molar teeth. There were no degenerative changes noted in either temporomandibular joint. The joint space was slightly wider on the right when compared to the left. No evidence of maxillary sinusitis was noted. Meniscal dislocation without reduction was strongly suspected. The patient was given a choice re: having an MRI or a procedure to reduce the meniscal dislocation. The patient chose a procedure rather than delaying treatment waiting for an MRI.

The patient was given three options for procedures: arthrocentesis, arthroscopy, and arthrotomy. After careful discussion of the three options, arthrocentesis was chosen. Right temporomandibular arthrocentesis was performed in the clinical setting with intravenous sedation. Arthrocentesis resulted in immediate increase in range of motion as well as decreased pain. She was placed on NSAIDs and soft diet. Her malocclusion resolved in the first week after treatment. At 4 weeks she was noted to be pain-free. Auscultation revealed no noise and full range of motion had been regained.

Alternative management that could have been considered would consist of occlusal splint therapy, but this is typically much better for extra-articular temporomandibular problems. Splint therapy has limited efficacy for acute internal derangement. Referral to physical therapy could also have been considered in an attempt to reduce the meniscal dislocation and reestablish disc mobility. Given the acute onset of the pain and limited range of motion, a diagnostic/therapeutic right temporomandibular block could have been offered as an initial procedure to reduce the dislocation.

Key Points

- Acute temporomandibular internal derangements should be managed as dislocations in the orthopedic sense, meaning that anatomic reduction as soon as practical should be attempted.
- Management by observation or splint therapy in this case would likely have resulted in a chronic internal derangement with a much poorer prognosis for relief of pain and return to normal mobility.
- The temporomandibular joint is unique in its envelope of motion because it both hinges and slides (translates). The first 25–30 mm of opening the mouth is a result of hinging within the glenoid fossa. Greater range of motion requires translation. Internal derangements typically compromise translation.
- When an acute internal derangement is suspected, prompt treatment or referral for treatment optimizes chances for successful resolution of the problem. If acute internal derangements are not properly managed, they become chronic internal derangements with a much poorer long-term prognosis.

References

1. Edens MH, Khaled Y, Napenas JJ. Intraoral pain disorders. Oral Maxillofacial Surg Clin N Am. 2016;28(3):275–88.
2. Okeson JP. Bell's oral and facial pain. 7th ed. Chicago: Quintessence Publishing Co, Inc; 2014.

Chapter 31
Pain of Dental Origin

John K. Jones

Case Presentation

A 34-year-old male presents with complaints of left facial pain. The pain was abrupt in onset and sharp in character. Over time it has become more of a dull aching pain that has gradually increased in intensity. There is no associated fever. The pain was initially well localized to the left upper quadrant of the maxillary dentition but has become rather diffuse and thus difficult to localize. It is somewhat positional in nature. The pain is worsened when bending over and also worsened with jarring such as walking down a flight of stairs. It is not exacerbated by eating. There is no significant history of trauma or recent dental intervention. The pain responds somewhat to NSAIDs but never resolves. A secondary complaint is that of nasal congestion and foul-tasting postnasal drip.

J. K. Jones
Department of Otolaryngology/Head and Neck Surgery/Oral and Maxillofacial Surgery, University of Arkansas for Medical Sciences, Little Rock, AR, USA
e-mail: jjones353f@uams.edu

J. Y. Suen, E. Petersen (eds.), *Diagnosis and Management of Head and Face Pain*, https://doi.org/10.1007/978-3-319-90999-8_31

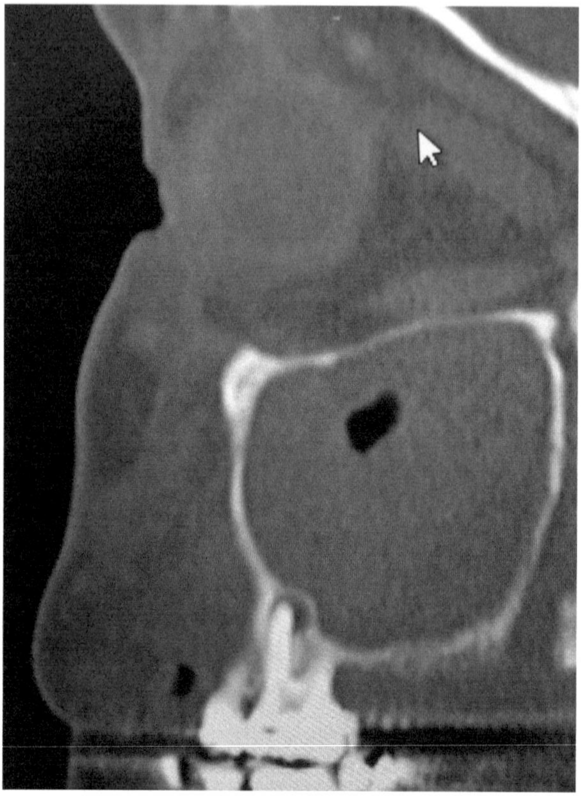

Overview

Orofacial pain is predominantly of dental origin. Odontogenic pain is so prevalent that it is important to rule out an odontogenic source of pain prior to diagnostic testing for other entities. Odontogenic sources of pain can mimic other painful conditions. Fortunately odontogenic pain has several helpful characteristics and routine diagnostic findings to help with accurate diagnosis. Odontogenic pain does not stay the same over time. It typically starts abruptly as a visceral pain response and evolves to a more musculoskeletal pain response over time. There are stereotypical radiographic findings associated with non-vital teeth as well as testing modalities to determine the presence or absence of pulpal vitality.

Differential Diagnosis

- Odontogenic pain
- Maxillary sinusitis

- Infraorbital neuropathic pain
- Referred pain
- Idiopathic or atypical facial pain

Diagnostic Work-Up

History should include:

- Time of onset and duration
- Character and consistency of pain
- Relieving or exacerbating factors
- Response to medication
- Associated findings such as fever, change in taste, odor, postnasal drip
- Date of last dental examination/treatment
- History of allergic rhinitis or sinusitis
- Prior history of similar presentation

Examination should include:

- General neurological exam
- Topographic examination of the face and neck for asymmetry, edema, erythema, or skin abnormalities, such as skin cancers
- Palpation of the affected area
- Intranasal examination
- Percussion of the maxillary sinuses
- Intraoral examination of the dentition and supporting structures with attention being paid to carious and heavily restored teeth, the presence of any edema, erythema, or fistulae

Imaging

Initial imaging can be accomplished with panoramic radiograph of the teeth or with a sinus series. A maxillofacial CT of the sinuses can also be used especially if the potential for sinus surgery is significant. This can be used to rule in or out sinus disease in the form of membrane edema, fluid accumulation, or both.

Referral

If pain of dental origin is suspected, referral to a dental healthcare professional is indicated.

Case Management

The patient was placed on antibiotic therapy empirically based on a provisional diagnosis of left maxillary sinusitis. Because the pain was consistent with maxillary sinusitis and the need for sinus surgery was likely, the patient was referred for a maxillofacial CT scan of the sinuses. The scan revealed a unilateral fluid level and membrane thickening in the left maxillary sinus. The other sinuses were clear, and no other remarkable findings were noted. The patient did not have a history of a recent dental examination or dental imaging. Because the fluid level was unilateral, the patient was referred to a dentist for evaluation of the left maxillary posterior dentition. The molar teeth were noted to be heavily restored. Extensive recurrent caries were noted. The maxillary left second molar tested non-vital and was deemed non-restorable. After discussion with the referring provider, the decision was made to extract the involved tooth with the reasoning that the chronic apical periodontitis associated with the tooth had contaminated the sinus [1]. Culture specimen was obtained at the time of extraction. The patient then underwent surgical irrigation of the maxillary sinus, and the maxillary ostium was enlarged surgically. If the sinus had been treated without resolving the dental cause, then recurrence was very likely [2]. Follow-up revealed complete resolution of the presenting pain.

Alternative Management Options

- Irrigation and debridement of the sinus without dental evaluation. Temporary resolution might have been possible, but recurrence would have been very likely.
- Extraction of the responsible tooth without appropriate management of the sinus. It is very likely that that sinusitis would have persisted as a result of the magnitude of involvement.

Key Points
- The upper posterior teeth can be the source of a maxillary sinus infection.
- Medical and dental interventions were necessary collaboratively to resolve the infection.

References

1. Edens MH, Khaled Y, Napenas JJ. Intraoral pain disorders. Oral Maxillofacial Surg Clin N Am. 2016;28(3):275–88.
2. Okeson JP. Bell's oral and facial pain. 7th ed. Chicago: Quintessence Publishing Co, Inc; 2014.

Chapter 32
Pain from Nasal Origin: Clinical Case

James Y. Suen and Chelsey Smith

Representative Case History

The patient is a 60-year-old white male with a history of severe headaches in the right lateral orbit and temple area for many years. The headaches occurred two to three times a month and would last for almost a week. About two to three times a year, his headaches would be so severe, he would have to be admitted to the hospital for 5–7 days to control his headaches. He was referred by his neurologist to see if we had anything to offer him to help or prevent the headaches.

While getting a detailed history, the patient said that at the onset of his headaches, he would notice discomfort in his right nostril, and over several hours, his right temple would begin hurting and the severe headaches would occur. He had nausea and vomiting with the headaches, and sumatriptan would help some if he took it early into the episode. He was also tried on several anticonvulsants and could not tolerate them. He would require large doses of narcotics in the hospital to control his pain and headaches.

J. Y. Suen (✉)
Department of Otolaryngology—Head and Neck Surgery, University of Arkansas for Medical Sciences, Little Rock, AR, USA
e-mail: suenjamesy@uams.edu

C. Smith
ENTcare, Dothan, AL, USA

J. Y. Suen, E. Petersen (eds.), *Diagnosis and Management of Head and Face Pain*, https://doi.org/10.1007/978-3-319-90999-8_32

Overview

There is a known medical entity called contact point headaches or "Sluder's neuralgia," which is pain in the face and head which originates in the nose [1, 2]. The pathophysiology is related to a "bony spur" on the nasal septum which can jut out and touch the middle or superior turbinate (Fig. 32.1) and compress the posterior-lateral branches of the palatine nerve off of the pterygopalatine ganglion (Fig. 32.2). This is a trigger point that can result in severe facial pain and headaches. The pain can be sharp, shooting and usually localized to one side. It usually starts in the cheek and radiates to other locations, especially the temple area. Decongestant medications can help prevent or treat the problem.

The diagnosis can be by a good physical exam but can also be recognized on a CT scan that can reveal a septal deviation which touches the turbinates on the side of the pain. Pain response to a nasal spray of decongestant and topical anesthetic can also be diagnostic. At the onset of the pain, a patient sprays a strong decongestant into the nose to shrink the turbinates and also uses a spray topical anesthetic, such as 4% lidocaine or 2% tetracaine. If the pain and headache are aborted, it is strong evidence of a contact point headache.

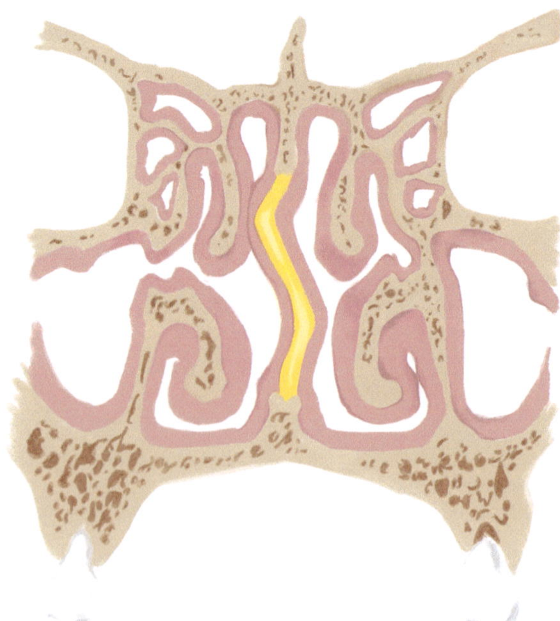

Fig. 32.1 A CT scan can give information regarding a septal spur impinging on the turbinate causing pain

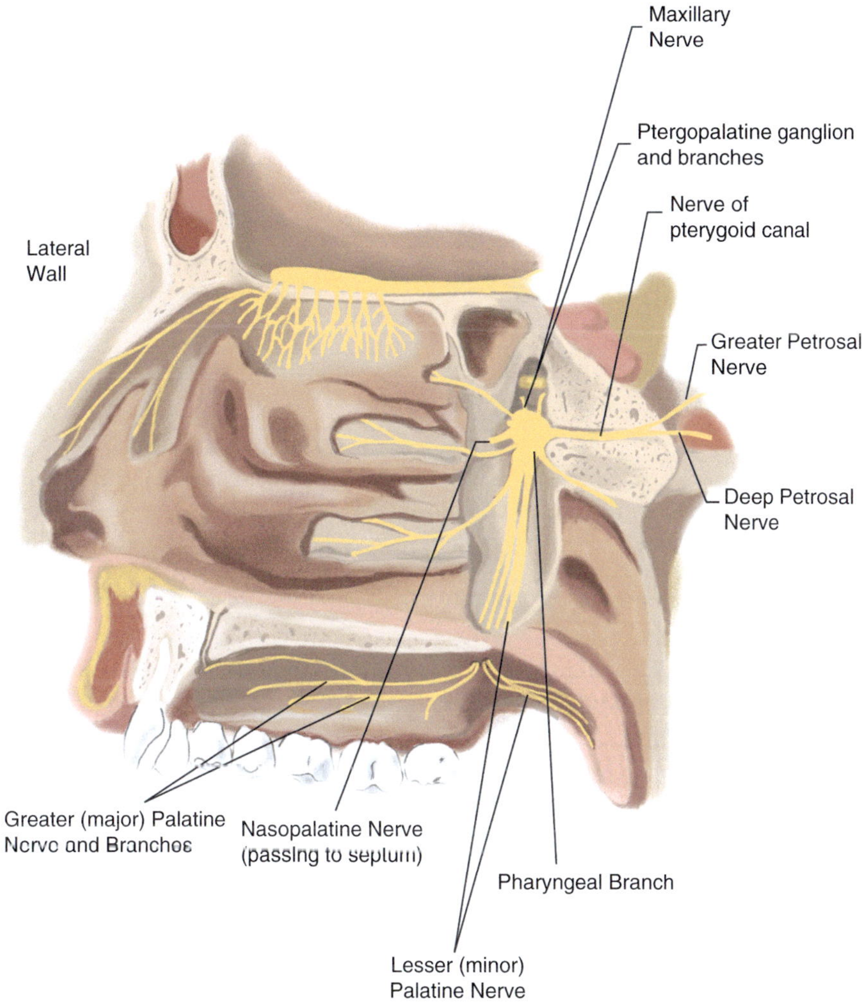

Fig. 32.2 Pterygopalatine ganglion with branches to the turbinates

The treatment is fairly simple and consists of a nasal septoplasty to remove the bony spur and straighten the septum [2, 3].

Differential Diagnosis

- Migraine headaches
- Peripheral trigeminal neuritis
- Sinusitis
- Dental origin pain

Diagnostic Workup

- A good history and physical exam is important to obtain the trigger point and whether nasal congestion from allergies or upper respiratory infections triggers the pain and also if cold medications, such as decongestants, help the pain.
- The physical exam should look carefully at the nose and especially the septum for "spurs" which touch the turbinates or are close.
- A CT scan can be helpful to identify the bony spur touching the turbinate [4].

Representative Case Management

The patient was evaluated and found to have a septal spur which jutted out and touched the middle turbinate on the right side. He was told to use oxymetazoline nasal spray at the onset of the facial pain, followed by spraying 4% lidocaine into the same nostril to see if the pain and headache would be aborted. He used this treatment and found that it would prevent the headaches.

The patient underwent a nasal septoplasty to remove the bony spur and straighten his septum. He was also told to use the oxymetazoline and lidocaine if he felt a headache starting. Since surgery, he has gone over 3 years without any facial pain or headaches.

Alternative Management Options

- Just use the decongestant and topical anesthetic at the onset of any pain.
- Do sphenopalatine ganglion blocks.
- Reduce the size of the nasal turbinates using various methods.
- Take medications such as pain medications or anticonvulsants.
- Workup and treat patients for allergies to try to prevent turbinate congestion.

Key Points

- A thorough history and physical exam is crucial to pinpoint the nose as the trigger point.
- If a nasal "contact point headache" is suspected, use decongestants and topical anesthetics to see if the headaches can be aborted. If it does, the diagnosis is pretty definite.
- If this entity is confirmed, a nasal septoplasty is usually curative for the headaches.

References

1. Oomen KP, Van Wijck AJ, Hordijk GJ, de Ru JA. Sluder's neuralgia: a trigeminal autonomic cephalalgia? Cephalalgia. 2010;30(3):360–4.
2. Giacomini PG, Alessandrini M, DePadova A. Septoturbinal surgery in contact point headache syndrome: long-term results. Cranio. 2003;21(2):130–5.
3. Tosun F, Gerek M, Ozkaptan Y. Nasal surgery for contact point headaches. Headache. 2000;40(3):237–40.
4. Pasha R, Soleja RQ, Ljaz MN. Imaging for headache: what the otolaryngologist looks for. Otolaryngol Clin North Am. 2014;47(2):187–95.

Chapter 33
Post Herpes Zoster Neuritis

James Y. Suen

Case Presentation

A 47-year-old white female had herpes zoster infection of her right V1 and V2 trigeminal nerve branches about 10 years previously. She had severe pain with her infection plus significant corneal ulceration. Her pain never resolved and caused a great deal of stress. Three years later, she had a nerve stimulator implanted over the right supraorbital nerve, and it helped about 75% of her pain. While the nerve stimulator helped a lot of her pain, it required frequent setting adjustments. The residual pain was located in the distribution of her right infratrochlear nerve, which was over the medial canthus of her right eye and bridge of her nose on the right side. This residual pain was severe and was aggravated by temperature changes, barometric weather changes, bright lights, and by wind blowing on her face. It affected her daily life significantly.

Overview

Herpes zoster infections usually cause a great deal of pain before and during the infection. About 10% of the patients who develop herpes zoster infections will have postherpetic neuritis, which can cause pain indefinitely. It has been shown that nerve blocks during the acute infection can help decrease the pain [1, 2], but there has not been much written about nerve blocks or nerve stimulators to help control long-term pain in these situations.

J. Y. Suen
Department of Otolaryngology—Head and Neck Surgery,
University of Arkansas for Medical Sciences, Little Rock, AR, USA
e-mail: suenjamesy@uams.edu

J. Y. Suen, E. Petersen (eds.), *Diagnosis and Management of Head and Face Pain*, https://doi.org/10.1007/978-3-319-90999-8_33

It is not uncommon for several divisions of the trigeminal nerve to be involved with herpes zoster infection. The virus can linger in the ganglion of nerves.

Most patients will be treated with various medications, including antivirals, anticonvulsants, amitriptyline, antianxiety medications, and narcotics, which can help the pain but do not usually control the pain. These patients are desperate for treatment to stop their pain.

Differential Diagnosis

- Post herpes zoster neuritis is an easy diagnosis, and there are not many other considerations for a differential diagnosis.

Diagnostic Evaluation

The history is important for diagnosis. When a patient describes a history of pain for several days, then an outbreak of a vesicular rash along one or more dermatomes lasting about 10–14 days is a certain diagnosis for herpes zoster infection. It is possible for patients to have a history of a previous herpes zoster infection. The critical question is whether the pain before and during the infection persisted after the rash cleared. If the pain persisted, the diagnosis is surely post herpes zoster neuritis.

Physical exam will commonly show residual scars from the rash. If the eye is involved, there may be corneal scars. Also it is common to find trigger points which are very sensitive to touch or pressure and can accentuate the pain.

Imaging studies are not usually necessary.

Representative Case Management

This patient had postherpetic neuritis in her V1 nerve distribution on her right side. After being treated for several years with medications, which did not control her pain, a right supraorbital nerve stimulator was suggested. After a successful trial with an externalized stimulator, she underwent the device implantation procedure (Fig. 33.1). The nerve stimulator helped a lot of her pain, but she continued to have severe pain in one area—the area supplied by the infratrochlear nerve on the same side. The pain was severe and increased with temperature changes, barometric weather changes, bright lights, and by wind blowing on her face. Also it was very sensitive to touch. The option for nerve blocks to augment the pain relief accomplished with the stimulator was recommended.

She had nerve blocks to the right medial canthus and bridge of nose areas using 3 mL of 1% xylocaine with epinephrine followed by 3 mL of 0.5% bupivacaine

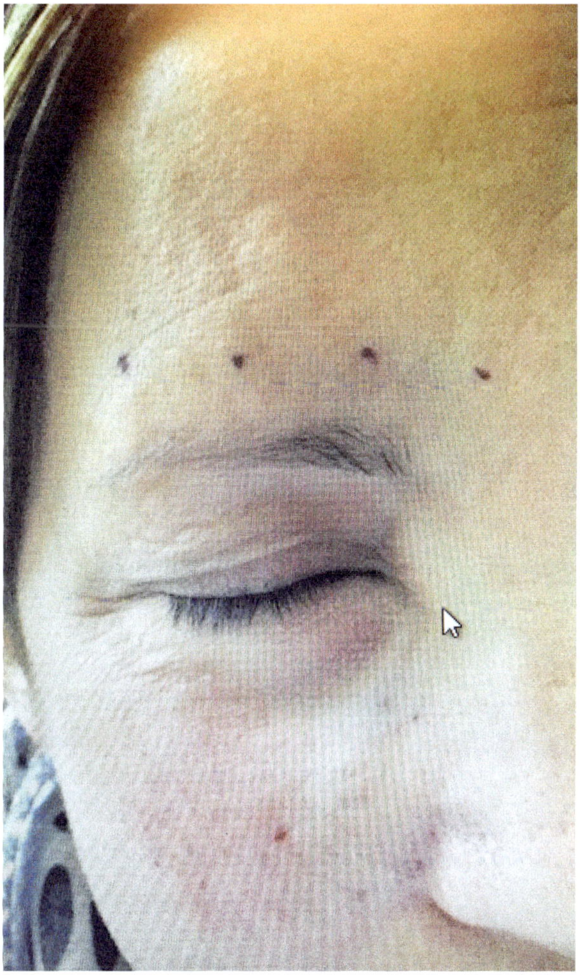

Fig. 33.1 Post herpes zoster neuritis of V1. Treated with a nerve stimulator implant (under the skin where dotted line is) and with nerve blocks where white arrow is pointing

subcutaneous (Fig. 33.1). She reported 50% relief for 2 weeks. Two and one half weeks later she had repeat injections, and Kenalog, 0.5 mL of 40 mg/mL, was added. She continued to have good pain relief for about 2 weeks each time. After about 1 year of repeated nerve blocks to help her pain, she requested a more permanent pain relief. She underwent surgical resection of the infratrochlear nerve by removing all of the tissue between her skin and bridge of her nose and orbital rim near the medial canthus.

She has had no significant pain in that area for over 10 months and is very pleased with the results. The small area of numbness does not bother her. She was able to decrease most of her medications she had been on for years. She does still have intermittent pain in her supraorbital nerve and continues to use the nerve stimulator to help control the pain in that area.

Alternative Management Options

- Continue nerve blocks.
- Inject alcohol into that area of her involved nerve, but it can cause severe pain and skin slough.
- Add another nerve stimulator electrode to the infratrochlear nerve area. This carries a higher risk for infection than non-implantable alternatives. The surgical implant also has a risk of device erosion and can be a less cost-effective option.

Key Points

- Post herpes zoster neuritis is very painful and causes major stress to the patient.
- Nerve blocks can help the pain during an acute infection with herpes zoster and also the postherpetic pain.
- If the nerve blocks are helpful, a nerve stimulator or resection of the involved nerves can help to control the pain.
- Insertion of nerve stimulators can be expensive compared to nerve resection.
- Patients rarely complain about the numbness and are happy to have less or no pain.

References

1. Blumenfeld A, Ashkenazi A, Napchan U, Bender SD, Klein BC, Berliner R, Ailani J, Schim J, Friedman DI, Charleston L IV, et al. Expert consensus recommendations for the performance of peripheral nerve blocks for headaches-a narrative review. Headache. 2013;53(3):437–46.
2. Evans RW, Pareja JA. Expert opinion: supraorbital neuralgia. Headache. 2009;49:278–81.

Chapter 34
Bilateral Face and Head Pain

Chelsey Smith and James Y. Suen

Representative Case History

This patient is a 52-year-old white female presenting to clinic for "migraine" headaches on both sides of her head. These symptoms began 8 years previously. Initially, the headaches had started in the "right face down to the chin" per the patient. She underwent dental evaluation and her problem was deemed unrelated to dentition. At an outside hospital, she was treated with a Gamma Knife for the pain, but the pain did not improve. The pain is daily and constant, affecting her quality of life to the point where she cannot get out of bed at times.

Overview

It is not uncommon for patients to present with a history of multi-location head and neck pain including bilateral pain. Pain in one nerve can trigger pain in other areas. This adds to the difficulty in treating this subset of patients. It is crucial to obtain a detailed history to try to determine where the pain or headache starts. This trigger point can help determine which nerves are the origin of the pain. There can be more

C. Smith
ENTcare, Dothan, AL, USA
e-mail: cjsmith2@aums.edu

J. Y. Suen (✉)
Department of Otolaryngology—Head and Neck Surgery,
University of Arkansas for Medical Sciences, Little Rock, AR, USA
e-mail: suenjamesy@uams.edu

J. Y. Suen, E. Petersen (eds.), *Diagnosis and Management of Head and Face Pain*, https://doi.org/10.1007/978-3-319-90999-8_34

than one trigger point. The history should include determining the trigger points, history of previous trauma, surgery, cancer, infections, or dental problems. Most of these patients will have been on many different medications and will be on narcotics for pain control.

Differential Diagnosis

- Brain tumors or intracranial vascular anomalies—history and imaging can rule this out.
- Head trauma from various causes. History is important to elicit.
- Skin cancer or other types of cancer.
- Entrapment from reconstructive plates/screws in bilateral locations.
- Migraine headaches.
- Tension headache.
- Sinus infections.
- Classic trigeminal neuralgia from vascular compression at the origins of the trigeminal nerves.
  - Bilateral neuralgia of unknown etiology.
  - Multiple sclerosis.
  - Psychogenic disorders.

Diagnostic Workup

Bilateral facial pain workup can be more tedious compared to unilateral pain patients. History and comprehensive physical evaluation are vital to optimum treatment of the patient along with detailed documentation. It is important to ascertain where the pain or headaches seem to begin and where the pain goes to from there. These trigger points can cause more diffuse pain. When pinned down, most patients will tell you where the pain starts. Past medical and surgical history should include medical conditions, systemic illnesses, central or peripheral nervous system pathology, prior cancers and their associated treatments, traumas, past surgeries, social risk factors, dental issues, and infections. Examine the overlying skin for any abnormalities and palpate the underlying bony structures and soft tissues, checking for masses, bony step-offs, or foreign bodies. Imaging can be very helpful in these patients, especially when trying to rule out central nervous system pathology that could be causing bilateral symptoms. We recommend MRI for this purpose. If bony structures such as reconstructed areas or sinuses need specific review, a CT scan can be performed as well.

Representative Case Management

While 8 years ago her pain had begun on the right side, currently her most significant pain was in the left auriculotemporal nerve distribution (temple) , but she also complained of pain in her left forehead and in her right temple area and in the right upper neck. The patient was currently medicating with cyclobenzaprine, gabapentin, amitriptyline, alprazolam, and hydrocodone. Both CT and MRI were obtained, each showing no underlying pathology. For diagnostic and therapeutic purposes, 1% lidocaine with 1/100,000 epinephrine (3 cc) was injected into the area of the left auriculotemporal nerve (ATN) (Fig. 34.1). This immediately caused her pain in that area to subside; however she still had pain in her right face and neck. This injection was followed by 0.5% bupivacaine (3 cc) injection in the ATN. We also did nerve blocks of her right auriculotemporal nerve and her right upper cervical plexus nerves with good pain relief of those areas.

The nerve blocks would control her pain for 2–3 weeks, and then she would return for repeat nerve blocks. Her most severe pain was in the left auriculotemporal nerve distribution. We tried 100 units of Botox into her left temporalis muscle, and it did not seem to help prolong her pain relief. It was noted that when her left-side pain was controlled, she had less pain in the right side. Because of the need for recurrent nerve blocks, discussion about nerve decompression of her left ATN versus nerve excision was recommended [1–3]. She opted for nerve excision, and this was performed 14 months after her visit to us. The superficial temporal artery was found to be looped around the auriculotemporal nerve and also abutting it for several

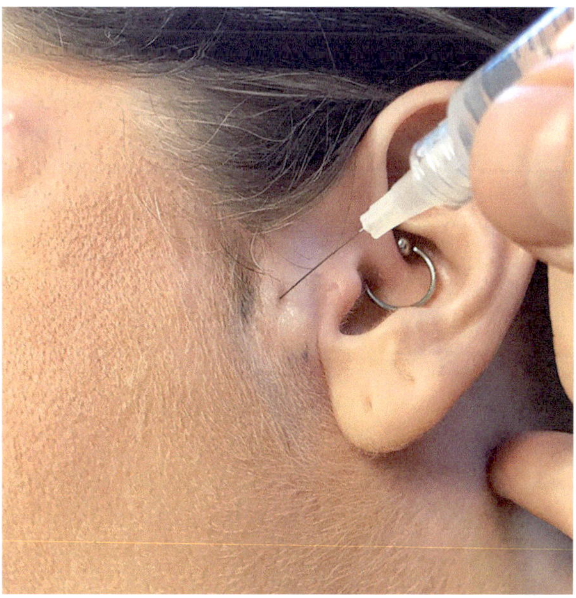

Fig. 34.1 Injection of the auriculotemporal nerve just posterior to the TMJ

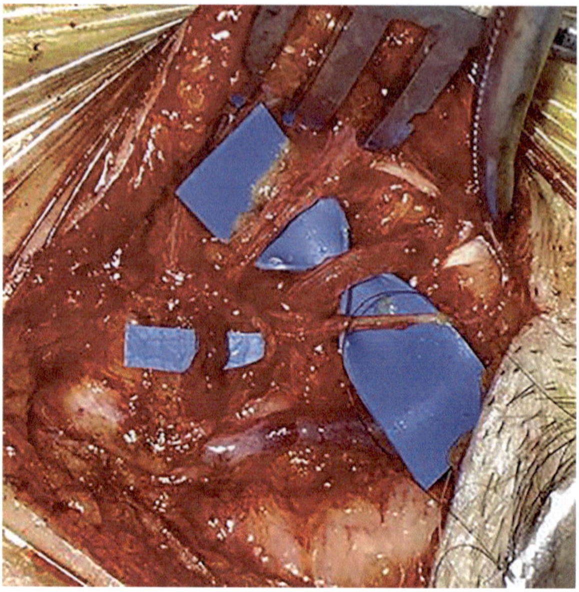

Fig. 34.2 Superficial temporal artery looping around the auriculotemporal nerve

centimeters (Fig. 34.2). The artery was excised, and 3 cm of the ATN and its branches were excised.

Postoperatively, she had resolution of pain in the left auriculotemporal region but had persistent complaint of pain in the left supraorbital nerve and zygomaticotemporal nerve distribution, right auriculotemporal distribution, and also her right cervical plexus distributions. Nerve block for all four of these locations was performed, each with immediate pain relief. Overall her pain was much better, and the severe pain in the left auriculotemporal nerve distribution is still gone after 8 months. She required nerve blocks in the other nerve areas about once a month to control her pain. She was interested in doing more nerve resections for long-term relief, so she underwent surgical resection of her left supraorbital, supratrochlear, and zygomaticotemporal nerves on the left and the auriculotemporal nerve on her right side. Over 5 months after these additional nerve excisions, the patient has had no pain or headaches since surgery, and she is very happy with the results. She was able to discontinue all pain meds.

Alternative Treatment Options

- Medical therapy for this patient could also include anticonvulsants, NSAIDs, and higher doses of narcotics. One must be wary of potential side effects with each of these classes of medications and understand the risk of addiction and intolerance.
- Nerve decompression instead of resection is an option but less chance for long-term relief.

- Ablation using alcohol or radiofrequency techniques could be utilized but, because of multiple nerves involved, would be difficult.
- Psychological evaluation and therapy might be useful.
- Resection of the other nerves causing her other pain could be performed.

Key Points

- Bilateral facial pain can be complex and also prove difficult to treat.
- Detailed history and physical evaluation is critical to locate trigger points and to identify which nerves are triggering the pain and headaches.
- Imaging should be performed to rule out other causes.
- Utilization of lidocaine/bupivacaine nerve blocks coupled with Botox and/or Kenalog can help achieve maximum time of pain control and help space out nerve injections.
- Unfortunately (as seen with this case report), when one area of pain is resolved, other locations of pain can surface. Do not be discouraged by this; these new areas are amenable to treatment as well. A step-wise approach to each problem area is paramount, and as seen in this particular patient, relief in her trigger point area (left auriculotemporal nerve) improved her quality of life.

References

1. Janis JE, Hatef DA, Ducic I, et al. Anatomy of the auriculotemporal nerve: variations in its relationship to the superficial temporal artery and implications for the treatment of migraine headaches. Plast Reconstr Surg. 2010;125:1422–8.
2. Guyuron B, Kriegler JS, Davis J, Amini SB. Five year outcome of surgical treatment of migraine headaches. Plast Reconstr Surg. 2011;127:603–8.
3. Janis JE, Dhanik A, Howard JH. Validation of the peripheral trigger point theory of migraine headaches: single-surgeon experience using botulinum toxin and surgical decompression. Plast Reconstr Surg. 2011;128:123–31.

Chapter 35
Anesthesia Dolorosa

Joshua M. Rosenow

Representative Case History

The patient is a 38-year-old right-handed woman who had the spontaneous onset of right facial pain. This original pain was intermittent "lightning electric pain" in the right V3 region. Over time this involved more of the right face. She tried several medications and, after a year without improvement, underwent microvascular decompression (MVD). She was pain-free for a week before the pain returned (the same quality as before the first MVD) primarily in the V2/V3 dermatomes. Twelve months later she had repeat MVD without any pain-free period postoperatively. She underwent stereotactic radiosurgery 6 months afterward without significant change in the pain but with a new "creepy crawly feeling" in the right V2/V3 dermatomes. She then underwent percutaneous balloon compression (PBC) rhizotomy. Following this procedure the pain changed and became constant burning, mostly in the right V1/V2 dermatomes "like a toothache" with improvement in the V3 distribution pain. She also developed new right corneal anesthesia. The shocking component was mostly relieved but replaced by the constant burning. She then underwent a second PBC several months later which magnified the burning and expanded the numbness in the face, as well as worsened her corneal sensory loss.

She next underwent right supraorbital neurectomy without change in the pain. After she had a trigeminal block which caused both temporary numbness and pain reduction, she underwent a total sensory rhizotomy (open sectioning of the trigeminal nerve root at the brain stem). She awoke from this with total right facial numbness and persistent V1/V2 burning pain, as well as new right occipital neuralgia. Removal of her cranioplasty plate and subsequent C1 and C2 ganglionectomy reduced but did not fully relieve the occipital pain.

J. M. Rosenow
Department of Neurosurgery, Northwestern Memorial Hospital, Chicago, IL, USA
e-mail: jrosenow@nm.org

J. Y. Suen, E. Petersen (eds.), *Diagnosis and Management of Head and Face Pain*, https://doi.org/10.1007/978-3-319-90999-8_35

Currently she continues to have constant burning pain in the right V1/V2 dermatomes. Running, swimming, significant continuous activity, and talking all increase the pain. She has tried to adjust her hours at work as a physical therapist to minimize exacerbations in pain.

She presented to our center using only nortriptyline and baclofen for pain reduction. In the past she had tried pregabalin, gabapentin, carbamazepine, hydrocodone/APAP, and multiple other opioids and neuromodulatory medications.

On physical and neurologic examination, she has healed incisions from her multiple prior procedures. She has a depression in the region of her prior right retrosigmoid procedures. She has a right occipital Tinel's sign. Her right face is completely anesthetic and she wears a right corneal prosthesis to protect her anesthetic cornea.

Overview

Anesthesia dolorosa (AD) is sometimes colloquially called "phantom face pain." It is the most severe form of trigeminal deafferentation pain and results from repeated intentional injury to the trigeminal nerve. As in this case, patients often initially present with uncomplicated pain such as trigeminal neuralgia, but the summation of numerous intentional injuries to the trigeminal nerve in the service of relieving the original pain can result in a numb face that remains painful.

Older statistics state the incidence of AD to be 2–4% among patients who undergo trigeminal rhizotomy [1].

Differential Diagnosis

Etiologies of anesthesia dolorosa can include [2–4]:

1. Intentional injury to the trigeminal nerve due to repeated ablative treatments for trigeminal neuralgia
2. Severe traumatic injury to the peripheral trigeminal nerve involving all three distributions
3. Unintentional injury to the trigeminal nerve during posterior fossa surgery for another condition such as acoustic neuroma, meningioma, or trigeminal neuroma

Diagnostic Workup

The diagnosis of anesthesia dolorosa is based on clinical examination and a history of injury to the trigeminal nerve. Patients have loss of sensation (most often complete) to fine touch and pinprick in the painful regions of the face.

Case Management

The patient had already failed numerous medical treatments, as well as percutaneous trigeminal blocks. In an attempt to begin with the least invasive surgical procedure, a trial of V1 and V2 peripheral stimulation was attempted. Not unexpectedly, the patient could perceive no stimulation-evoked paresthesias during the trial and obtained no pain relief.

She next underwent a 1-week trial of combined sensory thalamic (ventrocaudal nucleus—Vc) and periaqueductal gray (PAG) deep brain stimulation (DBS). Intraoperative microelectrode recording was performed. It was exceedingly difficult to locate the thalamic sensory region for the face due to (presumed) neuroplasticity in the face of chronic deafferentation. The thalamic sensory region for the arm had expanded to occupy the region normally subserving facial sensation. Despite multiple microelectrode tracks in more medial positions, very little facial sensory representation could be located, while there was abundant arm representation in all tracks. The thalamic electrode was implanted in the most medial position that still allowed PAG electrode placement without targeting conflicts. During the week of the inpatient trial, some facial paresthesias could be evoked, with accompanying arm paresthesias as well. The PAG stimulation caused a pleasant light-headed sensation. At the close of the trial, the patient felt that her pain had overall been decreased to an extent that merited permanent implant. However, over the course of the subsequent months, this pain reduction diminished to the point of being nonsignificant. Numerous programming changes failed to resolve this situation, and the device was removed approximately 9 months after implant.

The patient was subsequently offered either nucleus caudalis DREZ (dorsal root entry zone) lesioning or centrolateral thalamotomy, which she is considering.

Alternative Management Options

Like all central pain syndromes, anesthesia dolorosa is exceedingly difficult to treat. All surgical procedures have had mixed results. Deep brain stimulation has been employed with some success for AD, but not in this case [4]. This patient's stimulation targeted the ventrocaudal thalamus and the periaqueductal gray. The centromedian/parafascicular (CM/Pf) thalamic complex has also been used for deep brain stimulation with some success [5]. Another central neurostimulation option is epidural motor cortex stimulation. This has the advantage of not requiring awake mapping or implanting electrodes into the brain (with the concomitant risk of intracerebral hemorrhage). However, results of this therapy for AD have also been inconsistent [6]. Moreover, the programming of the device is time intensive, and there is a long-term risk of therapy-limiting seizures due to the electrical cortical stimulation [7, 8].

Other ablative procedures for AD include nucleus caudalis DREZ lesioning or central thalamotomy [3]. Again, neither of these procedures are certain to produce long-lasting pain relief, but both have shown some efficacy. Caudalis DREZ interrupts the second-order pathways in the brain stem that have lost afferent input as part of AD and may spontaneously generate pain impulses.

Central lateral (CL) thalamotomy has also been used to treat a variety of chronic pain states, including central pain such as AD [9]. Unlike other ablative treatments, some research has shown that patients who have pathologic elevations in EEG power spectra in certain frequency ranges may have a higher chance of benefitting from the procedure. While traditionally performed with radiofrequency lesioning, newer technologies such as MR-guided focused ultrasound (MRgFUS) have also been utilized for this purpose [10].

Key Points

- Anesthesia dolorosa (AD) is a chronic pain syndrome due to trigeminal nerve injury.
- AD may be caused by intentional or unintentional injury.
- Opioids and neuromodulatory medications may have little effect on AD symptoms.
- Both neuromodulatory (stimulation) and ablative surgical methods have been used to treat AD with some success, but results have been inconsistent.

References

1. Gorecki JP, Nashold BS. The Duke experience with the nucleus caudalis DREZ operation. Acta Neurochir Suppl. 1995;64:128–31.
2. Lazorthes Y, Sol JC, Fowo S, Roux FE, Verdie JC. Motor cortex stimulation for neuropathic pain. Acta Neurochir Suppl. 2007;97(Pt 2):37–44.
3. Sandwell SE, El-Naggar AO. Nucleus caudalis dorsal root entry zone lesioning for the treatment of anesthesia dolorosa. J Neurosurg. 2013;118(3):534–8.
4. Sims-Williams HP, Javed S, Pickering AE, Patel NK. Characterising the analgesic effect of different targets for deep brain stimulation in trigeminal anaesthesia dolorosa. Stereotact Funct Neurosurg. 2016;94(3):174–81.
5. Hollingworth M, Sims-Williams HP, Pickering AE, Barua N, Patel NK. Single electrode deep brain stimulation with dual targeting at dual frequency for the treatment of chronic pain: a case series and review of the literature. Brain Sci. 2017;7(1):9.
6. Fontaine D, Hamani C, Lozano A. Efficacy and safety of motor cortex stimulation for chronic neuropathic pain: critical review of the literature. J Neurosurg. 2009;110(2):251–6.
7. Henderson JM, Boongird A, Rosenow JM, LaPresto E, Rezai AR. Recovery of pain control by intensive reprogramming after loss of benefit from motor cortex stimulation for neuropathic pain. Stereotact Funct Neurosurg. 2004;82(5–6):207–13.
8. Henderson JM, Heit G, Fisher RS. Recurrent seizures related to motor cortex stimulator programming. Neuromodulation. 2010;13(1):37–43.
9. Jeanmonod D, Magnin M, Morel A. Chronic neurogenic pain and the medial thalamotomy. Schweiz Rundsch Med Prax. 1994;83(23):702–7.
10. Jeanmonod D, Werner B, Morel A, Michels L, Zadicario E, Schiff G, et al. Transcranial magnetic resonance imaging-guided focused ultrasound: noninvasive central lateral thalamotomy for chronic neuropathic pain. Neurosurg Focus. 2012;32(1):E1.

Chapter 36
Facial Pain Treated with Stellate Ganglion Block

Jordan Taylor MacNeil and Johnathan H. Goree

Representative Case History

The patient is a 51-year-old female who developed chronic facial pain following a radical neck dissection for T1N1 squamous cell carcinoma of the oral cavity, tongue, and right-sided cervical lymph nodes. She described her pain as a constant pulling sensation in the right side of her face. She also reported episodic sharp, shooting pain down her anterior and lateral neck with hyperalgesia of the surrounding skin. During her treatment course, she was unable to obtain control of pain with opioids, gabapentinoids, antidepressants (e.g., duloxetine), anxiolytics (e.g., alprazolam), or physical therapy.

Overview

Nociception, the sensory experience of pain, is mediated by the unmyelinated termini of primary afferent neurons and carried to the central nervous system by A-delta and C fibers [1]. These afferent neurons and their downstream connections can become sensitized resulting in chronic neuropathic pain disorders [2]. Symptoms may include hyperalgesia, a condition where a minimally painful stimulus results in an exaggerated pain response, and allodynia, a condition where a non-painful stimulus is perceived as painful. These primary afferent neurons

J. T. MacNeil · J. H. Goree (✉)
Department of Anesthesiology, University of Arkansas
for Medical Sciences, Little Rock, AR, USA
e-mail: jtmacneil@uams.edu; jhgoree@uams.edu

J. Y. Suen, E. Petersen (eds.), *Diagnosis and Management of Head and Face Pain*, https://doi.org/10.1007/978-3-319-90999-8_36

can begin to express receptors to catecholamines in a pathological condition known as sympathetically mediated pain [2, 3]. Examples include complex regional pain syndrome, trigeminal neuralgia, cancer pain, and phantom limb pain [4]. Patients with sympathetically mediated facial pain can be diagnosed and oftentimes treated with blockade of the afferent sympathetic cell bodies which reside in the sympathetic ganglion. An interventional pain block targeting the stellate ganglion would block the sympathetics of the inferior cervical ganglion and first thoracic ganglion, which supply the unilateral upper extremity, head, and neck [5]. An alternative to the global sympathectomy model is a microsympathectomy, which targets only the gray rami of spinal levels conveying pain and effectively reduces pain while not altering sympathetic outflow to unaffected areas. This procedure is not currently the standard of care, although studies in animal models are showing promise [6].

Differential Diagnosis

- Tumor recurrence, other regional tumors, or lymph node enlargement——Rule out with imaging. May also present with unilateral neurologic or vascular symptoms.
- Neuralgia (glossopharyngeal or trigeminal)——Commonly related to compression or infection. Pain commonly has a sudden onset, is usually described as sharp, and is provoked by sensory stimulation, such as touch.
- Postherpetic neuralgia——History would include a dermatomal rash consistent with previous acute herpes zoster.
- Posttraumatic trigeminal pain——May be suspected after surgical damage to trigeminal nerve with abnormal findings on qualitative sensory testing.
- Dental pain——Pain would be provoked by mastication and/or thermal stimuli, such as hot/cold foods. Imaging could assist in diagnosis.
- Cervical arterial dysfunction——Associated with manipulation of neck, such as in chiropractic practice, and may present with jaw claudication [7]. CT angiogram could be diagnostic.
- Infection (e.g., abscess)——Laboratory analysis would likely reveal a leukocytosis. Abscess could be seen with imaging.
- Craniocervical junction abnormalities——Symptoms may include vascular insufficiency, Horner's syndrome, or cranial nerve abnormalities. MRI or CT of upper spinal cord and brain can be used to rule out.
- Complex regional pain syndrome——Typical presentation originates in an extremity.
- Psychogenic pain——Presence of other comorbid psychiatric disorders is supportive. Pain or symptoms such as paralysis may be present. Pain often does not follow anatomic distributions such as a dermatome or myotome.

Diagnostic Workup

The workup should begin with a thorough patient history particularly focusing on the onset, location, duration, character, associated symptoms, radiation, timing, and severity of the pain. Focus should also be paid to a possible inciting event. In this patient, the onset of pain was after a major invasive procedure, which would raise concern for posttraumatic neuralgia or psychogenic causes. Since her history was remarkable for anxiety and depression, a psychogenic etiology is plausible. Postherpetic neuralgia should be ruled out without a history of acute herpes zoster. A dental history should be taken including previous caries, associated risk factors, and any history of oral procedures [8].

The physical exam will further narrow the differential. Simple observation of head and neck structures can provide evidence of inflammation or infection (e.g., erythema). Visualization of full dentition is important and can aid in diagnosis of dental pathology. Palpation of neck structures may reveal lymphadenopathy as a primary source of pain or compression of neuronal structures.

Imaging is effective in diagnosing many painful disorders of the head and neck, including craniocervical junction or anatomic abnormalities, abscess or local tissue inflammation (i.e., supporting infectious etiology), lymph node enlargement, or regional tumor. In our patient with a history of carcinoma, imaging revealed no abnormalities other than an enlarged lymph node, which was negative for cancer on fine needle aspiration. Laboratory investigation, such as a complete blood count, may rule out infectious etiologies. Our patient's laboratory investigations were unremarkable, further narrowing the differential. The patient's physical exam also revealed hyperesthesia of the shoulder and numbness of the face with symptoms relieved by gabapentin. This finding further supports a neuropathic origin. In a patient with neuropathic pain with a suspected sympathetically mediated component, stellate ganglion block can be performed for diagnostic purposes. On initial injection, this patient had abatement of pain confirming sympathetic contribution to her pathology.

Representative Case Management

The patient had undergone major surgery on the head and neck and was still having pain despite institution of appropriate pharmacotherapy. A stellate ganglion block was used for local sympathectomy. The block was achieved by injecting 0.25% bupivacaine with 1:200,000 epinephrine anterior to Chassaignac's tubercle under ultrasound and fluoroscopic guidance [9]. Both imaging modalities were used due to the high risk of intravascular injection due to surgically altered anatomy (see Fig. 36.1). This procedure proved both diagnostic and therapeutic for her condition. Within 1 month, the patient had a resolution of her symptoms for a duration of

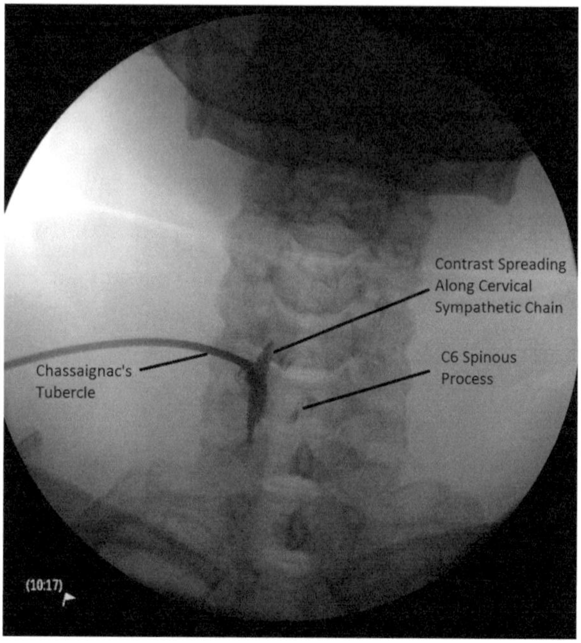

Fig. 36.1 Stellate ganglion block. Procedure view provided is anterior-posterior during fluoroscopic imaging. Chassaignac's tubercle at C6 is seen with contrast superior and inferior spreading through the sulcus of the stellate space

18 months. At this time, the symptoms returned, and another stellate ganglion block was performed, which resulted in a decline of symptoms within 1 month of the repeat procedure.

Alternative Management Options

- Trial of additional antineuropathic drugs (e.g., pregabalin). Uptitrate dose until at maximal dose or patient is unable to tolerate side effects.
- Trial of tricyclic antidepressants (e.g., amitriptyline) in combination with antineuropathic drugs can be more effective than either drug alone.
- Peripheral nerve stimulator implantation after failure of pharmacotherapy.
- Neurolysis of the sympathetic ganglion with chemical or radiofrequency ablation.

Key Points

- Homeostatic dysregulation at the level of the peripheral and central nervous system can lead to expression of adrenergic receptors on neurons, which can cause inappropriate stimulation of nociceptors. This disorder is called sympathetically mediated pain, and this mechanism to varying degrees underlies a number of chronic pain conditions.
- Characterizing the type of pain is crucial, because the presence of neuropathic pain symptoms, such as allodynia or hyperalgesia, suggests a neuropathic ori-

gin of the pain. Neuropathic pain can be amenable to pharmacotherapy, local anesthetic block, neurolysis, or neuromodulation. Opioids are usually avoided as they are generally not effective against neuropathic pain, and harm often outweighs potential benefits. Blockage of sympathetic ganglion is diagnostic and often therapeutic for sympathetically mediated pain.

References

1. Chambers D, Huang C, Matthews G. Chapter 57: Pain physiology. In: Basic physiology for anaesthetists. 1st ed. Cambridge: Cambridge University Press; 2015. p. 269–74.
2. Baron R. Mechanisms of disease: neuropathic pain—a clinical perspective. Nat Clin Pract Neurol. 2006;2(2):95–106.
3. Perl E. Causalgia, pathological pain, and adrenergic receptors. Proc Natl Acad Sci. 1999;96(14):7664–7.
4. Harden R, Oaklander A, Burton A, Perez R, Richardson K, Swan M, et al. Complex regional pain syndrome: practical diagnostic and treatment guidelines, 4th edition. Pain Med. 2013;14(2):180–229.
5. Bruehl S. Complex regional pain syndrome. BMJ. 2015;351:h2730.
6. Xie W, Chen S, Strong J, Li A, Lewkowich I, Zhang J. Localized sympathectomy reduces mechanical hypersensitivity by restoring normal immune homeostasis in rat models of inflammatory pain. J Neurosci. 2016;36(33):8712–25.
7. Kerry R, Taylor A, Mitchell J, McCarthy C, Brew J. Manual therapy and cervical arterial dysfunction, directions for the future: a clinical perspective. J Man Manip Ther. 2008;16(1):39–48.
8. Zakrzewska J. Differential diagnosis of facial pain and guidelines for management. Br J Anaesth. 2013;111(1):95–104.
9. Rathmell J. Chapter 10: Stellate ganglion block. In: Atlas of image-guided intervention in regional anesthesia and pain medicine. 1st ed. Philadelphia: Wolters Kluwer/Lippincott Williams & Wilkins Health; 2012. p. 151–61.

Chapter 37
Nonsurgical Management of Migraine

Nathaniel M. Schuster

Case History

A 26-year-old female biostatistics PhD student with history of motion sickness in childhood and no other significant past medical history presented for recurrent headaches. These headaches started during high school and were predominantly behind her left eye, throbbing, severe, and associated with light and sound sensitivity. Early in the course of a headache, she would experience nausea and would frequently vomit. Her headaches were worsened with routine activity and improved but did not completely remit with lying down in a dark room. They were not associated with visual disturbance. They could last days at a time. She noticed that most months she would have a debilitating headache starting 1 day prior to her menstrual periods (which were regular 28-day cycles on an oral contraceptive containing 20 mcg ethinyl estradiol). These were often more severe than her usual headaches and could often persist for 2–3 days despite treatment with ibuprofen 800 mg. She would often have one or two other headaches a month that would respond to ibuprofen 800 mg. She noticed that these often occurred in the setting of her rare chocolate consumption. In total, she had headaches about 4 days a month, all of them associated with light and sound sensitivity. Her sister had recently been diagnosed with migraines, and her mother recalled disabling headaches during the first trimester of her pregnancies and with her menstrual periods prior to menopause. During college, when her sleeping hours were less regular and alcohol consumption was more, she

---

N. M. Schuster
Center for Pain Medicine, Department of Anesthesiology,
University of California, San Diego, La Jolla, CA, USA
e-mail: nmschuster@ucsd.edu

J. Y. Suen, E. Petersen (eds.), *Diagnosis and Management of Head and Face Pain*, https://doi.org/10.1007/978-3-319-90999-8_37

recalled a stretch of time where her headaches became more frequent, and ultimately almost daily, with escalating use of aspirin/acetaminophen/caffeine (Excedrin). Her primary care doctor educated her about medication-overuse headache and encouraged her to limit her caffeine use to one cup a day, maintain better sleep habits, drink more water, limit alcohol consumption and aspirin/acetaminophen/caffeine, and use ibuprofen 800 mg no more than 2 or 3 days a week. With stopping aspirin/acetaminophen/caffeine and an effort toward these lifestyle modifications, her headaches returned to their prior pattern.

Overview

Migraine is a common neurologic disorder with cumulative lifetime incidence of 43% in women and 18% in men [1]. It is a common reason for presentation both in the clinic setting and emergency department and is often treated by practitioners from numerous different specialties, including primary care, OB/GYN, neurology, ophthalmology, otolaryngology, dentistry, neurosurgery, and emergency medicine.

Among primary headache disorders encountered in both outpatient and inpatient medicine, the most common is migraine. Migraine is defined in the International Classification of Headache Disorders-3 (ICHD-3; www.ichd-3.org) as a headache which if untreated or unsuccessfully treated lasts 4-72h h and is associated with nausea or with photophobia and phonophobia; and has at least 2 of the following 4 characteristics: 1) unilateral, 2) pulsating, 3) moderate/severe, and 4) worsened by routine physical activity.[2].

It exists in many subtypes, including migraine with and without aura, hemiplegic migraine, migraine with brainstem aura (formerly known as "basilar migraine"), retinal migraine, and others. Identifying migraine aura and other "migraine variants" is important due to concern for increased risk of vascular events in these patients. Of note, patients with migraine aura who are on estrogen-containing birth control and use tobacco are advised to either stop tobacco or discontinue estrogen-containing birth control due to their cumulative risk of vascular events. Triptans and ergots are contraindicated in patients with hemiplegic migraine due to theoretical risk of vasoconstriction, as well as in patients with prior vascular events or significant vascular risk factors.

It is important to quantify the frequency of headache days and migraine days per month. Patients are said to have "episodic migraine" if they have less than 15 headache days per month and "chronic migraine" if they have more than 15 headache days per month. Oral preventive medications are often initiated for patients with 4 or more migraine days per month, and onabotulinumtoxin A (Botox) is FDA indicated for patients with chronic migraine or at least 15 headache days and at least 8 migraine days per month.

For patients presenting with a migraine lasting longer than 72 h, they are said to have status migrainosus, which has its own treatments, sometimes called "rescue treatments."

Differential Diagnosis

There are a daunting number of headache disorders described in the ICHD-3 beta [2]. While most headaches are due to primary headache disorders (such as migraine or tension type headache), the first task in the evaluation of a new patient is excluding secondary headache disorders (such as vascular, infectious, and neoplastic causes). Practitioners are first charged to evaluate for "red flag" signs and symptoms concerning for secondary headache disorders, many of which represent medical emergencies. A helpful mnemonic is SNOOP (or S2NOOP4) [3]:

- Systemic signs or symptoms (fever, weight loss)
- Secondary risk factors (history of HIV or malignancy)
- Neurologic signs or symptoms (altered mental status, asymmetry on neurologic examination)
- Onset: Sudden or "thunderclap headache"
- Older: New onset headache at age >40
- Positional headache: Present upon awakening and improving with rising or present when sitting/standing and remitting with lying down
- (Change from) Prior headache in quality
- Papilledema
- Pregnancy

At initial visit, a thorough history and physical examination including neurologic examination should be performed. Funduscopic examination is important to evaluate for papilledema, which suggests increased intracranial pressure. If a secondary headache disorder is suspected, clinical judgment should be used to decide whether referral to the emergency department is warranted, or whether an outpatient consultation with a neurologist, neurosurgeon, or other specialist in appropriate.

Secondary headache disorders to consider include, but are not limited to:

- Subarachnoid headache
- Epidural, subdural, or intraparenchymal hematomas
- Cerebral venous thrombosis
- Carotid dissection
- Meningitis
- Temporal arteritis
- Brain tumor
- Idiopathic intracranial hypertension
- Spontaneous or iatrogenic CSF leak

Migraine is often diagnosed by ophthalmologists and otolaryngologists in patients concerned for eye or sinus pathology. An otolaryngology, neurology, allergy, and primary care consensus based on review of clinical trial data in 2006 stated that the majority of "sinus headache" is actually migraine [4].

A quick mnemonic for diagnosing migraine is "PIN," the mnemonic for the ID Migraine screening questionnaire: photophobia, incapacitating, and nausea. The validated questions that accompany the "PIN" mnemonic are about the incidence of certain features in association with headaches over a 3-month period:

1. Light bothered you (a lot more than when you don't have headaches)?
2. Your headaches limited your ability to work, study, or do what you needed to do for at least 1 day?
3. You felt nauseated or sick to your stomach when you had a headache?

If the patient answers "yes" to two of those three questions, the sensitivity and specificity for diagnosis of migraine are 81% and 75%, respectively [5].

This "PIN" mnemonic can help differentiate migraine from the other common primary headache disorder, tension-type headache, as well as less common primary headache disorders, most notably cluster headache. There are many other primary headache disorders on the differential as well, including the trigeminal autonomic cephalalgias and hypnic headache.

Diagnostic Workup

Laboratory testing is not always indicated. Labs should be considered if there is concern for an infectious etiology and in patients over the age of 50 with new-onset headache and/or visual disturbance, where giant cell (temporal) arteritis must be considered and evaluated for with erythrocyte sedimentation rate (ESR) and C-reactive protein (CRP).

Imaging may be warranted if secondary headache is suspected, but imaging is not routinely required for patients with headache [6]. Non-neurologists sometimes order CTs where MRI would be more helpful; discussion with radiology or neurology colleagues may help guide correct ordering. This is supported by the American Headache Society's Choosing Wisely campaign, which recommends against imaging in stable headaches meeting criteria for migraine and recommends MRI over CT except in case of emergency where MRI is not available [7].

Case Management

On evaluation by a neurologist, the patient had no "red flag" signs or symptoms and a normal neurologic examination, and she was reassured that an MRI of her brain was not necessary. She was diagnosed with episodic migraine without aura and was suggested to complete a 3-month headache diary given suspicion for menstrual-related migraine. The physician and neurologist discussed starting topiramate 25 mg nightly and titrating topiramate by 25 mg per day weekly up to 50 mg twice a day. While the patient was initially interested when she heard that topiramate might help her to lose a few unwanted pounds, she was dissuaded by topiramate's possible cognitive side effects. She opted instead to start magnesium oxide 400 mg daily for migraine prevention. Given her prominent nausea, she was given a trial of zolmitriptan nasal spray 5 mg for acute migraine treatment. She was educated about lifestyle modifications and trigger avoidance (in her case, chocolate). At 3-month follow-up, her headache diary confirmed migraines starting one day before her menstrual period in 2 of 3 months. She reported that her rare migraines between menstrual periods responded well to zolmitriptan nasal spray, but that her menstrual-related migraines did not. She was started on naproxen 550 mg twice a day starting 2 days prior to her menstrual period for menstrual-related migraine "mini-prophylaxis." She was educated that she could discuss with her primary care doctor switching from her current oral contraceptive to an "ultralow" dose oral contraceptive containing 10 mcg ethinyl estradiol, as this may help to prevent menstrual-related migraines as well.

Alternative Management Options

Migraine treatments can be divided into lifestyle modifications and trigger avoidance, pharmacologic treatments, and interventional treatments.

Lifestyle modifications include encouraging regular sleep and meal times, stable low dose of caffeine consumption, adequate hydration, regular exercise, and stress reduction and relaxation techniques. Patients report many triggers, some of which are more easily avoidable (such as alcohols or chocolate), others of which may be modifiable (such as irregular sleep and menstrual periods), and those which are least modifiable (such as weather changes and scents from others' perfume and tobacco smoke). Patients should be educated about medication-overuse headache; using acute migraine medications more than two or three times a week increases risk of headaches becoming more frequent and developing chronic migraine.

Pharmacologic migraine treatments can be divided into preventive (or prophylactic) treatments, acute (or abortive) treatments, and rescue treatments.

There are many oral preventive treatments for migraine; these should be used daily regardless of the presence of headache that day. An excellent resource is the 2012 guidelines from the American Academy of Neurology and American Headache Society (Table 37.1) [8]. The three classes of preventive medications most often used are antiepileptics (with evidence favoring topiramate and divalproex sodium), antidepressants (with evidence favoring amitriptyline and venlafaxine; nortriptyline is also commonly used in clinical practice), and antihypertensives (with evidence favoring propranolol, metoprolol, timolol, atenolol, and nadolol). Since these guidelines were published, newer positive studies have been published supporting the use of candes-

Table 37.1 Classification of migraine preventive therapies (available in the United States)

Level A: medications with established efficacy (≥2 class I trials)	Level B: medications are probably effective (1 class I or 2 class II studies)	Level C: medications are possibly effective (1 class II study)	Level U: inadequate or conflicting data to support or refute medication use	Others: medications that are established as possibly or probably ineffective
Antiepileptic drugs – Divalproex sodium – Sodium valproate – Topiramate	Antidepressants/SSRI/SSNRI/TCA – Amitriptyline – Venlafaxine	ACE Inhibitors – Lisinopril	Carbonic anhydrase inhibitor – Acetazolamide	Established as not effective
β-Blockers – Metoprolol – Propranolol – Timolol	β-Blockers – Atenolol – Nadolol	Antiotensin receptor blockers – Candesartan	Antithrombotics – Acenocoumarol – Coumadin – Picotamide	Antiepileptic drugs – Lamotrigine
Triptans (MRM[a]) – Frovatriptan[a]	Triptans (MRM[a]) – Naratriptan[a] – Zolmitriptan[a]	α-Agonists – Clonidine – Guanfacine	Antidepressants /SSRI/SSNRI – Fluvoxamine – Fluoxetine	Probably not effective – Clomipramine
		Antiepileptic drugs – Carbamazepine	Antiepileptic drugs – Gabapentin	Possibly not effective – Acebutolol – Clonazepam – Nabumetone – Oxcarbazepine – Telmisartan
		β-Blockers – Nebivolol – Pindolol	TCAs – Protriptyline	
		Antihistamines – Cyproheptadine	β-Blockers – Bisoprolol	
			Ca++ blockers – Nicardipine – Nifedipine – Nimodipine – Verapamil	
			Direct vascular smooth muscle relaxants – Cyclandelate	

From Silberstein et al. 2012 [8]

[a]For short-term prophylaxis of menstrually related migraine

artan, memantine, and simvastatin with vitamin D for migraine prevention. Nutraceuticals are natural treatments (including magnesium, riboflavin or vitamin B2, and melatonin) for migraine prevention, many of which have been demonstrated to be effective for migraine prevention in randomized controlled trials [9]. There are also four monoclonal antibodies targeting the calcitonin gene-related peptide (CGRP) or its receptor currently in clinical trials for migraine prevention. Some of these CGRP-targeted monoclonal antibodies have completed phase 3 trials with positive results recently being announced, while others are currently undergoing phase 3 trials.

Menstrual-related migraine, when supported by the patient's headache diary, may be treated preventively with 5-day courses of frovatriptan, naratriptan, zolmitriptan, or NSAIDs such as naproxen. These are usually dosed two or three times a day. The magnitude of the drop in estrogen (or ethinyl estradiol, if on oral contraceptives) with menstrual periods is believed to provoke menstrual-related migraine, and starting or changing to a very-low dose ethinyl estradiol oral contraceptive (10 mcg ethinyl estradiol) may help prevent menstrual-related migraine.

Acute (or abortive) migraine treatments are used as needed and should be used as early as possible during the course of migraine. An excellent resource is the 2015 American Headache Society assessment of evidence (Table 37.2) [10]. Treatments can be divided into simple analgesics (acetaminophen and NSAIDs), combination analgesics (such as aspirin/acetaminophen/caffeine, marketed as Excedrin), triptans, and ergots. Butalbital-containing compounds (marketed as Fioricet, Fiorinal, and Esgic) have been removed from the market in many countries, and the American Headache Society's Choosing Wisely recommendations advise against these compounds, as well as opioids, due to their risk of addiction, overdose, withdrawal, and medication-overuse headache (also known as rebound headaches) [7].

Medication overuse is a frequent cause of migraines becoming "chronic" or "transformed." In the AMPP study, overuse of butalbital-containing compounds and opioids conveyed an odds ratio of about 2 for episodic migraine transforming into chronic migraine at 1-year follow-up [11]. In clinical experience, many headache providers have found that frequent use of acetaminophen, NSAIDs, aspirin/acetaminophen/caffeine (Excedrin), and triptans all can cause medication-overuse headache and that with reducing overuse of these medications that patients can return to having episodic migraine.

There are seven triptans currently on the market: the fast-acting triptans are sumatriptan, zolmitriptan, rizatriptan, eletriptan, and almotriptan, and the long-acting triptans are naratriptan and frovatriptan. Fast-acting triptans are most often used for acute treatment of migraines, while the long-acting triptans are most often used for menstrual migraine prophylaxis or for the treatment of status migrainosus. Triptans and dihydroergotamine are also available in different formulations, including nasal sprays and injectables, which can be helpful for patients who experience nausea, vomiting, and gastric statis with their migraines. Lasmiditan, a novel 5HT-1F agonist, is currently being studied for acute treatment of migraine, with one positive phase 3 trial thus far. While triptans (5HT-1B/1D agonists) and ergots are contraindicated in patients with vascular risk factors due to concern for vasoconstriction, lasmiditan does not cause vasoconstriction in vitro and is being studied for

Table 37.2 Strength of the evidence

Level A	Level B	Level C	Level U	Others
Analgesic Acetaminophen 1000 mg (for non-incapacitating attacks)	**Antiemetics** [a]Chlorpromazine IV 12.5 mg Droperidol IV 2.75 mg [a]Metoclopramide IV 10 mg [a]Prochlorperazine IV/IM 10 mg: PR 25 mg	**Antiepileptic** Valproate IV 400–1000 mg	**NSAIDs** Celecoxib 400 mg	**Level B negative** **Other** Octreotide SC 100 µg
Ergots DHE [a]Nasal spray 2 mg Pulmonary inhaler 1 mg	**Ergots** DHE[a]IV, IM, SC 1 mg [a]Ergotamine/caffeine 1/100 mg	**Ergot** [a]Ergotamine 1–2 mg	**Others** [a]Lidocaine IV [a]Hydrocortisone IV 50 mg	**Level C negative** **Antiemetics** [a]Chlorpromazine IM 1 mg/kg [a]Granisetron IV 40–80 µg/kg
NSAIDs [a]Aspirin 500 mg Diclofenac 50, 100 mg Ibuprofen 200, 400 mg [a]Naproxen 500, 550 mg	**NSAIDs** [a]Flurbiprofen 100 mg Ketoprofen 100 mg Ketorolac IV/IM 30–60 mg	**NSAIDs** Phenazone 1000 mg		**NSAIDs** Ketorolac tromethamine nasal spray
Opioids [a]Butorphanol nasal spray 1 mg	**Others** $MgSO_4$ IV (migraine with aura) 1–2 g [a]Isometheptene 65 mg	**Opioid** [a]Butorphanol IM 2 mg [a]Codeine 30 mg PO [a]Meperidine IM 75 mg [a]Methadone IM 10 mg [a]Tramadol IV 100 mg		**Analgesic** Acetaminophen IV 1000 mg

Level A	Level B	Level C	Level U	Others
Triptans Almotriptan 12.5 mg Eletriptan 20, 40, 80 mg Frovatriptan 2.5 mg [a]Naratriptan 1, 2.5 mg [a]Rizatriptan 5, 10 mg Sumatriptan – [a]Oral 25, 50, 100 mg – [a]Nasal spray 10, 20 mg – Patch 6.5 mg – [a]SC 4, 6 m Zolmitriptan – Nasal spray 2.5, 5 mg – [a]Oral 2.5, 5 mg	**Combinations** [a]Codeine/acetaminophen 25/400 mg Tramadol/acetaminophen 75/650 mg	**Steroid** Dexamethasone IV 4–16 mg		
Combinations [a]Acetaminophen/aspirin/caffeine 500/500/130 mg Sumatriptan/naproxen 85/500 mg		**Others** [a]Butalbital 50 mg [a]Lidocaine intranasal		
		Combinations [a]Butalbital/acetaminophen/caffeine/codeine 50/325/40/30 mg [a]Butalbital/acetaminophen/caffeine 50/325/40 mg		

Level A: Medications are established as effective for acute migraine treatment based on available evidence
Level B: Medications are probably effective for acute migraine treatment based on available evidence
Level C: Medications are possibly effective for acute migraine treatment based on available evidence
Level U: Evidence is conflicting or inadequate to support or refute the efficacy of the following medications for acute migraine
Level B negative: Medication is probably ineffective for acute migraine
Level C negative: Medication is possibly ineffective for acute migraine
From Marmura et al. 2015 [10]
[a]Based on 2000 American Academy of Neurology evidence review

use in patients with vascular risk factors. Small-molecule CGRP antagonists are also currently in clinical trials for acute treatment of migraines.

Rescue treatments are used for migraines not responsive to the above acute medications as well as for status migrainosus. A series of three articles reviewed the evidence behind rescue treatments [12–14]. In the emergency room, intravenous therapy with ketorolac and a D2 antagonist (prochlorperazine or metoclopramide) together with diphenhydramine to prevent akisthesias due to D2 antagonists is most often used first and if ineffective is often followed with IV sodium valproate or IV dihydroergotamine. Other treatments commonly used in this situation include parenteral or oral steroids and IV magnesium.

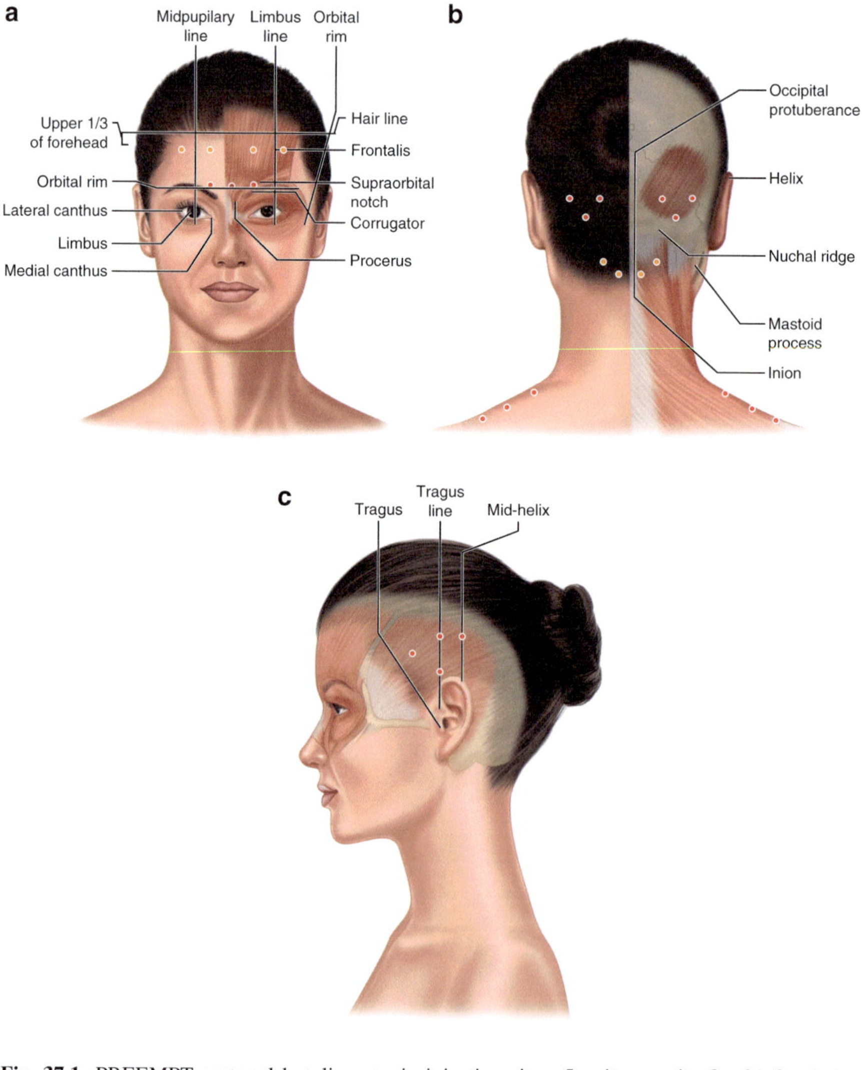

Fig. 37.1 PREEMPT protocol botulinumtoxin injection sites, 5 units per site for 31 fixed-site locations. (**a**) Red-Procerus (1 site), Purple- Corrugators (2 sites), Orange- Frontalis (4 sites). (**b**) Purple- Occipitalis (6 sites), Orange- Cervical Paraspinals (4 sites), Red- Trapezius (6 sites). (**c**) Temporalis (8 sites). [15]

Interventional treatments for migraine prevention include onabotulinumtoxin A (Botox) per PREEMPT protocol, an FDA-indicated treatment. Insurance companies generally require patients to have received adequate trials of two or three oral preventives from different pharmacologic classes prior to providing approval for onabotulintoxinA. The PREEMPT protocol consists of injections of 5 units of onabotulinumtoxin A to 31 standardized locations across the forehead, temples, occiput, and trapezeii (Fig. 37.1). Up to 40 additional units may be injected in a "follow the pain" manner, with the caveat that this must be mindful of avoiding areas where additional injections may have untoward cosmetic effects, eye ptosis, or neck drop. Pericranial peripheral nerve blocks are often performed for migraine prevention or for treatment of status migrainosus—greater occipital nerve blocks are the most common blocks performed. Supraorbital, supratrochlear, auriculotemporal, lesser occipital nerve blocks, and sphenopalatine ganglion blocks are also sometimes performed. Trigger point injections targeting the cervical paraspinals, trapezeii, levator scapulae, masseters, and other muscle groups may also be performed in patients for whom cervical myofascial pain is suspected of contributing to their headaches. Interventions targeting the temporomandibular joints, including injections and bite blocks, can be used when temporomandibular dysfunction is suspected of contributing to the patient's migraines.

Key Points

- Migraine is the most common primary headache disorder encountered in the outpatient and inpatient settings. Clinicians must first exclude secondary headache disorders before diagnosing migraine.
- Treatment should include education about lifestyle modifications including education about medication-overuse headache ("rebound headache").
- Pharmacologic treatments include preventive, acute, and rescue treatments.
- Oral preventive treatments are often started for patients with migraines 4 or more days a month, and onabotulinumtoxin A can be considered for patients with 8 or more migraine days a month and 15 or more headache days a month.

References

1. Stewart WF, Wood C, Reed ML, Roy J, Lipton RB. Cumulative lifetime migraine incidence in women and men. Cephalalgia. 2008;28(11):1170–8. https://doi.org/10.1111/j.1468-2982.2008.01666.x.
2. Headache Classification Committee of the International Headache Society (IHS). The International Classification of Headache Disorders, 3rd Edition (beta version). Cephalalgia. 2013;33(9):629–808. https://doi.org/10.1177/0333102413485658.
3. Dodick DW. Pearls: headache. Semin Neurol. 2010;30(1):74–81. https://doi.org/10.1055/s-0029-1245000.
4. Levine HL, Setzen M, Cady RK, et al. An otolaryngology, neurology, allergy, and primary care consensus on diagnosis and treatment of sinus headache. Otolaryngol Head Neck Surg. 2006;134(3):516–23. https://doi.org/10.1016/j.otohns.2005.11.024.

5. Lipton RB, Dodick D, Sadovsky R, et al. A self-administered screener for migraine in primary care: The ID Migraine validation study. Neurology. 2003;61(3):375–82. http://www.ncbi.nlm.nih.gov/pubmed/12913201. Accessed 16 May 2017.
6. Ross S, Wall E, Schierman B, et al. Quality improvement in neurology: primary headache quality measures. Neurology. 2015;84(2):200–3. https://doi.org/10.1212/WNL.0000000000001134.
7. American Headache Society | Choosing Wisely. http://www.choosingwisely.org/societies/american-headache-society/. 2013. Accessed 16 May 2017.
8. Silberstein SD, Holland S, Freitag F, Dodick DW, Argoff C, Ashman E. Evidence-based guideline update: pharmacologic treatment for episodic migraine prevention in adults report of the Quality Standards Subcommittee of the American Academy of Neurology and the American Headache Society. Neurology. 2012;78(17):1337–45. https://doi.org/10.1212/WNL.0b013e3182535d20.
9. Holland S, Silberstein SD, Freitag F, Dodick DW, Argoff C, Ashman E. Evidence-based guideline update: NSAIDs and other complementary treatments for episodic migraine prevention in adults: report of the Quality Standards Subcommittee of the American Academy of Neurology and the American Headache Society. Neurology. 2012;78(17):1346–53. https://doi.org/10.1212/WNL.0b013e3182535d0c.
10. Marmura MJ, Silberstein SD, Schwedt TJ. The acute treatment of migraine in adults: the American Headache Society evidence assessment of migraine pharmacotherapies. Headache. 2015;55(1):3–20. https://doi.org/10.1111/head.12499.
11. Bigal ME, Serrano D, Buse D, Scher A, Stewart WF, Lipton RB. Acute migraine medications and evolution from episodic to chronic migraine: a longitudinal population-based study. Headache. 2008;48(8):1157–68. https://doi.org/10.1111/j.1526-4610.2008.01217.x.
12. Kelley NE, Tepper DE. Rescue therapy for acute migraine, part 1: triptans, dihydroergotamine, and magnesium. Headache. 2012;52(1):114–28. https://doi.org/10.1111/j.1526-4610.2011.02062.x.
13. Kelley NE, Tepper DE. Rescue therapy for acute migraine, part 2: neuroleptics, antihistamines, and others. Headache. 2012;52(2):292–306. https://doi.org/10.1111/j.1526-4610.2011.02070.x.
14. Kelley NE, Tepper DE. Rescue therapy for acute migraine, part 3: Opioids, NSAIDs, steroids, and post-discharge medications. Headache. 2012;52(3):467–82. https://doi.org/10.1111/j.1526-4610.2012.02097.x.
15. Blumenfeld AM, Silberstein SD, Dodick DW, Aurora SK, Brin MF, Binder WJ. Insights into the functional anatomy behind the PREEMPT injection paradigm: guidance on achieving optimal outcomes. Headache. 2017;57(5):766–77.

Chapter 38
Surgical Techniques of Migraine Surgery

Eric J. Wright and William G. Austen Jr.

Frontal Migraine

Representative Case History

The patient is a 26-year-old white female who was referred to clinic for evaluation of her head pain. She has tried numerous pharmacologic treatments that have not alleviated her symptoms. She has been seen by numerous neurologists and has been given the diagnosis of chronic refractive frontal migraines. She currently does not work due to the almost daily migraines. She has no history of trauma. Her symptoms started approximately 10 years ago. Her pain starts at a constant location located above her right brow and spreads throughout the frontal area.

Overview

Patients found to be refractive to the current pharmacologic therapies of migraines can possibly benefit from surgical decompression of numerous peripheral nerves around the head and neck. It has been found that either the nerve irritation can act as a trigger for the migraines or a separate entity of a peripheral neuralgia. Patients

E. J. Wright (✉)
Division of Plastic and Reconstructive Surgery, Department of Surgery, University of Arkansas for Medical Sciences, Little Rock, AR, USA
e-mail: plasticsurgery@drericwright.com

W. G. Austen Jr.
Division of Plastic and Reconstructive Surgery, Harvard Medical School, Massachusetts General Hospital, Boston, MA, USA
e-mail: wausten@mgh.harvard.edu

J. Y. Suen, E. Petersen (eds.), *Diagnosis and Management of Head and Face Pain*, https://doi.org/10.1007/978-3-319-90999-8_38

frequently have been treated with numerous pharmacologic therapies yet continue to have symptoms. The pain will start at the area of nerve compression but will spread. This range of pain location can confuse the diagnosis of a single nerve etiology.

Differential Diagnosis

- Chronic frontal migraine with a peripheral trigger
- Supratrochlear/supraorbital neuralgia
- Intracranial process
- Frontal sinus pathology

Diagnostic Workup

As has been described, the success of the surgery will depend upon the correct patient selection. Migraines are a pathologic condition of the brain that, when triggered by peripheral nerve irritation or compression, can be treated with extracranial surgery. A thorough history and physical are performed at the initial patient encounter. If patients take a preventative medication, they are asked to stop several days before the clinic visit. Ideally, the patient will be experiencing a migraine at the time of the clinic visit. Patients evaluated are those who have been labeled as experiencing chronic migraines that are not successfully prevented or treatment with pharmacologic therapies or have not tolerated the treatment medications due to side effects.

Medical records from the neurologist are reviewed along with any imaging that has previously been performed. A migraine questionnaire is completed assessing the number of migraine per month, duration, intensity, location, and triggers.

Neurologists are with increasing frequency performing nerve blocks and administering botulinum toxin type A. A positive history of improvement or resolution of symptoms, even if temporary, is an indication that surgery could benefit the patient.

Patients are asked to point with one finger to the exact location of the onset of pain. It is at this location bupivacaine or lidocaine can be injected, 1–2 cc. Large amounts of anesthetic are not needed, as it is beneficial to isolate to the exact location as possible the area of nerve irritation. Patients are reevaluated in 10–15 min. If they have had a significant improvement or complete resolution of their pain, then it is believed that surgical intervention can offer a more permanent treatment solution. If the pain continues, this does not exclude surgery. Patients can have more than one peripheral trigger. Blocking of one area can unmask a second area. The areas are blocked sequentially until they have all been addressed. If the patient experiences numbness in the nerve distribution yet continues to have no significant improvement, at this point, surgery is not recommended.

The surgical procedures that have been described continue to evolve as our experience and understanding of the anatomical basis improves. Here, we describe the authors' preferred method of migraine surgery.

Representative Case Management

The patient has failed to achieve migraine control with medical management under direction of a neurologist. After office injection of lidocaine, her symptoms significantly improved; therefore she was offered surgical decompression of her supraorbital and supratrochlear nerves. Given the location of the trigger point areas, surgical access must be considered to avoid unsightly scarring on the face. Though endoscopic procedures can be successfully performed, the authors use an open approach for all decompression areas [1].

Under general anesthesia, the forehead and upper eyelid areas are injected with lidocaine 1% with 1:100,000 epinephrine. A transpalpebral incision at the supratarsal crease is made. The orbicularis oculi muscle elevated superiorly staying superficial to the septum. This is continued until the lateral orbital rim is encountered. By staying lateral, the target nerves will not be accidently injured in the exposure. Blunt dissection is performed medially until the supraorbital nerve is identified (Fig. 38.1). The nerve is released from either the bony foramen or notch. The nerve is then followed as it traverses the glabellar muscle unit. The depressor supercilii, corrugator supercilii, and procerus muscle fibers that surround the nerve as it travels superiorly are resected, completely freeing the nerve until it enters the subcutaneous tissue plane. The supraorbital artery, if found to be in close proximity of the nerve, is coagulated and resected. Once the nerve has been completely released, in order to prevent nerve scarring and contour irregularities, a fat flap is created from the medial fat pad and is sutured around the nerve. The skin is then closed. No drain is needed for the procedure.

Alternative Management Options

- Continued local anesthetic injection with long-acting or liposomal formula.
- Botulinum toxin type A has been shown to be a successful treatment for frontal migraines. However, this has been found to have decreasing efficacy in some patients. The neurologist before referral usually tries this option.
- Nerve resection can be performed if the patient continues to have symptoms following the decompression. This is reserved to secondary surgery due to the numbness of the forehead and anterior scalp. There is also concern that a neuroma can develop at the site of transection. In the authors' experience, this is typically not required.

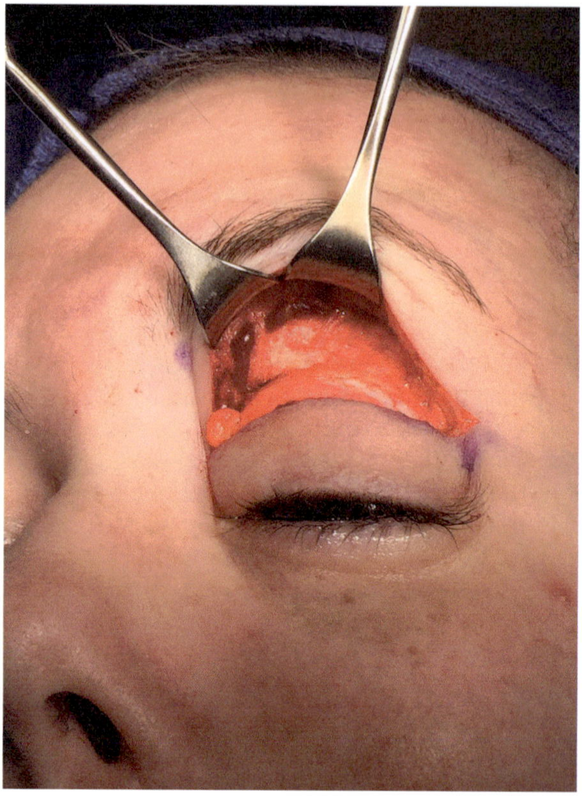

Fig. 38.1 Intraoperative view of the transpalpebral (upper blepharoplasty) approach to the orbital rim. The supratrochlear and supraorbital nerves are seen. The supraorbital nerve is seen exiting a tight bony foramen

Key Points

- Patients have failed medical management under the supervision of a neurologist.
- Upon injection of local anesthesia in the supraorbital area, patients' symptoms significantly improve. These patients can be expected to benefit from nerve decompression.
- Surgical approach is performed through a transpalpebral supratarsal crease incision to minimize any visual scarring.
- Complete release of the nerves is carried out along with resection of any muscle that could cause compression. The supraorbital artery is resected.

Conclusion

With careful patient selection, patients diagnosed with refractive chronic migraines can find symptomatic improvement with surgical decompression of the involved nerves. The described surgical procedures are performed via an open approach with thorough anatomical exploration for any areas of compression or irritation of the affected nerves. The field of migraine surgery will continue to evolve with ongoing research and experience.

Reference

1. Gfrerer L, Maman DY, Tessler O, Austen WG. Nonendoscopic deactivation of nerve triggers in migraine headache patients: surgical technique and outcomes. Plast Reconstr Surg. 2014;134(4):771–8. https://doi.org/10.1097/PRS.0000000000000507.

Chapter 39
Representative Clinical Case: Occipital Neuralgia

Michael D. Staudt and Jennifer A. Sweet

Representative Case History

The patient is a 44-year-old African-American female who presented with severe, lancinating occipital pain. Her medical history was notable for a motor vehicle collision resulting in a whiplash injury and a Chiari malformation for which she underwent decompression surgery. The pain was predominantly right-sided and described as constant, stabbing, and sharp and made worse with palpation and neck movement. The patient was neurologically intact on physical examination, although had a positive Tinel's sign with exquisite tenderness to palpation over the greater occipital nerve on the right side predominantly, as well as the left side to some degree. She achieved notable but transient pain relief with selective occipital nerve blocks and transcutaneous electrical nerve stimulation. Anticonvulsant medications resulted in pain relief initially, but were less effective over time.

Overview

Occipital neuralgia (ON) is a pain disorder described by the International Headache Society as sharp, shooting, or stabbing pain which manifests along the distribution of the greater (GON), lesser (LON) , or third occipital nerves [1]. It can be unilateral

M. D. Staudt
Department of Neurological Surgery, Case Western Reserve University, University Hospitals Cleveland Medical Center, Cleveland, OH, USA
e-mail: Michael.staudt@londonhospitals.ca

J. A. Sweet (✉)
Department of Neurosurgery, Case Western Reserve University, University Hospitals Cleveland Medical Center, Cleveland, OH, USA
e-mail: Jennifer.sweet@uhhospitals.org

J. Y. Suen, E. Petersen (eds.), *Diagnosis and Management of Head and Face Pain*, https://doi.org/10.1007/978-3-319-90999-8_39

or bilateral and presents with recurring paroxysmal episodes lasting for a few seconds to a minute. The pain is often elicited with palpation of the affected nerve branches or even with certain movements of the head and neck. It may also be associated with dysesthesias or allodynia. Frequently, nerve blocks will be done and produce temporary relief of symptoms, but lack of efficacy of the block does not necessarily exclude ON as a diagnosis [2, 3].

Knowledge of the anatomy of the occipital nerves is essential to understanding the diagnosis and treatment of ON. The dorsal ramus of C2 emerges between the atlas and axis and curves inferiorly and obliquely before giving off a medial branch, the GON [4]. The GON then pierces the semispinalis capitis and trapezius to supply the occipital skin toward the scalp vertex and is often accompanied by the occipital artery. The LON similarly arises from the C2 dorsal ramus, with an occasional contribution from the C3 dorsal ramus, and ascends the posterior border of the sternocleidomastoid before piercing the posterior triangle of the neck to innervate the mastoid region [4, 5]. The third occipital nerve arises from the superficial medial branch of the C3 dorsal ramus and innervates the suboccipital region [6]. A variable pain distribution in ON may be explained by the convergence between cervical and trigeminal afferents in the pars caudalis of the spinal trigeminal nucleus [4].

There are a variety of potential etiologies of ON, although most presentations are idiopathic [5]. However, ON can occur as a result of trauma or compression of the occipital nerves or upper cervical dorsal root ganglion. Thus, a thorough history and physical exam are important, as are radiographic imaging such as flexion/extension x-rays or occasionally a cervical MRI. ON may also arise from a neoplastic process. In addition, pain in the posterior scalp can be associated with a number of headache and non-headache disorders, although ON tends to be distinguished by the localized tenderness in the distribution of the occipital nerves.

Initial treatment measures are conservative and include alternating warm or cold compresses and physical therapy or massage to alleviate muscle tension [7]. Medications such as antiepileptics and antidepressants may decrease the frequency and severity of ON pain when taken regularly, and anti-inflammatories may alleviate pain during acute episodes [7]. Local anesthetic blocks and steroid injections can be both diagnostic and therapeutic, although the benefit is usually transient. Pulsed radiofrequency has gained popularity as an effective nondestructive treatment, but these effects are also short-lived [8]. There are numerous surgical treatment options for ON, including occipital neurectomy, C2 ganglionectomy, and rhizotomy, although these procedures tend to be invasive and destructive and confer variable benefit [9]. As such, occipital nerve stimulation (ONS) has emerged as an additional treatment modality for patients with medically refractory ON and has been demonstrated to provide excellent and sustained pain relief with low complication rates [10, 11]. ONS is also a reversible and adjustable treatment that does not produce numbness, unlike the lesioning procedures described above.

Differential Diagnosis

- Tension headache
- Cluster headache
- Migraine headache
- Hemicrania continua
- Cervicogenic headache
- Myofascial pain
- Chiari malformation
- C1–C2 degenerative arthritis
- Neoplasm involving the posterior fossa or C2 nerve root
- Systemic vasculitis or inflammatory lesions of the C2 nerve root or greater occipital nerve
- Giant cell arteritis involving the occipital arteries
- Postherpetic neuralgia involving the C2 nerve root or greater occipital nerve
- Metabolic disorders including diabetes
- Infection

Diagnostic Workup

The clinical history is important to distinguish ON from other headache disorders, primarily based on the distribution and characteristics of pain. Pain from true ON tends to be sharp and stabbing with paroxysmal attacks. It can be elicited with palpation of the neck and/or occiput and triggered with neck movements. In contrast, dull, aching, and throbbing pain that is more diffuse and harder to localize to the occipital nerves is less likely to be ON. Patients may report avoiding washing or brushing their hair, or wearing hats. Although the majority of ON cases are idiopathic, it is important to ask about prior head or neck trauma, neck surgery, or other systemic disorders.

A physical exam should demonstrate pain on palpation of the occipital region. There may also be allodynia with stimulation of other regions of the scalp or hair. A positive Tinel's sign is frequently elicited over the affected nerve that reproduces the patient's pain. The neck and occipital region should be examined for irregularities or scars from previous head or neck trauma or surgery.

An initial diagnostic workup includes head and neck imaging (MRI or CT) to rule out a structural cause for the patient's symptoms, such as a tumor, degenerative cervical spine disease, or a Chiari malformation, as well as flexion/extension cervical X-rays to rule out instability. Additional testing may include blood work for systemic inflammatory or metabolic processes, if the clinical history is suggestive of these etiologies. Local anesthetic block of the GON and/or LON is both diagnostic and therapeutic. However, it is important to recognize that other headache types may also respond to occipital nerve blocks [12].

Case Management

The patient had a history of a whiplash injury and Chiari decompression prior to the onset of her symptoms, which may complicate the diagnosis of ON as these pathologies can present with neck pain and posterior headaches. However, the characteristics of her occipital pain and physical exam findings were most consistent with a diagnosis of ON. Conservative management was first attempted with medications, including gabapentin (800 mg TID) and amitriptyline (25 mg daily). Topiramate was tried but was ineffective. Local anesthetic blocks and transcutaneous electrical nerve stimulation resulted in significant but transient benefit. A decision was then made to proceed with an occipital nerve stimulation trial.

After a pain psychology evaluation confirmed the patient's candidacy for surgical intervention, a trial stimulator lead was placed. The patient was positioned supine with a shoulder bump, under MAC and local anesthesia, and an 8-contract trial percutaneous spinal cord stimulator electrode was inserted from a stab incision in the right posterior auricular region, extending across the occiput bilaterally at the level of the posterior arch of C1, as confirmed with intraoperative fluoroscopy. The lead position also corresponded with the location of the patient's positive Tinel's sign, which was marked preoperatively. The patient was awoken during the trial procedure and tested to confirm adequate coverage of her pain. The trial leads were externalized and secured, and she was sent home with multiple stimulation program options for 7 days. Trial stimulation resulted in greater than 50% pain relief (Fig. 39.1).

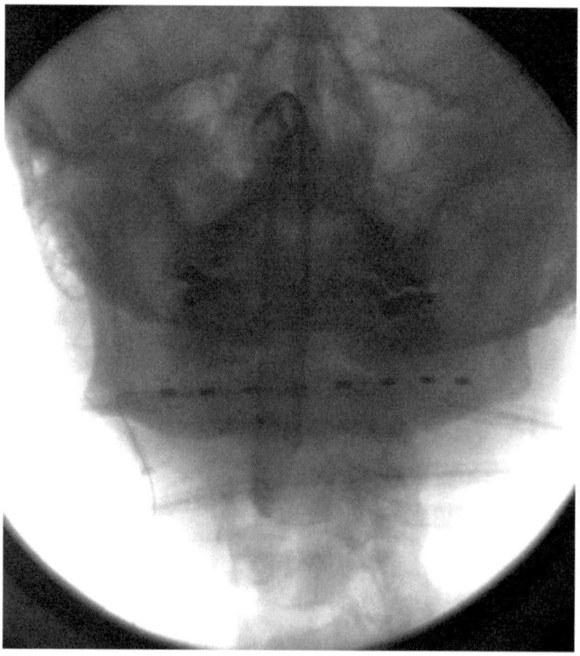

Fig. 39.1 Intraoperative x-rays during trial occipital nerve stimulator electrode implantation. The electrode is inserted through the right side and extends to the contralateral side as well, corresponding with the patient's pain distribution

One month later, the patient underwent permanent ONS lead implantation, performed in the same manner described above. Again, an 8-contact percutaneous spinal cord stimulator electrode was inserted through a small incision in the right posterior auricular region of the scalp. The lead was secured with an anchor, which was sutured to the fascia, and a strain relief loop was placed. The lead was then tunneled to the right infraclavicular region and connected to a rechargeable, implantable pulse generator. Impedances were checked, the generator was secured to the fascia, and the wounds were irrigated and closed in sequential layers. Postoperative x-rays confirmed good positioning of the lead (Fig. 39.2).

The patient maintained the same benefit from her permanent stimulator as from the trial and was able to be more active in her daily life. In follow-up, she has described significant and near-complete resolution of her pain, without requiring oral pain medications.

Alternative Management Options

- Conservative therapy with anticonvulsants and antidepressants was first tried and failed, despite adjustments in medication types and dosages. Further medical therapy alone would likely be ineffective.
- Occipital neurectomy of the greater and/or lesser occipital nerves could be attempted, although would be difficult due to the previous scar tissue from the Chiari decompression. These procedures also have a high rate of pain recurrence, and the proximal nerve stump may develop a painful neuroma.

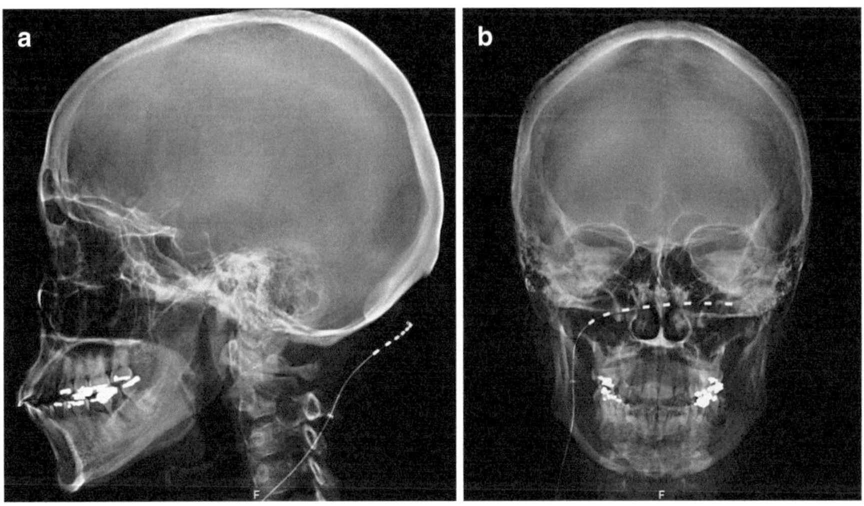

Fig. 39.2 Postoperative lateral (**a**) and anterior-posterior (**b**) skull x-rays demonstrate appropriate occipital nerve stimulator electrode placement

- C2 ganglionectomy avoids the issues of nerve regeneration and neuroma formation that occur with neurectomy and would result in complete sensory loss in the C2 distribution. This procedure is more invasive and technically complicated and may result in a painful deafferentation syndrome.
- Rhizotomy could be attempted as a last resort, although it is more invasive and technically complicated than all other therapeutic measures. Selective dorsal rhizotomies are usually attempted to minimize sensory loss.

Key Points

- Occipital neuralgia is characterized by severe, paroxysmal, sharp, and stabbing pain in the distribution of the greater, lesser, and/or third occipital nerves.
- Diagnosis is confirmed by occipital tenderness and a positive Tinel's sign along the occipital nerve and is relieved with local anesthetic blocks.
- First-line treatment consists of medical management with antiepileptic and/or antidepressant medications.
- Medically refractory occipital neuralgia is best managed with occipital nerve stimulation, a procedure that is relatively easy to perform, is associated with low surgical risk, and confers excellent and lasting clinical benefit.
- Surgical lesioning procedures may be considered as alternative therapies but are much more invasive and technically challenging. They tend to produce permanent numbness but can also result in painful deafferentation syndromes.

References

1. The International Classification of Headache Disorders, 3rd edition (beta version). Cephalalgia. 2013;33:629–808. https://doi.org/10.1177/0333102413485658.
2. Tobin JA, Flitman SS. Occipital nerve blocks: effect of symptomatic medication: overuse and headache type on failure rate. Headache. 2009;49:1479–85. https://doi.org/10.1111/j.1526-4610.2009.01549.x.
3. Tobin J, Flitman S. Occipital nerve blocks: when and what to inject? Headache. 2009;49:1521–33. https://doi.org/10.1111/j.1526-4610.2009.01493.x.
4. Johnstone CS, Sundaraj R. Occipital nerve stimulation for the treatment of occipital neuralgia-eight case studies. Neuromodulation. 2006;9:41–7. https://doi.org/10.1111/j.1525-1403.2006.00041.x.
5. Cesmebasi A, Muhleman MA, Hulsberg P, Gielecki J, Matusz P, Tubbs RS, Loukas M. Occipital neuralgia: anatomic considerations. Clin Anat. 2015;28:101–8. https://doi.org/10.1002/ca.22468.
6. Bogduk N. Cervicogenic headache: anatomic basis and pathophysiologic mechanisms. Curr Pain Headache Rep. 2001;5:382–6.
7. Vanelderen P, Lataster A, Levy R, Mekhail N, van Kleef M, Van Zundert J. 8. Occipital neuralgia. Pain Pract. 2010;10:137–44. https://doi.org/10.1111/j.1533-2500.2009.00355.x.
8. Cohen SP, Peterlin BL, Fulton L, Neely ET, Kurihara C, Gupta A, Mali J, Fu DC, Jacobs MB, Plunkett AR, Verdun AJ, Stojanovic MP, Hanling S, Constantinescu O, White RL, McLean BC, Pasquina PF, Zhao Z. Randomized, double-blind, comparative-effectiveness study comparing pulsed radiofrequency to steroid injections for occipital neuralgia or migraine with occipital nerve tenderness. Pain. 2015;156:2585–94. https://doi.org/10.1097/j.pain.0000000000000373.

9. Slavin KV, Nersesyan H, Wess C. Peripheral neurostimulation for treatment of intractable occipital neuralgia. Neurosurgery. 2006;58:112–119; discussion 112-119.
10. Weiner RL, Reed KL. Peripheral neurostimulation for control of intractable occipital neuralgia. Neuromodulation. 1999;2:217–21. https://doi.org/10.1046/j.1525-1403.1999.00217.x.
11. Sweet JA, Mitchell LS, Narouze S, Sharan AD, Falowski SM, Schwalb JM, Machado A, Rosenow JM, Petersen EA, Hayek SM, Arle JE, Pilitsis JG. Occipital nerve stimulation for the treatment of patients with medically refractory occipital neuralgia: congress of neurological surgeons systematic review and evidence-based guideline. Neurosurgery. 2015;77:332–41. https://doi.org/10.1227/NEU.0000000000000872.
12. Bovim G, Sand T. Cervicogenic headache, migraine without aura and tension-type headache. Diagnostic blockade of greater occipital and supra-orbital nerves. Pain. 1992;51:43–8.

Chapter 40
Head and Neck Cancer Pain: A Case Study

Vinita Singh and Johnathan H. Goree

Representative Case History

The patient is a 53-year-old male with T3N2c squamous cell carcinoma of the left supraglottis who is now 4 weeks into a 7-week course for radiation and chemotherapy. He presents with constant, uncontrolled throat pain described as burning and shooting. He remarks that this began shortly after the onset of his radiation therapy and chemotherapy treatments. Of note, the patient does have a history of chronic pain secondary to failed back surgery treated with tricyclic antidepressants and low-dose opiates.

Overview

Radiation-induced mucositis is defined as mucosal damage to the oral and pharyngeal cavity as a result of cancer therapy. This is a common and treatment-limiting side effect of radiotherapy, and this risk is increased in patients who are receiving concurrent chemotherapy. Sonis et al. estimate the occurrence of mucositis with cancer of the head and neck to be 42%, while others have estimated these numbers to be much higher [1]. While it was previously believed that this disease is simply a loss of the epithelium due to the destruction of epithelial stem cells, current models

V. Singh (✉)
Department of Anesthesiology, Emory University School of Medicine, Atlanta, GA, USA
e-mail: vinita.singh@emory.edu

J. H. Goree
Department of Anesthesiology, University of Arkansas for Medical Sciences, Little Rock, AR, USA
e-mail: jhgoree@uams.edu

J. Y. Suen, E. Petersen (eds.), *Diagnosis and Management of Head and Face Pain*, https://doi.org/10.1007/978-3-319-90999-8_40

of disease pathophysiology now suggest a much more complex, five-stage mechanism [2]. First is *initiation* where oxidative stress and reactive oxygen species are generated by chemotherapeutic agents and radiation. Second is the *generation of messenger signals*. During this phase, reactive oxygen species through various mechanisms begin to generate secondary mediators of injury including TNF-α and others. Third is *amplification*, in which these mediators like TNF-α and other pro-inflammatory cytokines begin to activate a number of pathways that result in tissue injury and apoptosis. This leads to *ulceration* which includes the bacterial colonization of growing lesions where epithelial death has recently occurred. The last phase is *healing* which is associated with re-epithelialization and reestablishment of oral flora [1, 2]. Symptoms of mucositis include oral pain, restricted speech, secondary infections, and difficulty swallowing often leading to reduced oral intake [2–4].

Differential Diagnosis

- Neoplasm-related pain
- Oral thrush
- Candidiasis
- Scarring secondary to radiation
- Herpes simplex virus
- Oral mucositis secondary to radiation therapy or chemotherapy

Diagnostic Workup

Diagnosis is mostly clinical based on history and physical exam. Radiation-induced mucositis may be associated with burning sensation and pain. Clinical exam often reveals redness, edema, or ulceration of the affected area [5, 6]. Difficulty with speech, difficulty swallowing (even saliva) and decreased oral opening may be observed. Multiple scoring systems for the severity of mucositis have been developed, but none are universally accepted. One example is the National Cancer Institute Common Terminology Criteria. This includes elements of pain, erythema, ulceration, function, and dietary intake. There are also more specific scales for patients who are undergoing radiation and chemotherapy for treatment of head and neck cancer.

Case Management

Since the pain onset coincided with radiation treatment, it was more likely radiation-induced mucositis-related pain as opposed to primary neoplasm-related pain. Physical exam revealed erythema of left oropharyngeal area and tenderness to palpation over erythematous area. The patient was advised to do frequent saline flushes throughout the day to keep the oral cavity clean and avoid superimposed infection. He was also prescribed magic mouthwash which contained Maalox (aluminum hydroxide, magnesium hydroxide, and simethicone), nystatin, diphenhydramine, and lidocaine to swish and swallow 10 mL by mouth every 4–6 h as needed. He was prescribed liquid gabapentin for neuropathic pain. This patient was opioid tolerant and had to be maintained on high dose of opioids as well for acute pain control. Fentanyl patch was chosen as a long-acting opiate to avoid issues with swallowing. Liquid oxycodone was chosen as breakthrough medication for ease of administration. Medication dosage was titrated on various occasions as his pain increased during the continued treatment, but we were able to wean opiates to his baseline after he finished his treatment. Superior laryngeal nerve block was considered, given the location of his tumor, but could not be pursued as he developed systemic infection involving his peripherally inserted central catheter shortly after initiation of his therapy.

Alternative Management Options

- Superior laryngeal nerve block
- Keratinocyte growth factor-1
- 0.5% doxepin mouthwash
- 2% morphine mouthwash
- Zinc supplementation

Key Points

- Early speech and occupational rehabilitation are crucial when a patient is receiving head and neck radiation.
- Medications may be difficult to swallow, and oral liquid and transdermal pain medications should be considered.
- Nutrition can become challenging if swallowing becomes an issue.
- Oral hygiene is of utmost importance to reduce severity of oral mucositis and avoid complications such as infection

References

1. Sonis A, et al. Perspectives on cancer therapy-induced mucosal injury. Cancer. 2004;100:1995–2025.
2. Lalla R, et al. MASSC/ISOO clinical practice guidelines for the management of mucositis secondary to cancer treatment. Cancer. 2014;120:1453–61.
3. Mallick S, Benson R, Rath GK. Radiation induced oral mucositis: a review of current literature on prevention and management. Eur Arch Otorhinolaryngol. 2016;273:2285–93.
4. Epstein JB, Schubert MM. Oropharyngeal mucositis in cancer therapy. Review of pathogenesis, diagnosis, and management. Oncology (Williston). 2003;17:1767–79; discussion 1779–1782.

5. Rahman S, Maillou P, Barker D, Donachie M. Radiotherapy and the oral environment the effects of radiotherapy on the hard and soft tissues of the mouth and its management. Eur J Prosthodont Restor Dent. 2013;21:80–7.
6. Moslemia D, et al. Management of chemo/radiation-induced oral mucositis in patients with head and neck cancer: a review of the current literature. Radiother Oncol. 2016;120:13–20.

Chapter 41
Cervical Plexus Pain Case Report

Chelsey Smith and James Y. Suen

Representative Case

This patient is a 66-year-old white female presenting with severe pain in the right upper neck and jaw area. The pain has been present since being weaned off of a ventilator during an ICU stay for sepsis. She had a tracheostomy placed during her stay in the ICU because of a prolonged need for ventilation. The tracheostomy tube has been removed. Constant in nature, the pain is debilitating for her. She also has pain on both sides of her upper neck and jawline area. She has been on gabapentin, hydrocodone, and alprazolam, and the pain is not controlled.

Overview

The upper cervical plexus sensory innervation covers several topographic areas with its three named branches: lesser occipital, greater auricular, and the anterior cervical nerves (Fig. 41.1). The branches wrap around the posterior border of the sternocleidomastoid muscle (SCM) approximately 1–2 cm superior to the midpoint of the sternocleidomastoid muscle between the mastoid and clavicle. The branches extend radially like the spokes of a bicycle wheel. The *lesser occipital branch* supplies

C. Smith
ENTcare, Dothan, AL, USA
e-mail: cjsmith2@aums.edu

J. Y. Suen (✉)
Department of Otolaryngology—Head and Neck Surgery,
University of Arkansas for Medical Sciences, Little Rock, AR, USA
e-mail: chelseyjsmith5@gmail.com

J. Y. Suen, E. Petersen (eds.), *Diagnosis and Management of Head and Face Pain*, https://doi.org/10.1007/978-3-319-90999-8_41

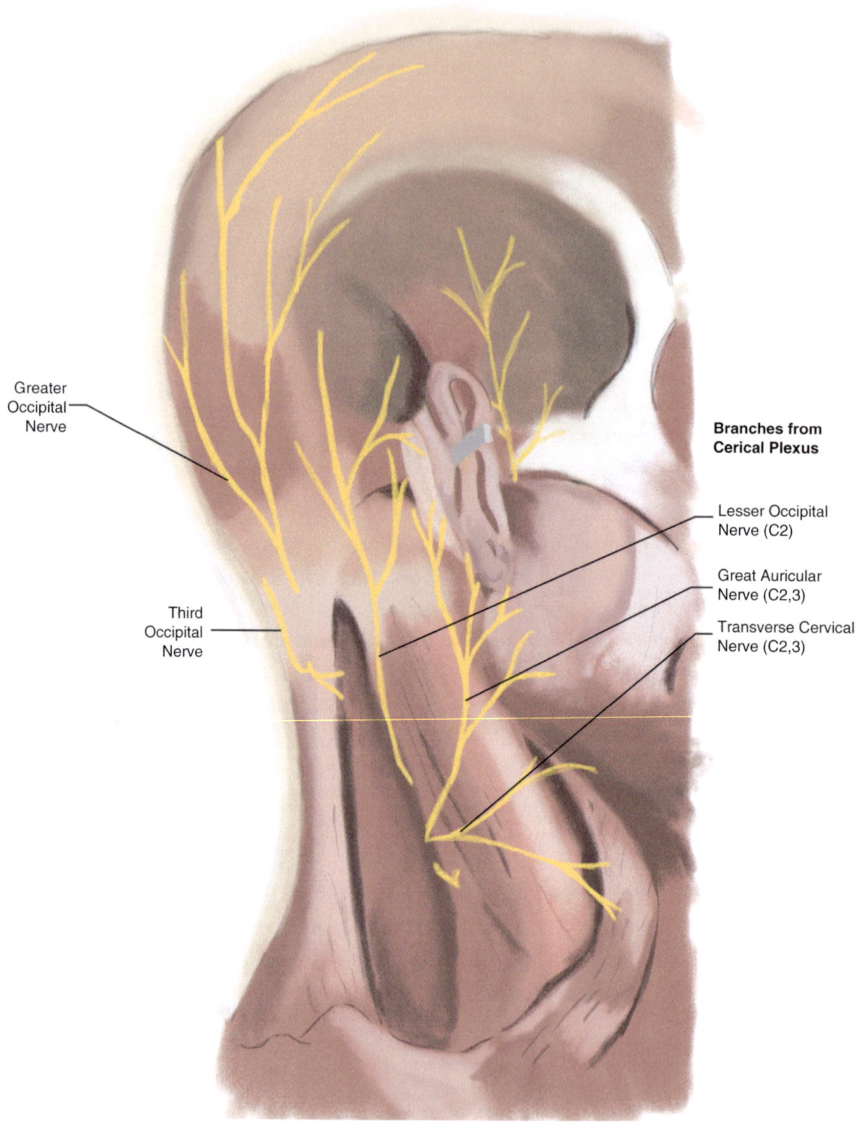

Fig. 41.1 The upper cervical plexus nerves innervate the areas behind the ear to the top, the lower one half of the ear, the parotid, and angle of the jaw

sensation to the postauricular area to above the ear. The *greater auricular nerve* ascends around the SCM muscle and supplies the lower earlobe and the skin over the parotid gland. The *transverse cervical nerve* supplies sensation to the angle of the jaw area. Due to its wide distribution, it can be the culprit for head, neck, and facial pain. The patient will often denote a trigger point within this dermatome with accompanying radiation of pain in one or more nerve branch regions. Chief complaints associated with cervical plexus neuralgia can range from ear pain to jaw pain to scalp pain to neck pain, and commonly the patient has previously been misdiagnosed.

Differential Diagnosis

- Trauma—can compress nerves or cause neuromas.
- Skin cancer or other cancers with perineural invasion and lymph node metastasis.
- Postoperative after neck dissection.
- Brain tumors—history and imaging can rule this out.
- Migraine headaches.
- Neck musculature pain.
- Eagle's syndrome.
- Cervical plexus neuralgia of unknown etiology.

Diagnostic Workup

In addition to the timeline of pain in the cervical plexus region, quality, radiation, consistency, and triggers are important. Trigger points are significant and can convey which branches are most impacted by the pain. Previous history of cancers, surgeries, infections, and traumas are also pertinent. Ask about risk factors such as tobacco and alcohol use, along with any signs of neck masses. Comprehensive head and neck exam is paramount for cervical plexus dermatomal pain, particularly in those patients with cancer risk factors. Ear exam, mirror exam of the pharynx and larynx, and palpation of the neck for lymphadenopathies, masses, and thyroid pathology should be performed on these patients also. Imaging for this subset of patients may include cervical CT scan to work up masses/pathology in the neck or to aid in the workup of any suspicious lesions in the upper aerodigestive tract. MRI can be used to rule out cervical spine pathology and also to better delineate any vascular or lymphatic malformations that are found.

Representative Case Management

The patient's neck and face pain was debilitating for her. Daily medications such as tramadol, hydrocodone, and gabapentin were being utilized multiple times daily with little effect. She was also on anticonvulsants chronically for a history of seizures. CT and MRI were performed to rule out any underlying pathology related to cervical plexus pain for this patient. No specific findings were found on MRI, but she was noted to have a right-sided elongated styloid process adjacent to her right carotid artery. Initially, nerve injections were tried in the clinic setting for diagnosis and pain control. The primary injection of 1% lidocaine with 1/100,000 epinephrine (3 cc) into the right cervical plexus would relieve her pain, and this was followed with 0.5% bupivacaine (3 cc) injection [1]. Liposomal bupivacaine injection were also used at times. With the nerve blocks, she would experience immediate pain relief that lasted from 1 day to 1 week. Due to the findings of elongated styloid process, we discussed excision of her elongated styloid process to help with her pain, and she underwent the procedure. After resection of the styloid process, her seizures stopped, and she indicated that her neck pain was less but still persistent. Nerve blocks were resumed for residual pain. Because the residual pain persisted, we discussed with her resection of the greater auricular and transverse cervical nerve branches (pain distribution was in these areas primarily). After the resection of these nerve branches was performed, she had some mild residual pain and soreness for the first 4 weeks postoperatively, but she has been pain-free except for some tolerable soreness and had not taken any narcotic pain medication in over 10 months. Her quality of life was greatly improved, as this was the first time in 3 years she had not been reliant on narcotic medications. She continues to do well at subsequent follow-up visits and maintains discontinuation of narcotic medications. Also the pain on the opposite side of her jaw area and upper neck has resolved since surgery.

Alternative Management Options

- Cervical plexus nerve decompression could have been initially performed in lieu of nerve resection, but the patient was not concerned about permanent numbness in the jawline and neck, so nerve resection was pursued.
- Ablation using alcohol or radiofrequency techniques can be utilized for pain relief, but these techniques can be painful.

Key Points
- Nerve blocks aided in diagnosis and short-term management of her symptoms.
- Treatment of her pain was multifaceted in that imaging (CT) indicated that the elongated styloid process could be linked to her pain, but after surgical resection of the styloid process, only a portion of her pain was relieved.
- Post styloid resection, her pain was controllable with nerve blocks but only for short intervals.
- If nerve blocks do not give prolonged pain relief, then nerve resection can be an option.
- Nerve resection can give prolonged or permanent pain relief.

Reference

1. Dash KS, Janis JE, Guyuron B. The lesser and third occipital nerves and migraine headaches. Plast Reconstr Surg. 2005;115:1752–8. discussion 1759–1760

Chapter 42
Head Pain in Pediatrics

Natalie Strickland and Yuanxu Dong

Representative Case History

John is a 12-year-old otherwise healthy white male who is brought in by his mother. She is concerned with a history of intermittent changes in his vision as well as complaints that he is often fatigued, complaining of neck stiffness, poor sleep, and irritab. She has been going through a divorce and is concerned he is making this up to get attention.

When asked he describes the changes to his vision as objects being bigger or smaller than he knows they should be. Sometimes stationary objects will appear to move. The changes in his vision usually last about 30–60 minutes. He said this normally only happens about twice a year since he was 5 but now it is happening twice a month. Upon further questioning he reports right-sided frontal pain that he says hurts very bad after his vision gets better. Sometimes he also wants to vomit. He states improvement with going to a quiet dark room and taking ibuprofen. If he can't lie down and take medicine, the pain has a 2-day duration.

N. Strickland (✉)
Department of Anesthesiology, University of Arkansas Medical Sciences,
Little Rock, AR, USA
e-mail: nataliestrickland1@icloud.com

Y. Dong
Department of Pediatric Anesthesiology, Arkansas Children's Hospital,
Little Rock, AR, USA

J. Y. Suen, E. Petersen (eds.), *Diagnosis and Management of Head and Face Pain*, https://doi.org/10.1007/978-3-319-90999-8_42

Overview

Headache is a common pediatric pain syndrome in the head and neck area. Since brain tissue is insensate, headache is the result of stimulation of pain-sensitive nerve fibers in large cerebral blood vessels, periosteum, and soft tissues within the scalp, sinuses, the temporomandibular joints, dentition, or the gingiva. Stimulation of these pain-sensitive nerve fibers can result from many primary and secondary causes, including predisposition due to family history, an intracranial process, trauma, vascular disease, or sinusitis. Headaches can have significant impact on the lives of pediatric patients, resulting in missed school days, poor academic performance, loss of social interactions, missed extracurricular activities, and psychosocial issues. Studies vary in the epidemiology of childhood headaches. There is an overall prevalence of 58% of patients reporting some form of headache in the past year. Headaches are more common in boys in children under 7 years, but as puberty approaches, the ratio changes. 27% of adolescent females and 20% of adolescent males have frequent or severe headaches. This same sex differentiation applies for migraines. In the past year, 5% of boys and 8% of girls have had a migraine. Recognition of the cause for the pediatric headaches is crucial to the success of their treatment.

Differential Diagnosis

The most common pediatric primary headaches are migraine and tension-type headaches. Both types can be classified by temporal pattern: acute, acute recurrent, chronic nonprogressive, and chronic progressive. See Table 42.1 for examples of the four temporal patterns of headaches.

The International Headache Society (IHS) has classified headaches into three groups on the basis of etiology and has provided diagnostic criteria to facilitate proper evaluation and treatment. The three main classifications are as follows:

- Primary headaches
  - Migraine
  - Tension type
  - Trigeminal autonomic cephalalgias (cluster and paroxysmal hemicranias)
  - Others (i.e., exercise primary cough, new daily persistent headache)
- Secondary headaches such as head/neck trauma, vascular disorders, infection, or psychiatric disorders
- Cranial neuralgias, facial pain, and others

Table 42.1 Causes of pediatric headaches

Acute headache causes	
Infection: sinusitis, pharyngitis, meningitis, or upper respiratory tract Migraine Intracranial hemorrhage Hypertension Substance abuse (e.g., cocaine, alcohol) Hydrocephalus	Ventriculoperitoneal shunt malfunction Brain tumor Trauma Stroke Vasculitis Intoxicants (e.g., lead, carbon monoxide)
Acute recurrent headache causes	
Migraine Fasting/eating disorders Mitochondrial disease Trigeminal autonomic cephalalgias	Tension headache Recurrent toxin: alcohol, illicit drugs, medications Seizure-associated headache
Chronic nonprogressive headache causes	
Tension headache Chronic posttraumatic headache Chronic trigeminal autonomic cephalalgias Thyroid disease Dental disease	Sleep apnea Chronic migraine New daily persistent headache Chronic sinus disease Idiopathic intracranial hypertension Fasting/eating disorders
Chronic-progressive headache causes	
Brain tumor Brain abscess/infection Aneurysm or vascular malformation Hydrocephalus or other elevated causes of intracranial hypertension Thyroid disease Parathyroid disease	Pseudotumor cerebri Medications (birth control, tetracycline, high-dose vitamin A) Intoxication (lead poisoning) Sinus venous thrombus Chiari malformation Vasculitis

Diagnostic Workup

For primary pediatric headaches, a thorough history and physical examination is often sufficient to obtain the diagnosis. Laboratory, radiographic imaging, and electroencephalographic studies are not useful to establish the diagnosis of a primary pediatric headache. They can be helpful in excluding secondary causes of headache such as an electroencephalogram for a child with migraine variants that is concerning for seizure activity.

Neuroimaging should be performed if there is any suspicion of a structural etiology to the headache in question. Table 42.2 provides red flags for causes of secondary headaches that warrant imaging. Given the broad differential of structural causes for headache and the wide array of imaging modalities that are available, imaging studies must be chosen judiciously in order to yield the greatest amount of clinical information in a cost-effective manner. However, routine imaging studies often are

Table 42.2 Red flags for secondary headache

Worst headache of life
Acute headache with exploding or sudden severe onset
Thunderclap headache
Progressive chronic headache
Increased headache with straining, coughing, or sneezing
Focal neurologic symptoms: altered mental status, papilledema, ataxia, abnormal reflexes, abnormal eye movements, other abnormalities, or asymmetric neurologic exam
Age less than 3 years old
Presence of ventriculoperitoneal shunt
Neurofibromatosis or tuberous sclerosis or other neurocutaneous syndrome
Systemic symptoms: fever, weight loss, rash, or joint pain
Secondary risk factors: immunosuppression, genetic disorder, rheumatologic disorder, cancer, hypercoagulable state
Change in headache pattern: new or different change in frequency, severity, or clinical features
Morning headache or vomiting upon awakening
Headache waking the patient up from sleep
Meningeal signs

not necessary for pediatric patients with long-standing stable headache symptoms and normal neurologic examination, since the likelihood of these patients having any significant structural pathology is low.

John does not have a history of any intracranial abnormalities or seizure disorder. His 14-point review of systems is negative except as described in the representative case above. He saw an ophthalmologist 1 week ago and had a normal visual exam. There is no family history of seizures or brain tumors. His mother, sister, and aunt all have migraines. On exam, John is not in distress. He is slightly overweight with normal vital signs for his age. A complete neurologic exam is normal. The rest of his physical exam was unremarkable.

Representative Case Management

Pathophysiology

Migraine headaches make up the majority of primary pediatric headaches. Prevalence is around 1–3% in children 3–7 years old and 8–23% in adolescence. The exact etiology of migraine headaches still remains unclear, but it is felt that the cause is multifactorial. One proposed contributing mechanism of migraine pain suggests the stimulation of the trigeminovascular system. The initial triggers for the activation of the trigeminovascular system remain unclear. The release of pro-inflammatory mediators such as substance P, calcitonin gene-related peptide, and vasoactive intestinal peptide from the synaptic boutons of the perivascular branches of the trigeminal nerve at the meningeal and basal cerebral vessel level leads to neurogenic inflammation such as rupture of local blood vessel and disruption of blood-brain barrier. The subsequent vasodilatation further stimulates the trigeminovascular system thus creating a positive feedback loop within the system.

Another proposed contributing mechanism of migraine headaches is abnormal central transmission of afferent pain signals in these patients. Evidence exists that patients with migraine headaches can exhibit a defect in the central catecholaminergic system that leads to cortical hyperexcitability. Abnormal magnesium metabolism, more specifically low magnesium level, can also contribute in the abnormal afferent central transmission of pain.

Radiographically white matter hyperintensities in the posterior circulation territories on MRI T2-weighted images are observed at a higher frequency in patients with migraines accompanied by aura. The exact role of this phenomenon in the pathophysiology of migraines still needs further elucidation.

An other proposed mechanism of migraine headache has its origin within the brain stem. The aura in a migraine headache is thought to be mediated by neuronal activation followed by suppression, otherwise known as cortical spreading depression, throughout the cortical surface. At the same time, changes occur in cerebral blood flow resulting in hyperperfusion followed by hypoperfusion. This process of cortical spreading depression is thought to be due to either trauma or changes in the local concentration of potassium, hydrogen ions, and glutamate. Possibly through the release of nitric oxide, atrinatriuretic peptide, noradrenergic pathways activation, and/or alterations to cerebral blood flow, cortical spreading depression activates the nociceptive pathway within the central nervous system. Cortical spreading depressions can also lead to neurogenic inflammation, which can stimulate several neurotransmitters that cause cerebral blood flow alteration and nociceptor activation within the central nervous system.

Migraine headaches may also exhibit a genetic predisposition. Almost 70% of pediatric migraine patients have at least one family member with migraine headache. In familial hemiplegic migraine, a rare migraine subtype, several genetic mutations were found in ion channels that are responsible for neurotransmitter release within the CNS. These mutations may ultimately change cortical excitability.

Classification of Migraines

Pediatric migraines can be divided into two groups: with aura and without aura. They are often bilateral in nature and the precise location is often difficult to obtain from children. The duration is often shorter when compared to adults, can be only 30–60 min. Migraine without aura is more common in pediatrics. Aura is seen in 14–30% of children with migraines. Like adult patients, pediatric patients also experience premonitory symptoms. The most common symptoms include neck stiffness, fatigue, irritability, face changes, and mood changes. Other premonitory symptoms included yawning, nausea, phonophobia, photophobia, cacosmia, hyperactivity, sleep problems, increased anxiety, food cravings, and difficulty concentrating.

Migraine without aura is identified by at least five episodes meeting the following criteria:

Duration under 72 h

- At least two of the following:
  - Unilateral or bilateral
  - Pulsating
  - Moderate to severe in intensity
  - Aggravated by or causing avoidance of routine physical activity
- At least one of the following must be present during the episodes:
  - Nausea and/or vomiting
  - Photophobia and/or phonophobia
- Not attributed to any other cause

Symptoms of dizziness, blurry vision, difficulty reading, stomach pain, flushing, sweating, limb pain, pallor, and dark circles of the eye may also be present during a migraine. Children will often have loss in appetite, be quitet, and want to be left alone. They may have intolerance to light, noise, smells, and physical activity.

Common migraine triggers include stress, "let up" from stress, dehydration, fasting, illness, and lack of sleep. Other lifestyle factors affecting migraines include obesity, lack of physical exercise, regular consumption of alcohol or caffeine, dysfunctional family situation, physical or emotional abuse, bullying, unfair treatment at school, and insufficient leisure time.

Migraine with aura consists of migraine headaches episodes that meet IHS criteria for migraine without aura along with visual, sensory, or speech symptoms or combination of the three. The onset of the aura is gradual and the aura lasts no more than 60 min. Auras usually occur less than 30 min before the onset of headache. See Table 42.3 for common pediatric auras. Both positive and negative features can be

Table 42.3 Auras

Motor (rare)	Weakness or hemiplegia
Retinal	Sudden loss of vision or photopsia or scintillations in only one eye
Sensory (less common than visual)	Numbness or tingling
Visual	Scotomata Blurry vision Tunnel vision Scintillations Zigzag lines Alice in Wonderland syndrome

experienced with the aura and the symptoms are completely self-limited. Migraine with aura includes the following types of headaches:

- Typical aura with migraine
- Typical aura with nonmigraine headache
- Typical aura without headache
- Familial hemiplegic migraine
- Sporadic hemiplegic migraine
- Basilar type migraine

Some less common migraines are characterized by prominent sensory aura such as vision disturbances and distorted sense of space and time. Patients may experience sensory hallucinations such as micropsia and/or metamorphopsia.

Hemiplegic migraine is seen more commonly in pediatric patients than in adult patient. It is characterized by sudden onset of hemiparesis and/or hemianesthesia with the headache to follow shortly after. Other associated symptoms include numbness, aphasia, and confusion. This can be familial or sporadic.

Basilar artery migraines are more common in female pediatric patients. These headaches are usually characterized by dizziness, ataxia, nystagmus, dysarthria, tinnitus/hyperacusis, bilateral paresthesias, diplopia or other vision disturbance, vomiting, and severe occipital headache. There is no motor weakness. The auras can be unilateral or bilateral.

Our case patient John meets the definition of pediatric migraine with a visual aura. He describes the Alice in Wonderland syndrome visual aura about 30–60 min before he has unilateral, moderate/severe intense frontal headache associated with nausea, photophobia, and phonophobia. He has a history of these headaches in the past with recent exacerbation. It may be alarming to have had an increase in the frequency of his headaches; however, his stress levels are elevated with his parents' divorce. This is the likely explanation for the exacerbation and neuroimaging is not necessary. Now let's discuss treatment options.

Treatment Goals and Guidelines

The short-term goals of treatment for migraines in pediatric patients are analgesia, prevent associated symptoms such as nausea, and promote proper sleep. The long-term goals for these patients and their caretakers are to improve their quality of life by decreasing the severity and frequency of each headache episodes.

Agents employed in the symptomatic treatment of primary pediatric headaches should be chosen carefully according to the headache type, frequency of occurrence, associated symptoms, and potential adverse-effect profile of the chosen agent. It is also important to consider the patient's other comorbidities when choosing a pharmacologic therapeutic agent in order to achieve the greatest clinical effect while avoiding poly-pharmacy.

Given the availability of multiple levels of therapeutic agents for symptomatic treatment, the stratified care approach is preferred over a stepwise treatment approach. Rather than beginning therapy with the agent of the lowest cost and gradually escalating care as needed, the severity of the patient's clinical situation and needs are assessed up front. The level of therapy is then chosen based on the patient's specific clinical needs in an overall cost-effective manner.

Adjustment to the treatment plan is recommended in order to achieve the most effective regimen. The goals of an effective regimen should aim at treating the headache but also targeting other associated symptoms such as nausea, vomiting, photophobia, or phonophobia. Medication use should be under the supervision of a physician in order to avoid misuse that may result in exacerbation of headache symptoms. Parents should also closely monitor therapy in pediatric patients.

Treatment Agents

Analgesic therapy such as NSAIDs is the first-line treatment for these types of headaches, especially in the setting of recent development of these headache syndromes. Other helpful adjunctive agents include analgesics both opioid based and non-opioid based, sedatives, and antiemetics. It is important to recognize that an opioid is an agent of last resort especially in migraine headaches when all other avenues of treatment have been exhausted and should not be withheld due to fear of misuse. The use of opioids in these patients should be handled by healthcare professionals who are experienced in proper opioid management.

Non-pharmacologic modalities such as adequate sleep, darkness, and a quiet room are essential in the proper management of acute and tension-type headaches. Regularly scheduled meal times, proper sleep hygiene, relaxation techniques such as meditation or diaphragmatic breathing, and adequate physical activity are all adjunct activities that should be encouraged in addition to prescription treatment plan. The treatment plan should be individualized based on the age of the child and his/her ability for behavior modification since behavioral techniques can be very effective in the treatment of primary headache disorders. Complementary or alternative medicine such as acupuncture can also be considered for some patients.

Headaches that are acute in nature are often responsive to relatively mild analgesic agents such NSAIDS. Acetaminophen and ibuprofen are recommended as first-line treatment for symptomatic relief. Opioids and other medication with addictive potential such as benzodiazepines should be avoided. Appropriate lifestyle changes can reduce the occurrences of headaches by identifying and eliminating headache triggers such as alcohol, excessive caffeine, and triggering drugs such as nitrates and hormone therapy. Table 42.4 lists common medications that are associated with potentially causing headaches.

The goal of abortive therapy is to interrupt a headache and its progression after its onset. In patients with frequent headaches, all abortive agents carry the risk of overuse that may lead to more headaches. See Table 42.5 for a list of abortive agents.

Table 42.4 Medications associated with headaches

Acid blockers: famotidine and ranitidine	Corticosteroids
Amiodarone	Ergotamine
Angiotensin-converting enzyme inhibitors	Estrogen
Alpha- and beta-adrenergic agonists and blockers	Immunoglobulin
Anti-arrhythmics	Methylxanthines
Antimicrobials: amoxicillin, metronidazole, sulfamethoxazole, trimethoprim, ciprofloxacin, gentamicin, nitrofurantoin, ofloxacin, tetracyclines	Nitrates
Calcium channel blockers	Opioids
Caffeine	Oral contraceptives
	Phosphodiesterase inhibitors
	Sympathomimetics
	Thyroid hormone replacement
	Vitamin A and retinoic acid

Table 42.5 Abortive headache and migraine agents

Drug	Starting dose	Max daily dose	Comment	FDA approved for pediatric headaches
Single agents				
Acetaminophen (Tylenol)	15 mg/kg	75 mg/kg	Avoid with severe liver disease	Yes, age >6
Ibuprofen (Motrin)	10 mg/kg	40 mg/kg	Avoid with aspirin triad	Yes, age >12
Naproxen (Aleve)	2.5–5 mg/kg	1000 mg	Avoid with aspirin triad	Yes, age >12
Combination				
Fiorinal (aspirin-butalbital-caffeine)	1–2 capsules q4hr	6 capsules	Salicylate sensitivity	No
Midrin (isometheptene mucate-dichloralphenazone-acetaminophen)	2 capsules, followed by 1 capsule every hour until relief	5 capsules in 12 h	Avoid if recent MI, stroke, or MAOI use	No
5-HT1 receptor agonists				
Almotriptan	6.25–12.5 mg, may repeat after 2 h	2 doses/day	Contains sulfa	Yes, age >12
Rizatriptan (Maxalt)	<40 kg–5 mg >40 kg–10 mg	Dosing not established	If taking propranolol: 40 kg do not use >40 kg–5 mg	Yes, age 6–17
Sumatriptan (Imitrex)	25–50 mg, may repeat after 2 h	200 mg		Yes, age >12
Zolmitriptan Nasal Spray (Zomig)	2.5–5 mg, may repeat after 2 h	10 mg	If taking cimetadine max single dose 2.5 mg, daily 5 mg	Yes, age >12

Triptans such as sumatriptan are an effective class of abortive agents for migraine headaches. Several triptans are approved for pediatric patients with acute migraine headaches by the US Food and Drug Administration. Triptans' primary mechanism of action is through vasoconstriction via serotonin 5-HT1 receptor agonist activities. As a result of this vasoconstrictive property, the use of triptans is contraindicated in patients with heart diseases, poorly controlled hypertension, pregnancy, or patients with hemiplegic and basilar migraines. In addition to clinical efficacy, triptans are very easy to administer due to their various formulations. Triptans can be delivered as an oral tablet, nasal spray, transdermally, subcutaneous injection, or parenterally. Some adverse effects of triptans include flushing/warm sensations, dizziness, chest pain, and cardiac arrhythmias. However, overuse of triptans (>10 times per months for 3 months) or frequent acute migraine headaches episodes (>15 episodes per month) requiring the use of triptans can lead to rebound or withdrawal headaches.

Isometheptene and ergotamines can also be used as abortive agents for pediatric patients with migraine headaches. They are most effective when given at the beginning of a migraine attack or at the onset of an aura if present. They are less effective in young pediatric patients due to the fact that they are less able to effectively communicate the early symptoms of a headache or the beginning of an aura, both of which make the administration of these agents at the appropriate time more difficult. Same as triptans, rebound or withdrawal headaches can occur with overuse of these agents.

The long-acting formulation of NSAIDs such as naproxen is less likely to cause medication overuse headaches when compared to other abortive agents. They are readily available over the counter, but such availability can result in improper use and systemic toxicity due to inadequate medical supervision. To avoid rebound or withdrawal headaches, the general recommendation is to keep use less of NSAIDs and acetaminophen to less than 10 days per month.

Since John has some relief with an NSAID, he can add acetaminophen to his regimen. Given his moderate nausea, an antiemetic agent is also appropriate. If his migraines do not break or become intolerable in severity with the addition of acetaminophen, he should be prescribed a 5-HT1 receptor agonist to take at aura onset.

Prophylactic therapy is usually considered for pediatric patients with migraine headaches when the headaches occur at such frequency to significantly interfere with patient's lifestyle and regular activities. There is currently no agreed consensus on specific criteria to start prophylactic therapy. Frequency and severity of acute migraine headaches episodes are important considerations in the decision to start a prophylactic regimen and the agents used. In addition, the decision to start a prophylactic regimen must also weigh the potential risks associated with long-term drug use against the potential for headache relief. Like abortive agents, several classes of medication are available.

The effects of a prophylactic regimen are not immediate. Generally speaking, it takes several weeks for prophylactic therapy to yield significant clinical response of decreased frequency and/or severity of acute migraine headache episodes. Discussion of this important aspect of prophylactic therapy with the patient and

Table 42.6 Prophylaxis treatment for pediatric headaches

Drug	Starting dose	Max dose	Comments	FDA-approved for pediatric headaches
Anticonvulsant				
Carbamazepine (Tegretol)	20 mg/kg/day (100–200 mg twice daily)	35 mg/kg/day	Monitor for blood dyscrasias and depression	No. Usually used if ≥6 years old
Topiramate (Topamax)	5–10 mg/kg/day Start 25 mg qHS. Increase by 25 mg/day	100 mg divided BID	Monitor for metabolic acidosis, depression and hyperammonemia	Yes, age >12 years old
Valproic acid (Depakote)	20 mg/kg/day (max, 250 mg twice daily)	Titrate up to 40–45 mg/kg/day in BID dosing over 4–6 weeks Max 1000 mg/day	Monitor for pancreatitis, depression, or hyperammonemia	Yes, age >12 years old
Antidepressant				
Amitriptyline	0.1–0.2 mg/kg/day	2 mg/kg/day	Monitor for arrhythmias and depression	No
Antihistamine				
Cyproheptadine (Periactin)	0.25–1.5 mg/kg	2–8 mg	Avoid with MAOI use	No. Usually use if >3 years old
Beta-blocker				
Metoprolol tartrate (Lopressor)	2 mg/kg/day	6 mg/kg/day or 200 mg	Increase at weekly intervals	No
Propranolol (Inderal)	0.5 mg/kg/day (10–40 mg TID)	4 mg/kg/day	Increase at weekly intervals	No. Usually use if >3 years old

caregivers leads to more realistic expectations and better compliance. Frequent adjustment to a prophylactic regimen is not recommended. All prophylactic therapy should be given a sufficiently long trial period before dosing adjustment or cross titration of medications except in the case when patient is experiencing significant adverse effects from the treatment. Table 42.6 provides common examples of prophylactic pediatric headache agents.

Migraine headache patterns are known to change and even remit spontaneously in some pediatric patients. Thus the need for continuous prophylactic therapy should be reassessed at a regular interval. Once the decision is made to discontinue prophylactic therapy, the medication used should taper off slowly to avoid potential withdrawal symptoms. If the patient's headaches resume during the tapering process, then the patient should remain on the lowest headache-free dose of the prophylactic agent used. Patients and their caregivers also need to be cognizant of the fact that the patient may never be headache-free or the headaches may return in the future despite appropriate therapy.

Nonselective beta-blockers such as propranolol and nadolol are effective as prophylactic therapy for childhood migraines. Nadolol is easier to administer due to its longer half-life that results in less frequent daily dosing. Beta-blockers are contraindicated in asthmatics and diabetics as B-blockers may cause bronchospasm and hypoglycemia. In adolescent patients, beta-blockers may cause symptoms of depression. Beta-blockers may also interfere with athletic performance by causing bradycardia and hypotension and infrequently cause sexual dysfunction in adolescent males who are sexually active. Some beta-blockers may cause AV block and anaphylactic reactions.

Tricyclic antidepressants are frequently used for prophylactic therapy in pediatric migraine patients. Amitriptyline is especially known to be effective in migraine prevention. One significant drawback of tricyclic antidepressants is potential excessive sedation.

The antihistamine/antiserotonin agent cyproheptadine is also commonly used especially in younger patients. Its side effects include sedation, increased appetite, and weight gain. Cyproheptadine is contraindicated in patients taking monoamine oxidase inhibitors or those who have glaucoma.

Anticonvulsants valproic acid, carbamazepine, and topiramate are another prophylactic agents that have been used with reasonable success in pediatric migraine patients. They are particularly useful if the patient has a coexisting seizure disorder. The mechanism of action for these agents is not well understood. The administration should be closely monitored due to potentially serious side effects such as blood dyscrasias, somnolence, dizziness, hyponatremia, metabolic acidosis, glaucoma, depression, pancreatitis, and hepatic failure.

Although calcium channel blockers such as verapamil have been used for migraine prophylaxis in adults, their efficacy in pediatric migraine patients have not been validated.

Prophylactic therapy may become appropriate for John in the future if his headaches continue to increase in frequency and cause significant impairment of function. There are no specific criteria to follow to determine when to start a prophylactic agent. Appropriate follow-up to monitor his symptoms and potential functional impairment will be needed.

Alternative Management Options

The exact role of diet in primary headache disorders remains unclear. Foods rich in tyramine or phenylethylamine such as chocolate and fermented cheese are common triggers. Other dietary triggers include nitrates, citrus fruits, caffeine, aspartame, and monosodium glutamate. If a dietary trigger for headaches is identified, the avoidance of such trigger can have an obvious positive impact.

Table 42.7 Hours of sleep needed in pediatric patients

Age	Hours of sleep needed on average
2	13
3–4	12
5	11
6–12	10–11
13–18	9

Lack of physical activity and childhood obesity has been linked to pediatric primary headache disorders. Lifestyle changes that lead to healthy weight loss and increased physical activity will lead to an improvement of overall health for these patients with the potential for relief from their headache disorder.

Patients suffereing form primary headches, especially teenager, who are prone to sleep debt, a regular sleep schedule with proper sleep hygiene and avoidance of sleep deprivation or oversleeping and adequate amounts of sleeps can have a significant impact on headache control. Table 42.7 lists the average hours of sleep children need according to their age in a 24-h period.

Children experience stress just like adults. Stress, both as a trigger for and a consequence of a headache disorder especially for patients with tension-type headache, is another important focus for nonpharmacologic treatment of pediatric headache disorders. General stress reduction itself can lead to improvement in headache disorders.

Cognitive behavior therapy can benefit patients whose headaches are triggered by stress. For patients who are under significant stress, psychotherapy should be prescribed to reduce the negative effects. Family therapy is indicated if stressors in the home environment such as a divorce or an ill family member are contributing factors.

Relaxation techniques with biofeedback through cutaneous temperature measurements or muscular contraction monitoring with an electromyography can be very useful in modifying the bodies response to stress and can prevent headache occurrence by itself in older and cooperative pediatric patients. Done by a psychologist trained in cognitive-behavior therapy, the treatment is usually performed several times a week over a period of 1–2 months.

John should start to keep a migraine diary. This diary should focus on finding patterns to his symptoms. He should monitor his sleep and stress levels as well as any known food triggers to find out what his specific headache triggers may be. I would also have John start a graduated walking program to improve his activity and reduce stress.

Key Points

- Pediatric migraines have different criteria for diagnosis than adult migraines.
- Diagnostic workups in pediatric headaches are indicated if red flags for secondary headaches are present.
- Lifestyle modifications including decreased stress, improved sleep hygiene, cognitive behavioral therapy, and avoiding food triggers are the first-line treatments in pediatric headache management.

- Single agents such as acetaminophen and NSAIDs are frequently effective in treating pediatric migraines.
- If significant distress and functional impairment occur, starting prophylactic medications is indicated.

Suggested Reading

1. Abu-Arefeh I, Russell G. Prevalence of headache and migraine in schoolchildren. BMJ. 1994;309(6957):765–9.
2. Blume H. Pediatric headache: a review. Pediatr Rev. 2012;33(12):562–75.
3. Chakravarty A, Mukherjee A, Roy D. Migraine pain location: how do children differ from adults? J Headache Pain. 2008;9(6):375–9.
4. Cuvellier JC, Mars A, Vallee L. The prevalence of premonitory symptoms in paediatric migraine: a questionnaire study in 103 children and adolescents. Cephalalgia. 2009;29(11):1197–201.
5. Davis K, Parker K, Montgomery G. Sleep in infants and young children: part one: normal sleep. J Pediatr Health Care. 2004;18(2):65–71.
6. Graf WD, Kayyali HR, Alexander JJ, Simon SD, Morriss MC. Neuroimaging-use trends in nonacute pediatric headache before and after clinical practice parameters. Pediatrics. 2008;122(5):e1001–5.
7. Lewis D. Headaches in children and adolescents. Am Fam Physician. 2002;65(4):625–32.
8. Milde-Busch A, Blaschek A, Borggräfe I, Heinen F, Straube A, von Kries R. Associations of diet and lifestyle with headache in high-school students: results from a cross-sectional study. Headache. 2010;50(7):1104–14.
9. Mortimer MJ, Kay J, Jaron A. Childhood migraine in general practice: clinical features and characteristics. Cephalalgia. 1992;12(4):238–43; discussion 186.
10. Olesen J, Goadsby PJ, Ramadan NM, Tfelt-Hansen P, Welch M. The headaches. 3rd ed. Philadelphia: Lippincott Williams & Wilkins; 2006.
11. Russo A, Bruno A, Trojsi F, Tessitore A, Tedeschi G. Lifestyle factors and migraine in childhood. Curr Pain Headache Rep. 2016;20(2):9.
12. Taheri S. Effect of exclusion of frequently consumed dietary triggers in a cohort of children with chronic primary headache. Nutr Health. 2017;23(1):47–50.
13. Wöber-Bingöl C, Wöber C, Karwautz A, Vesely C, Wagner-Ennsgraber C, Amminger GP, et al. Diagnosis of headache in childhood and adolescence: a study in 437 patients. Cephalalgia. 1995;15(1):13–21; discussion 4.
14. Wöber C, Wöber-Bingöl C. Clinical management of young patients presenting with headache. Funct Neurol. 2000;15(Suppl 3):89–105.
15. Zee P. The normal duration of daily sleep for different age groups. Medscape. 2017.
16. Headache Classification Subcommittee of the International Headache Society. The international classification of headache disorders: 2nd edition. Cephalalgia. 2004;24(Suppl 1):9–160.
17. International Headache Society Classification ICHD-II. March 23, 2012.
18. Lexicomp online pharmacology database.

Index

J. Y. Suen, E. Petersen (eds.), *Diagnosis and Management of Head and Face Pain*, https://doi.org/10.1007/978-3-319-90999-8

B

N

O

P

MIX
Papier aus verantwortungsvollen Quellen
Paper from responsible sources
FSC® C105338

If you have any concerns about our products,
you can contact us on
ProductSafety@springernature.com

In case Publisher is established outside the EU,
the EU authorized representative is:
Springer Nature Customer Service Center GmbH
Europaplatz 3, 69115 Heidelberg, Germany

Printed by Libri Plureos GmbH
in Hamburg, Germany